Update on Open Vascular Surgery

Editor

MICHAEL T. LAWTON

NEUROSURGERY
CLINICS OF NORTH AMERICA

www.neurosurgery.theclinics.com

Consulting Editors
RUSSELL R. LONSER
DANIEL K. RESNICK

October 2022 • Volume 33 • Number 4

ELSEVIER

1600 John F. Kennedy Boulevard • Suite 1800 • Philadelphia, Pennsylvania, 19103-2899

http://www.theclinics.com

NEUROSURGERY CLINICS OF NORTH AMERICA Volume 33, Number 4
October 2022 ISSN 1042-3680, ISBN-13: 978-0-323-98665-6

Editor: Stacy Eastman
Developmental Editor: Ann Gielou Posedio

Neurosurgery Clinics of North America (ISSN 1042-3680) is published quarterly by Elsevier Inc., 360 Park Avenue South, New York, NY 10010-1710. Months of issue are January, April, July, and October. Business and Editorial Offices: 1600 John F. Kennedy Blvd., Suite 1800, Philadelphia, PA 19103-2899. Customer Service Office: 11830 Westline Industrial Drive, St. Louis, MO 63146. Periodicals postage paid at New York, NY, and additional mailing offices. Subscription prices are $447.00 per year (US individuals), $1,043.00 per year (US institutions), $479.00 per year (Canadian individuals), $1,074.00 per year (Canadian institutions), $556.00 per year (international individuals), $1,074.00 per year (international institutions), $100.00 per year (US students), $255.00 per year (international students), and $100.00 per year (Canadian students). International air speed delivery is included in all *Clinics* subscription prices. All prices are subject to change without notice. **POSTMASTER:** Send address changes to *Neurosurgery Clinics of North America*, Elsevier Periodicals Customer Service, 11830 Westline Industrial Drive, St. Louis, MO 63146. **Customer Service: 1-800-654-2452 (US and Canada). From outside the US and Canada, call: 1-314-453-7041. Fax: 1-314-453-5170. E-mail: JournalsCustomerService-usa@elsevier.com (for print support) and journalsonlinesupport-usa@elsevier.com (for online support).**

Reprints. For copies of 100 or more, of articles in this publication, please contact the Commercial Reprints Department, Elsevier Inc., 360 Park Avenue South, New York, NY 10010-1710. Tel. 212-633-3874; Fax: 212-633-3820; E-mail: reprints@elsevier.com.

Neurosurgery Clinics of North America is covered in *MEDLINE/PubMed (Index Medicus), EMBASE/Excerpta Medica,* and *Current Contents/Clinical Medicine (CC/CM).*

Contributors

CONSULTING EDITORS

RUSSELL R. LONSER, MD
Professor and Chair, Department of
Neurological Surgery, The Ohio State
University Wexner Medical Center, Columbus,
Ohio, USA

DANIEL K. RESNICK, MD, MS
Professor and Vice Chairman, Program
Director, Department of Neurosurgery,
University of Wisconsin-Madison School of
Medicine and Public Health, Madison,
Wisconsin, USA

EDITOR

MICHAEL T. LAWTON, MD
President and CEO, Department of
Neurological Surgery Chair, Robert F. Spetzler
Neuroscience Chair, Department of
Neurosurgery, Barrow Neurological Institute,
St. Joseph's Hospital and Medical Center,
Phoenix, Arizona, USA

AUTHORS

HUSSAM ABOU-AL-SHAAR, MD
Department of Neurological Surgery, University
of Pittsburgh Medical Center, Pittsburgh,
Pennsylvania, USA

PATRICK W. ALFORD, PhD
Department of Biomedical Engineering,
University of Minnesota Twin Cities,
Minneapolis, Minnesota, USA

HANNA ALGATTAS, MD
Department of Neurological Surgery, University
of Pittsburgh Medical Center, Pittsburgh,
Pennsylvania, USA

JOÃO PAULO ALMEIDA, MD, PhD
Department of Neurosurgery, Mayo Clinic,
Jacksonville, Florida, USA

OMID AMILI, PhD
Mechanical, Industrial, and Manufacturing
Engineering, The University of Toledo, Toledo,
Ohio, USA

ARNAU BENET, MD
Resident Physician, Division of Neurosurgery,
Barrow Neurological Institute, Phoenix, Arizona

DIMITRI BENNER, BS
Neuroscience Publications, Barrow
Neurological Institute, St. Joseph's Hospital
and Medical Center, Phoenix, Arizona, USA

JOSHUA BURKS, MD
Department of Neurosurgery, University of
Miami Miller School of Medicine, Lois Pope Life
Center, Miami, Florida, USA

JOSHUA S. CATAPANO, MD
Department of Neurosurgery, Barrow
Neurological Institute, St. Joseph's Hospital
and Medical Center, Phoenix, Arizona, USA

CASEY A. CHITWOOD, PhD
Department of Biomedical Engineering,
University of Minnesota Twin Cities,
Minneapolis, Minnesota, USA

PHILIPP DAMMANN, MD
Department of Neurosurgery and Spine Surgery, University Hospital Essen, Essen, Germany

JASON M. DAVIES, MD, PhD
Departments of Neurosurgery and Biomedical Informatics, Jacobs School of Medicine and Biomedical Sciences, University at Buffalo, Research Director, Jacobs Institute, Buffalo, New York, USA

OMER DORON, MD
Cerebrovascular Surgery Fellow, Department of Neurosurgery, Lenox Hill Hospital, Donald and Barbara Zucker School of Medicine at Hofstra/Northwell, New York, New York, USA

JASON A. ELLIS, MD
Associate Professor and Director of Cerebrovascular Surgery Fellowship, Department of Neurosurgery, Lenox Hill Hospital, Donald and Barbara Zucker School of Medicine at Hofstra/Northwell, New York, New York, USA

PAUL A. GARDNER, MD
Department of Neurological Surgery, University of Pittsburgh Medical Center, Pittsburgh, Pennsylvania, USA

MOLECA M. GHANNAM, MD
Department of Neurosurgery, Jacobs School of Medicine and Biomedical Sciences, University at Buffalo, Buffalo, New York, USA

VAIDYA GOVINDARAJAN, BS
Department of Neurosurgery, University of Miami Miller School of Medicine, Lois Pope Life Center, Miami, Florida, USA

CHRISTOPHER S. GRAFFEO, MD
Department of Neurosurgery, Barrow Neurological Institute, St. Joseph's Hospital and Medical Center, Phoenix, Arizona, USA

ANDREW W. GRANDE, MD
Department of Neurosurgery, University of Minnesota Twin Cities, Stem Cell Institute, Minneapolis, Minnesota, USA

BENJAMIN K. HENDRICKS, MD
Department of Neurosurgery, Barrow Neurological Institute, St. Joseph's Hospital and Medical Center, Phoenix, Arizona, USA

SPYRIDON KARADIMAS, MD, PhD
Department of Surgery, Temerty Faculty of Medicine, University of Toronto, Division of Neurosurgery, Sprott Department of Surgery, University Health Network

MOHAMED A. LABIB, CM, MD
Department of Neurosurgery, Barrow Neurological Institute, St. Joseph's Hospital and Medical Center, Phoenix, Arizona, USA

MICHAEL J. LANG, MD
Department of Neurosurgery, University of Pittsburgh Medical Center, Pittsburgh, Pennsylvania, USA

DAVID J. LANGER, MD
Chairman and Professor, Department of Neurosurgery, Lenox Hill Hospital, Donald and Barbara Zucker School of Medicine at Hofstra/Northwell, New York, New York, USA

ANTHONY S. LARSON, MD
Department of Neurosurgery, University of Minnesota Twin Cities, Minneapolis, Minnesota, USA

MICHAEL T. LAWTON, MD
President and CEO, Department of Neurological Surgery Chair, Robert F. Spetzler Neuroscience Chair, Department of Neurosurgery, Barrow Neurological Institute, St. Joseph's Hospital and Medical Center, Phoenix, Arizona, USA

VICTOR LU, MD, PhD
Department of Neurosurgery, University of Miami Miller School of Medicine, Lois Pope Life Center, Miami, Florida, USA

EVAN LUTHER, MD
Department of Neurosurgery, University of Miami Miller School of Medicine, Lois Pope Life Center, Miami, Florida, USA

ARKA N. MALLELA, MD, MS
Department of Neurological Surgery, University of Pittsburgh Medical Center, Pittsburgh, Pennsylvania, USA

JUSTIN MASCITELLI, MD, FAANS
Department of Neurosurgery, The University of Texas Health Science Center at San Antonio, San Antonio, Texas

DAVID J. MCCARTHY, MD, MS
Department of Neurological Surgery, University of Pittsburgh Medical Center, UPMC Presbyterian, Pittsburgh, Pennsylvania, USA

MICHAEL M. MCDOWELL, MD
Department of Neurological Surgery, University of Pittsburgh Medical Center, Pittsburgh, Pennsylvania, USA

ALI TAYEBI MEYBODI, MD
Resident Physician, Department of Neurosurgery, Rutgers New Jersey Medical School, Newark, New Jersey

MIKA NIEMELÄ, MD, PhD
Department of Neurosurgery, Helsinki University Hospital, University of Helsinki, Töölö Hospital, Helsinki, Finland

BRENDA M. OGLE, PhD
Department of Biomedical Engineering, University of Minnesota Twin Cities, Stem Cell Institute, Minneapolis, Minnesota, USA

ANEEK PATEL, BS
Department of Neurological Surgery, University of Pittsburgh Medical Center, Pittsburgh, Pennsylvania, USA

IVAN RADOVANOVIC, MD, PhD
Baxter and Alma Ricard Chair in Neurosurgery, Associate Professor, Department of Surgery, Temerty Faculty of Medicine, University of Toronto, Active Staff, Division of Neurosurgery, Sprott Department of Surgery, Toronto Western Hospital, University Health Network, Senior Scientist, Krembil Brain Institute

REDI RAHMANI, MD
Department of Neurosurgery, Barrow Neurological Institute, St. Joseph's Hospital and Medical Center, Phoenix, Arizona, USA

IAN RAMSAY, BS
Department of Neurosurgery, University of Miami Miller School of Medicine, Lois Pope Life Center, Miami, Florida, USA

ROBERT C. RENNERT, MD
Department of Neurological Surgery, Center for Neurorestoration, Keck School of Medicine, University of Southern California, Los Angeles, California, USA

BEHNAM REZAI JAHROMI, MD
Department of Neurosurgery, Helsinki University Hospital, University of Helsinki, Töölö Hospital, Helsinki, Finland

HOWARD RIINA, MD
Department of Neurosurgery, New York University, New York, New York

KAVELIN RUMALLA, MD
Department of Neurosurgery, Barrow Neurological Institute, St. Joseph's Hospital and Medical Center, Phoenix, Arizona, USA

JONATHAN J. RUSSIN, MD
Associate Professor, Department of Neurological Surgery, Associate Director, Center for Neurorestoration, Director, Cerebral Revascularization Center, The Keck School of Medicine of USC, University of Southern California Neurorestoration Center, Los Angeles, California, USA

ALEJANDRO N. SANTOS, MD
Department of Neurosurgery and Spine Surgery, University Hospital Essen, Essen, Germany

HUSAIN SHAKIL, MD, MSc
Department of Surgery, Temerty Faculty of Medicine, University of Toronto, Division of Neurosurgery, Sprott Department of Surgery, University Health Network

ELIZABETH D. SHIH, BS
Department of Biomedical Engineering, University of Minnesota Twin Cities, Minneapolis, Minnesota, USA

MICHAEL SILVA, MD
Department of Neurosurgery, University of Miami Miller School of Medicine, Lois Pope Life Center, Miami, Florida, USA

CARL H. SNYDERMAN, MD, MBA
Department of Otolaryngology, University of Pittsburgh Medical Center, Pittsburgh, Pennsylvania, USA

VISISH M. SRINIVASAN, MD
Department of Neurosurgery, Barrow Neurological Institute, St. Joseph's Hospital and Medical Center, Phoenix, Arizona, USA

ROBERT M. STARKE, MD, MS
Department of Neurosurgery, University
of Miami Miller School of Medicine,
Lois Pope Life Center, Miami, Florida,
USA

ULRICH SURE, MD
Department of Neurosurgery and Spine
Surgery, University Hospital Essen, Essen,
Germany

MICHAEL TYMIANSKI, MD, PhD, FRCSC
Krembil Brain Institute

XUE-YAN WAN, MD
Department of Neurosurgery and Spine
Surgery, University Hospital Essen, Essen,
Germany

ERIC W. WANG, MD
Department of Otolaryngology, University of
Pittsburgh Medical Center, Pittsburgh,
Pennsylvania, USA

MATTHEW WEBB, DO
Department of Neurosurgery, The University of
Texas Health Science Center at San Antonio,
San Antonio, Texas

GEORGIOS A. ZENONOS, MD
Department of Neurological Surgery, University
of Pittsburgh Medical Center, Pittsburgh,
Pennsylvania, USA

YUAN ZHU, MD
Department of Neurosurgery and Spine Surgery,
University Hospital Essen, Essen, Germany

Contents

Wide-neck aneurysms (WNA) often require advanced open surgical and endovascular techniques to achieve adequate aneurysm occlusion. Microsurgical treatment often requires advanced clip configurations. Occasionally, more complex open surgical techniques are required. Advancements in endovascular therapies (EVT) and devices have expanded endovascular treatment options for WNAs and have improved aneurysm occlusion rates compared with primary coiling. Certain EVT require dual antiplatelet therapy, limiting their use in the ruptured setting. Evidence suggests that microsurgical treatment should remain a consideration for treatment of ruptured WNAs, but perhaps with novel endovascular techniques and devices, EVT should be first-line treatment in the unruptured setting.

 Video content accompanies this article at http://www.neurosurgery.theclinics.com.

Anterior circulation aneurysms have classically been treated using the pterional (PT) craniotomy. Minimally invasive alternatives to the PT craniotomy have been successfully used to treat vascular pathologies of the anterior circulation. These approaches offer smaller incisions and reduced tissue dissection, resulting in shorter hospital stay, improved cosmetic results, and comparable outcomes for aneurysm treatment compared with classic open approaches. The supraorbital, lateral supraorbital (LSO), mini-PT, minimal interhemispheric, and endoscopic transpterional port approach (ETPA) are each best suited for different aneurysm targets. Outpatient aneurysm surgery has been possible with the use of minimally invasive approaches.

Cerebrovascular bypass has undergone a remarkable evolution since its initial description. Recent developments have required the conceptualization of a fourth generation in bypass techniques, encompassing both unconventional suturing techniques (type 4A; eg, intraluminal suturing) and atypical vascular constructs (type 4B; eg, middle communicating artery bypass). This cohort study reports 44 bypass operations performed by a single cerebrovascular neurosurgeon from 1997 to 2021 among a total cohort of 750 bypasses. Most bypasses were for the treatment of complex aneurysms (36 of 44 cases, 89%). Although challenging, these operations empower novel approaches to a variety of otherwise untreatable lesions.

Cavernous malformations (CMs) are low-flow vascular lesions of the central nervous system prone to symptomatic hemorrhage. CMs are estimated to be present in approximately 0.5% of the population. Usually, they are characterized by a relatively benign clinical course, staying asymptomatic in many patients. However, depending on the anatomic location, CMs can cause significant morbidity due to symptoms such as seizures or focal neurologic deficits (most of the time caused by symptomatic hemorrhage). This nonsystematic review aims to summarize important recent clinical research focusing on the biology and surgical management of CMs published since 2017.

Significant progress has been made in the use of artificial intelligence (AI) in clinical medicine over the past decade, but the clinical development of AI faces challenges. Although the spectrum of AI applications is growing within clinical medicine, including in subspecialty neurosurgery, applications focused on cerebral cavernous malformations (CCMs) are relatively scarce. The recently introduced brainstem cavernous malformation (BSCM) grading scale, approach triangles, and safe entry zone systems provide a discrete framework to explore future machine learning (ML) applications of AI systems. Given the immense scalability of these models, significant resources will likely be allocated to pursuing these future efforts.

Big data studies are on the rise in vascular neurosurgery. Advanced computer processing power combined with vast amounts of digitized data collected and stored by electronic medical records have led to studies using machine learning, deep learning algorithms, and their applications—artificial intelligence. Big data is challenging the gold standard model of randomized controlled trials introducing more pragmatic research designs including registries and registry-based randomized trails. There is a maturation of cerebrovascular disease studies. Studies have larger patient sample sizes allowing for more compelling conclusions that we reach with higher confidence. This pertains to diagnosis, treatment, outcomes, and a more nuanced understanding of less common presentations of illnesses. The following review will critically discuss big data applications in vascular neurosurgery as well as its implications in quality improvement, innovation, and global neurosurgery.

The exoscope is the technological successor to the operating microscope in cerebrovascular neurosurgery. It offers advantages including improved operative field magnification, resolution, lighting, ergonomics, team cohesiveness, and microsurgical training However, these advantages of using the exoscope must be weighed against the learning curve during its adoption, especially for senior microneurosurgeons. As exoscope technology is refined, seamless integration of robotics, automation, augmented reality, and hands-free real-time neuronavigation is anticipated.

NEUROSURGERY CLINICS OF NORTH AMERICA

SERIES OF RELATED INTEREST

Neurologic Clinics
https://www.neurologic.theclinics.com/
Neuroimaging Clinics
https://www.neuroimaging.theclinics.com/

THE CLINICS ARE AVAILABLE ONLINE!
Access your subscription at:
www.theclinics.com

Preface
A Lasting Future for Open Vascular Neurosurgery

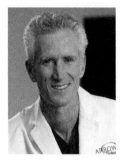

Michael T. Lawton, MD

Editor

Open vascular neurosurgery has been transformed by the widespread implementation of endovascular techniques and stereotactic radiosurgery. Aneurysms once treated with microsurgical clipping are now coiled, pipelined, or treated with intravascular flow diverters. Aneurysms at the basilar bifurcation and paraclinoid internal carotid artery, which helped incorporate orbitozygomatic craniotomies and anterior clinoidectomies into open vascular neurosurgery, are no longer routinely clipped, and many trainees have never seen these skull base surgical techniques. Similarly, arteriovenous malformations (AVMs), once resected microsurgically, are now typically embolized and treated with radiosurgery or managed conservatively. Open vascular case volume has decreased, and more neurosurgeons use a hybrid open and endovascular approach focused on the specific disease rather than on particular operative techniques. These trends, combined with the advent of mechanical thrombectomy for treating acute ischemic stroke, economic pressures, and convenience, have led many cerebrovascular neurosurgeons to favor endovascular therapies.

This issue of *Neurosurgery Clinics of North America* is an update on how open vascular neurosurgery has responded to these developments. First, microneurosurgeons have focused on complex cases that are less favorable for endovascular therapy, for which microneurosurgery is more efficacious, or that require a multimodal approach. Articles in this issue on wide-neck and bifurcation aneurysms, giant aneurysms, and dolichoectatic vertebrobasilar aneurysms exemplify this willingness to tackle the most challenging aneurysms. Second, microneurosurgeons continue to innovate and advance open techniques. Articles on novel bypasses and fourth-generation constructs, as well as transcavernous approaches, exemplify this increasing technical sophistication. Third, microneurosurgeons have redoubled efforts to treat pathologies for which endovascular therapy is limited, namely cerebral cavernous malformations and AVMs. Articles in this update examine the state of surgical practice for these two key lesions. Fourth, open vascular neurosurgery is changing with the integration of technology and its delivery to patients. This update addresses minimally invasive aneurysm surgery performed in the outpatient setting, endoscopic techniques, use of the exoscope, and the application of big data and artificial intelligence. Last, microneurosurgeons are conducting laboratory research to identify novel therapies for aneurysms and other vascular lesions, both technical and pharmacologic. This research includes studies on the hemodynamics and biology of aneurysm rupture and AVM formation and anatomical studies as the basis for new surgical approaches and devices.

Open microsurgery has a lasting role in vascular neurosurgery. As this issue demonstrates, open microsurgery may be superior to endovascular therapies in treating patients with complex aneurysms. Brainstem cavernous malformations exemplify how fresh insights and the application of open microsurgical skills can expand vascular neurosurgery. AVMs demonstrate that, even as other modalities minimize invasive interventions, occlusive and obliterative therapies remain inferior to resective therapies. Open microsurgery is and should remain a cornerstone of neurosurgical culture because it offers anatomical insights that result from direct contact with pathology, which is difficult to obtain from radiography alone. Instruments under the microscope respond to the hands with precision, and we should not relinquish this power. Our very best neurosurgeons must be capable of repairing complex lesions that cannot be managed in any other way. Manual dexterity and technical skill still matter. Anastomoses that have existed for decades produce some of neurosurgery's most artful constructs, and we resort to old-fashioned techniques when cutting-edge devices fail. Modern neurosurgery has been shaped by endovascular technology, radiosurgery, endoscopy, minimally invasive techniques, and biologic therapies that demand little of the neurosurgeon. Open microsurgery resists these trends by emphasizing a few simple instruments, steady hands, and meticulous technique. The craft will last and remain relevant if enough creative surgeons continue to engage our hands, heads, and hearts in treating our most complex and difficult lesions.

Michael T. Lawton, MD
Department of Neurosurgery
Neuroscience Publications
Barrow Neurological Institute
St. Joseph's Hospital and Medical Center
350 West Thomas Road
Phoenix, AZ 85013, USA

E-mail address:
neuropub@barrowneuro.org

Wide-Neck and Bifurcation Aneurysms
Balancing Open and Endovascular Therapies

Matthew Webb, DO[a], Howard Riina, MD[b], Justin Mascitelli, MD[a],*

KEYWORDS

- Intracranial aneurysm • Endovascular therapies • Microsurgical clipping • Wide-neck aneurysm
- Bifurcation aneurysm • Aneurysm coiling

KEY POINTS

- Wide-neck and bifurcation aneurysms (neck >4 mm or a dome-to-neck ratio <2) often require more advanced open vascular and endovascular therapies to achieve aneurysm occlusion.
- Microsurgical clipping of WNAs often necessitates complex clip configurations to occlude the aneurysm neck, such as fenestrated, intersecting, stacked, overlapping, and tandem clips.
- Primary coiling of WNAs is often unsuccessful and advanced techniques and devices are required to achieve aneurysm occlusion including balloon-assisted coiling, stent-assisted coiling, flow diversion, flow disruption, and neck reconstruction.
- Novel endovascular devices and techniques have improved occlusion rates for endovascular treatment of WNAs; however, the risk and timing of dual antiplatelet therapy must be considered.
- A balanced approach between microsurgery and endovascular therapy is reasonable, especially in the ruptured setting.

Wide-neck aneurysms (WNA), most commonly defined as aneurysms with a neck width greater than or equal to 4 mm or a dome-to-neck ratio less than 2, are of clinical interest because they are challenging to treat and require more advanced techniques compared with narrow-neck aneurysms.[1] From the microsurgical (MS) standpoint, complex clipping techniques (eg, stacked clips, intersecting clips, and fenestrated tubes) are frequently required to completely obliterate the aneurysm neck. Occasionally, bypass techniques are needed for large/giant, thrombotic, and highly calcified/atheromatous aneurysms, all of which tend to fall into the WNA category. From the endovascular therapy (EVT) standpoint, adjunctive techniques, such as balloon-assisted coiling (BAC), stent-assisted coiling (SAC), flow diversion (FD), use of intrasaccular devices, and novel neck support devices, have been developed specifically for WNAs. Certainly, this subset of intracranial aneurysms draws more attention than narrow-neck aneurysms for which simple clipping and stand-alone coiling are straightforward options. Like any aneurysm, WNAs can occur of the side-wall of an intracranial vessel or at a bifurcation (WNBA), the latter which is generally considered even more challenging to treat given the need for preservation of two efferent branches.[2]

MICROSURGICAL TECHNIQUES

MS clipping has long been a treatment option for WNAs with a high degree of durability but certainly is the most invasive option. Since the advent of endovascular coiling, however, there has been an overall shift in the treatment of intracranial

[a] Department of Neurosurgery, University of Texas Health Science Center at San Antonio, 7703 Floyd Curl Drive, MC 7843 San Antonio, TX 78229, USA; [b] Department of Neurosurgery, New York University, 530 1st Avenue Skirball Suite 8R, New York, NY 10016, USA
* Corresponding author
E-mail address: mascitelli@uthscsa.edu
Twitter: twitter@jmascite (J.M.)

Neurosurg Clin N Am 33 (2022) 359–369
https://doi.org/10.1016/j.nec.2022.05.002
1042-3680/22/© 2022 Elsevier Inc. All rights reserved.

aneurysms from MS to EVT. Despite the advancement of EVT technology over the last three decades, specifically aimed at treating WNAs, there remain certain instances when MS remains a safe and effective option for WNAs. There may be circumstances that are irrespective of the aneurysm neck status, such as young patient age, cranial neuropathy, very small or very large aneurysms, and contraindications to EVT. There are also circumstance specific to WNAs, such as the ruptured setting, when the use of dual antiplatelet therapy (DAPT), which is often required for certain EVT options for WNAs, may increase hemorrhagic complications.

Simple clipping is performed for uncomplicated WNAs without high-risk features or challenging anatomy. An example is using a standard, right-angled clip for a typical middle cerebral artery WNAB. Frequently, however, more complex clipping strategies are required for WNA neck reconstruction, including fenestrated clips for the stronger closing force and multiple clips in a stacked, intersecting, overlapping, or tandem configuration (**Fig. 1**). Multiple/fenestrated clips may be advantageous because single, long, non-fenestrated clips have a lower closing force at the distal tip and may potentiate aneurysm refilling.[3]

Furthermore, WNAs that are very large/giant, calcified, atheromatous, or thrombotic, all of which tend to fall within the WNA category, are even more challenging to treat with MS because of incomplete clip closure across the aneurysm neck. Advanced techniques, such as aneurysm thrombectomy, mobilization of existing coils, or transection of the aneurysm dome, may be necessary to facilitate complete neck closure when treating thrombotic aneurysms. If these maneuvers fail or are anticipated to fail, then a revascularization strategy accompanied by complete trapping, distal, or proximal occlusion of the aneurysm should be considered (**Fig. 2**).[4]

ENDOVASCULAR TREATMENT OF WIDE-NECK ANEURYSMS

There are numerous EVT options for WNAs, each with their own efficacy and safety profile. Stand-alone coiling of WNAs carries the risk of coil exposure, coil prolapse, and occasionally complete inability to coil, making it generally a less ideal EVT treatment strategy. The only scenario where stand-alone coiling is reasonable option for WNAs is in the ruptured setting when the aneurysm has a dome-to-neck ratio close to but still less than 2. Many advances in EVT have been developed to facilitate treatment of WNAs

including BAC, SAC, FD, intrasaccular flow disruptors, neck bridging devices, and other novel adjuncts.

Balloon-Assisted Coiling

BAC is the oldest EVT adjunct for treating WNAs, in which a balloon is temporarily inflated across the aneurysm neck while coils are deployed and then ultimately removed at the end of the procedure (**Fig. 3**). BAC has been proven safe and effective in the ruptured and unruptured setting with higher reported occlusion rates than stand-alone coiling.[5–10] BAC is advantageous in the ruptured setting because the risk of DAPT is avoided and the balloon is temporarily inflated in the setting of intraoperative rupture or perforation. Multiple techniques exist for balloon remodeling and newer dual-lumen balloons allow for simultaneous inflation and coiling through a single catheter.[11]

Stent-Assisted Coiling

SAC involves placement of a stent within the parent vessel to support coils within the aneurysm and prevent coil herniation into the parent vessel. A systematic review and meta-analysis comparing aneurysms treated with BAC versus SAC reported higher complete occlusion rates in patients treated with SAC with similar complication rates.[12] SAC requires DAPT to avoid thrombosis of the permanent implant and therefore its use is often limited in the ruptured setting. Several studies have reported higher periprocedural and postprocedural hemorrhagic complications for SAC of ruptured versus unruptured aneurysms.[13,14] SAC is performed simply with placement of one stent within the parent vessel or with more complex techniques including Y, X, T, and H configurations with multiple stents, or by a transcirculation approach (**Fig. 4**).[15]

Advances in stent technology continue to improve deliverability, metal coverage, and deployment into smaller parent vessels. Recent studies of the low-profile intraluminal support device LVIS (Microvention, Terumo, CA), and the Neuroform Atlas stent (Stryker Neurovascular, Fremont, CA) reveal high efficacy and safety for the treatment of WNAs.[16–19] There has also been suggestion that SAC results in somewhat of an FD effect and allows some aneurysms to progress from incomplete occlusion immediately after the procedure to complete occlusion at follow-up.[20] Although SAC is a safe and effective treatment of WNAs, it may be associated with a higher complication rate in the ruptured setting. Despite excellent technology, such as BAC and SAC, there was still a need for advancement of novel EVT

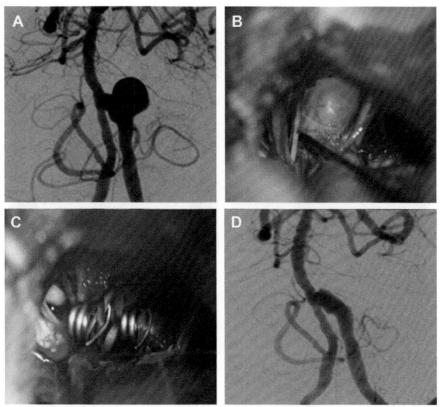

Fig. 1. Patient with an unruptured large, wide-neck vertebral artery (VA) aneurysm who was not a candidate for EVT treated with surgical clipping through an extended retrosigmoid craniotomy. (*A*) Digital subtraction angiography (DSA) demonstrating a wide-neck left VA aneurysm. (*B*) Surgical view of the aneurysm dome through the glossopharyngeal-cochlear triangle. (*C*) Surgical view of the stacked fenestrated clip configuration. (*D*) Postoperative DSA revealing complete occlusion of the aneurysm and patency of the VA and posterior inferior cerebellar artery.[59]

for treatment of WNBAs. This is exemplified by studies, such as the 2018 BRANCH study, which investigated 115 unruptured wide-neck basilar apex and middle cerebral artery aneurysms, and used core laboratory adjudicated angiographic outcomes, and demonstrated low complete occlusion and moderate complication rates.[21]

Flow Diversion

FD was originally indicated for giant cavernous and paraclinoid internal cerebral artery aneurysms. More recently, the indications have expanded to include aneurysms of the communicating segment of the internal cerebral artery, and more distal aneurysms (**Fig. 5**).[22,23] Most recently, the 5-year results of the Pipeline for Embolization of Uncoilable or Failed Aneurysm Trial (PUFS) demonstrated favorable long-term safety and aneurysm occlusion.[24] The indications for FD continue to expand as advancements in technology improved navigability, deployment,

flow-diverting properties, and smaller sizes in the latest generation of devices including the Surpass Evolve (Stryker) and the Flow Redirection Intraluminal Device (FRED, Microvention).

Similarly to SAC, FD requires DAPT, which has been associated with higher rate of treatment-related complications in the ruptured setting.[25–27] New surface-modified flow diverters, currently the Pipeline with Shield Technology (Medtronic, Minneapolis, MN), use a phosphorylcholine polymer to reduce thrombogenicity of the device and therefore may be advantageous in the ruptured setting. Initial studies have reported high efficacy and safety of the Pipeline Shield device and less in-stent stenosis than non-surface-modified devices.[28] Several reports describe single antiplatelet regimens and highlight the earlier time-to-treatment than with traditional FD in the ruptured setting.[29] Although initial data on surface-modified FD are promising, further long-term studies are required because a consensus on timing and antiplatelet therapy does not yet

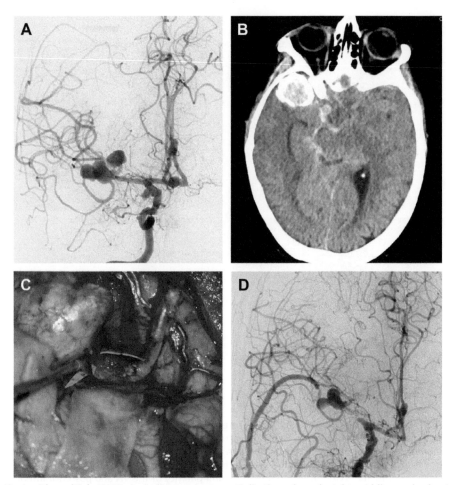

Fig. 2. Patient with multiple WNAs including a giant, partially thrombosed, right middle cerebral artery (MCA) bifurcation aneurysm. (*A*) DSA demonstrating partial filling of a giant right MCA bifurcation aneurysm, and additional wide-neck MCA aneurysm, a wide-neck anterior communicating aneurysm, anterior choroidal aneurysm, and pericallosal aneurysm. (*B*) Computed tomography head (CTH) showing the entire, largely thrombosed and calcified right MCA bifurcation aneurysm. (*C*) Intraoperative view showing a high flow bypass from the right external carotid artery (ECA) to the right temporal M2 and the giant right MCA aneurysm with proximal clip occlusion of the right M1 (not seen in view). Patient also underwent clipping of multiple additional WNAs during the surgery. (*D*) Postoperative DSA demonstrating patency of the bypass and retrograde filling of the entire MCA territory and base of the MCA aneurysm.

exist. With that said, surface modification of intracranial stents (FD and SAC) has the potential to shift the treatment of ruptured WNAs even further from MS as the concerns for DAPT are removed from the equation.

Intrasaccular Flow Disruption

A new treatment option for WNAs is termed intrasaccular flow disruption and there are a few devices available, most notably the Woven EndoBridge (WEB) device (Microvention, Aliso Viejo, CA). The WEB device is a globular-shaped braided nitinol wire device that is deployed within the aneurysm and promotes aneurysm thrombosis. The WEB does not require DAPT (although DAPT is sometimes used). The Clinical Assessment of WEB device in Ruptured aneurYSms (CLARYS) trial demonstrated short- and long-term safety of the WEB device for use in ruptured WNBA because no rebleeding events occurred at 1 month or at 1 year.[30] Although the safety profile of the WEB device is favorable, modest rates of complete occlusion (53%) were reported at 2-year follow-up by three prospective trials (WEBCAST, WEBCAST-2, and the French Observatory Study). Adequate occlusion (Raymond Roy I or II) was reported in 81% (98/121) with a retreatment rate of 9.3%.[31] Furthermore, early studies reported treatment failure rates up

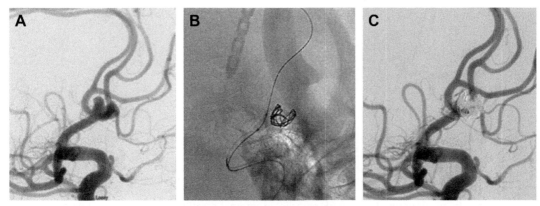

Fig. 3. Patient with a ruptured, bilobed, wide-neck anterior communicating artery (Acomm) aneurysm treated with BAC. (*A*) DSA of the internal carotid artery demonstrating a bilobed anterior communicating artery aneurysm. (*B*) Unsubtracted view demonstrating placement of the balloon across the aneurysm neck allowing coiling of both aneurysm lobes. (*C*) Postoperative DSA revealing occlusion of the aneurysm after removal of the balloon.

to 17% and device compression in up to 30% leading to more specific case selection and improved device sizing to prevent treatment failure.[32–34] The WEB device remains a safe and effective treatment option for ruptured and unruptured WNAs (especially WNBAs), although the modest complete occlusion rates and potential for retreatment must be considered for each patient.

Other novel intrasaccular devices including the Contour (Cerus Endovascular, Freemont, CA), the Artisse (formerly LUNA, Medtronic, Fremont, CA), and the Nautilus (Endostream Medical, Tel Aviv, Israel) exist with limited but favorable initial safety and efficacy data. The Contour device targets and deploys within the aneurysm neck and does not depend on the aneurysm dome morphology, making it advantageous for asymmetric WNBA. The Artisse device has reports of similar adequate occlusion and complication rates compared with the WEB device, with faster time to deployment than with primary coiling.[35–38] The Nautilus device's unique tornado design bridges the aneurysm neck to facilitate coiling.[39–41] In summary, intrasaccular flow disruption of WNA potentially avoids complications associated with DAPT and improvement in device technology has expanded the indications and success of intrasaccular flow disruption. However, lower complete occlusion rates may warrant closer radiographic follow-up.

Novel Devices

The PulseRider (Cerenovus, Fremont, CA) device is an extrasaccular neck reconstruction device with a support component placed within or

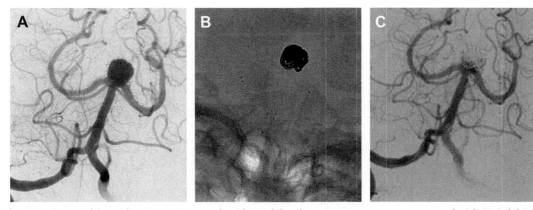

Fig. 4. Patient with an enlarging, unruptured, wide-neck basilar artery apex aneurysm treated with SAC. (*A*) DSA of the right VA demonstrating wide-neck basilar artery apex aneurysm. (*B*) Unsubtracted view demonstrating Y-stent configuration and placement of coils into the aneurysm. (*C*) Postoperative DSA demonstrating occlusion of the aneurysm after SAC.

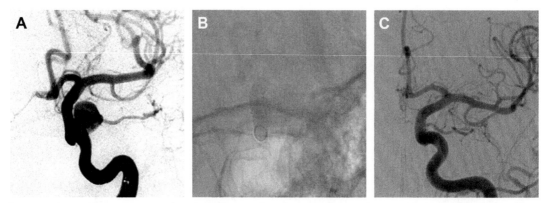

Fig. 5. Patient with an unruptured wide-neck paraclinoid internal carotid artery (ICA) aneurysm treated with flow diversion. (*A*) DSA of the left ICA demonstrating a wide-neck paraclinoid ICA aneurysm. (*B*) Unsubtracted view demonstrating placement of a Pipeline flow diverter across the aneurysm neck. (*C*) Six-month postoperative DSA revealing complete aneurysm occlusion.

outside the aneurysm neck allowing for adjunctive coiling or deployment of an intrasaccular device (**Fig. 6**). A 2018 systematic review and meta-analysis of three available PulseRider studies investigated 63 total unruptured WNBA aneurysms (37/63 located at basilar apex), and reported a 7.9% intraoperative complication rate, a 66.7% complete occlusion rate, and one recanalization at 6-month follow-up.[42] The PulseRider contains significantly less metal than traditional stents; however, its initial use has largely been in the setting of DAPT with the exception of several case reports successfully using antiplatelet monotherapy and its limited use in the ruptured setting.[43–45]

Similar to PulseRider, pCONUS (Phenox, Bochum, Germany) is a stent-like implant with intrasaccular petals that facilitates adjunctive coiling of WNBA. Currently, only retrospective studies exist; however, a systematic review and meta-analysis of 203 patients with unruptured WNBA

treated with pCONUS reveals a high technical success rate, a 60% complete occlusion rate, a 14% retreatment rate and favorable safety profile at long-term follow-up (average, 9.9 months).[46] Limited data exist for pCONUS use in the ruptured setting; however, several studies reported thrombus formation in the setting of antiplatelet monotherapy requiring further antiplatelet dosing, infusion, or intervention and therefore DAPT continues to be recommended.[47,48]

The endovascular clip system, eCLIPS (Evasc Neurovascular, Vancouver, Canada) is a leaf-shaped intraluminal device with neck bridging and flow-diverting properties that facilitates adjunctive coiling. Currently, a multicenter prospective trial of the device is underway; however, initial studies report comparable safety and efficacy to other EVT and increased flow diverting properties compared with pCONUS and PulseRider. Because of its high metal coverage, DAPT is required and its use in the ruptured setting is unknown.[49,50]

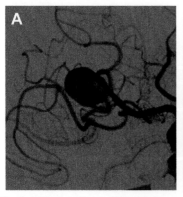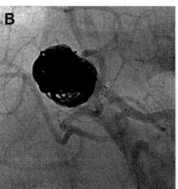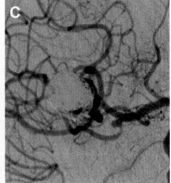

Fig. 6. Elderly patient with a large unruptured wide-neck MCA aneurysm treated with PulseRider assisted coiling. (*A*) DSA of the right ICA demonstrating a large wide-neck right MCA bifurcation aneurysm. (*B*) Unsubtracted view demonstrating the PulseRider device within the parent vessel and coils within the aneurysm. (*C*) Postoperative DSA revealing aneurysm occlusion and patent bifurcation vessels.

The Comaneci temporary embolization assist device (Rapid Medical, Yokneam, Israel) is a unique hybrid between BAC and SAC consisting of a radiopaque expandible temporary stent that serves to buttress the aneurysm neck and facilitate coil embolization (**Fig. 7**). The Comaneci avoids arrest in blood flow that occurs during BAC; however, it cannot be used for temporary occlusion in the setting of an intraoperative rupture. The device is removed following coil embolization making it a useful adjunct in the ruptured setting because the risks associated with DAPT are avoided. Initial use of the Comaneci for ruptured and unruptured WNAs has demonstrated satisfactory occlusion and complication rates at follow-up; however, further long-term prospective trials are necessary to elucidate its overall safety and efficacy.[51–53]

BALANCING MICROSURGERY AND ENDOVASCULAR THERAPY

Previous randomized controlled trials have shown improved outcomes for EVT of all ruptured intracranial aneurysms, although these results may not apply to WNAs because few studies have directly compared MS with EVT specifically for WNAs.[54,55] A 2017 systematic review and meta-analysis of 2794 aneurysms by Fiorella and colleagues[2] concluded that conventional methods of EVT (coiling, BAC, SAC) and MS for WNBA resulted in low complete occlusion rates of 39.8% and 52.5% at 1-year follow-up, respectively. However, the higher rate of complete occlusion in the MS group was accompanied by an increase in periprocedural complication rate (21.1% vs 24.3% for EVT and MS cases, respectively).[2]

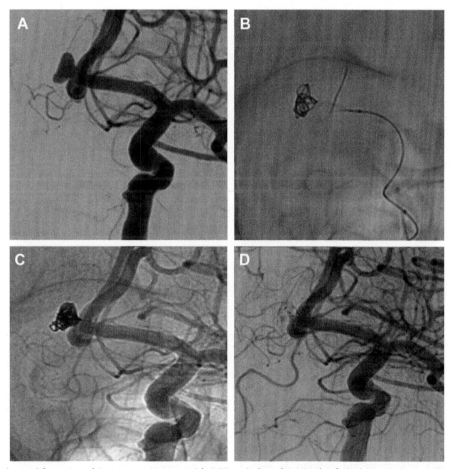

Fig. 7. Patient with ruptured Acomm aneurysm with DTR ratio less than 2 who failed stand-alone coiling and was treated with Comaneci assisted coiling. (*A*) DSA of the left ICA demonstrating a bilobed Acomm aneurysm. (*B*) Unsubtracted view demonstrating expansion of the Comaneci device to support the aneurysm neck during coiling. (*C*) Unsubtracted view of the coils after removal of the Comaneci device. (*D*) Postoperative DSA demonstrating aneurysm occlusion.

A post hoc analysis of WNAs in the Barrow Ruptured Aneurysm Trial (BRAT WNA) revealed that WNA status significantly impacted the treatment strategy with a high percentage of patients in the EVT to MS crossover group having a WNA. Clinical outcomes were similar when comparing MS with EVT at all time points using intent-to-treat and as-treated analyses.[56] The Endovascular Therapy versus Microsurgical Clipping of Ruptured Wide Neck Aneurysms (EVERRUN Registry) is a multicenter prospective propensity score analysis of 87 ruptured WNAs with MS and EVT compared using propensity score analysis. Similar to BRAT WNA, there was no difference in clinical outcome at 1 year. Additionally, 12.7% of patients required retreatment in the EVT group, whereas no patients in the MS group required retreatment.[57] BRAT WNA and EVERRUN provide evidence that MS should remain a viable treatment option for ruptured WNAs.

In the unruptured arm of the same WNA registry from which EVERRUN was published, although there was no difference in the primary outcome using propensity score analysis, improved clinical outcomes and less complications were seen with EVT cohort and better angiographic outcomes were seen in the MS cohort in the unadjusted analysis.[58] Thus, for unruptured aneurysms, EVT may be a better first-line approach compared with MS, keeping in mind that angiographic outcomes may be worse and that retreatment over time may be more common.

SUMMARY

WNAs are often more challenging to treat and often require EVT adjuncts or advanced clipping techniques to reconstruct the aneurysm neck. This is especially true for WNBAs, which tend to be more challenging to treat, although many of the new EVT technologies are focused on WNBAs. The safety and efficacy profile of each treatment option should be considered when making treatment decisions for patients with WNAs. High-quality comparative studies are required to assist in evidence-based clinical decision making.

CLINICS CARE POINTS

- Wide-neck aneurysms are defined as neck width greater than 4 mm and dome-to-neck ratio less than 2.
- WNBA have historically lower adequate occlusion rates and higher rates of retreatment.

- Advanced surgical clipping techniques are often required to achieve adequate occlusion.
- Open microsurgical clipping should be considered, especially in the ruptured setting.
- Advanced endovascular therapies exist to treat WNAs but often necessitate dual antiplatelet therapy.
- EVT may be associated with improved clinical outcomes versus microsurgery in the unruptured setting.

DISCLOSURE

Dr J. Mascitelli is a consultant to Stryker. No funding was received for this article.

REFERENCES

1. Hendricks BK, Yoon JS, Yaeger K, et al. Wide-neck aneurysms: systematic review of the neurosurgical literature with a focus on definition and clinical implications. Available at: https://thejns.org/view/journals/j-neurosurg/133/1/article-p159.xml.
2. Fiorella D, Arthur AS, Chiacchierini R. How safe and effective are existing treatments for wide-necked bifurcation aneurysms? Literature-based objective performance criteria for safety and effectiveness. J Neurointerv Surg 2017. Available at: https://pubmed.ncbi.nlm.nih.gov/28798268/. Accessed November 15, 2021.
3. Horiuchi T, Rahmah NN, Yanagawa T, et al. Revisit of aneurysm clip closing forces: comparison of titanium versus cobalt alloy clip. Neurosurg Rev 2013–;36(1): 133–8. https://doi.org/10.1007/s10143-012-0398-x. https://pubmed.ncbi.nlm.nih.gov/22699927/. Accessed November 15, 2021.
4. Lawton MT. Section I: The Tenets . In: Seven Aneurysms: Tenets Und Techniques for Clipping. New York, NY: Thieme; 2011:11-54.
5. Santillan A, Gobin YP, Mazura JC. Balloon-assisted coil embolization of intracranial aneurysms is not associated with increased periprocedural complications. J Neurointerv Surg 2006. Available at: https://pubmed.ncbi.nlm.nih.gov/22730337/. Accessed December 14, 2021.
6. Shapiro M, Babb J, Becske T, et al. Safety and efficacy of adjunctive balloon remodeling during endovascular treatment of intracranial aneurysms: a literature review. Am J Neuroradiol 2008. Available at: http://www.ajnr.org/content/29/9/1777. Accessed December 8, 2021.
7. Lowe SR, Bhalla T, Tillman H. A comparison of diffusion-weighted imaging abnormalities following balloon remodeling for aneurysm coil embolization in the ruptured vs unruptured setting. Neurosurgery

2018. Available at: https://pubmed.ncbi.nlm.nih.gov/28520916/. Accessed December 8, 2021.

8. Pierot L, Cognard C, Anxionnat R, et al, Clarity Investigators. Remodeling technique for endovascular treatment of ruptured intracranial aneurysms had a higher rate of adequate postoperative occlusion than did conventional coil embolization with comparable safety. Radiology 2011. Available at: https://www.ncbi.nlm.nih.gov/pubmed/21131582. Accessed December 11, 2021.

9. Pierot L, Spelle L, Leclerc X. Endovascular treatment of unruptured intracranial aneurysms: comparison of safety of remodeling technique and standard treatment with coils. Radiology 2009. Available at: https://pubmed.ncbi.nlm.nih.gov/19318586/. Accessed November 15, 2021.

10. Pierot L, Cognard C, Anxionnat R. Remodeling technique for endovascular treatment of ruptured intracranial aneurysms had a higher rate of adequate postoperative occlusion than did conventional coil embolization with comparable safety. Radiology 2011. Available at: https://pubmed.ncbi.nlm.nih.gov/21131582/. Accessed November 21, 2021.

11. Pierot L, Cognard C, Spelle L. Safety and efficacy of balloon remodeling technique during endovascular treatment of intracranial aneurysms: critical review of the literature. AJNR Am J Neuroradiol 2012. Available at: https://pubmed.ncbi.nlm.nih.gov/21349960/. Accessed November 21, 2021.

12. Wang F, Chen X, Wang Y. Stent-assisted coiling and balloon-assisted coiling in the management of intracranial aneurysms: a systematic review & meta-analysis. J Neurol Sci 2016. Available at: https://pubmed.ncbi.nlm.nih.gov/27084238/. Accessed November 15, 2021.

13. Ryu CW, Park S, Shin HS, et al. Complications in stent-assisted endovascular therapy of ruptured intracranial aneurysms and relevance to antiplatelet administration: a systematic review. AJNR Am J Neuroradiol 2015. Available at: https://www.ncbi.nlm.nih.gov/pmc/articles/PMC7968784/. Accessed November 15, 2021.

14. Zhang X, Zuo Q, Tang H. Stent assisted coiling versus non-stent assisted coiling for the management of ruptured intracranial aneurysms: a meta-analysis and systematic review. J Neurointerv Surg 2018. Available at: https://pubmed.ncbi.nlm.nih.gov/30842307/. Accessed November 15, 2021.

15. Mascitelli JR, Levitt MR, Griessenauer CJ, et al. Trans-circulation approach for stent-assisted coiling of intracranial aneurysms: a multicenter study. J Neurointerv Surg 2021;13(8):711–5. https://doi.org/10.1136/neurintsurg-2020-016899. https://pubmed.ncbi.nlm.nih.gov/33203763/. Accessed December 5, 2021.

16. Fiorella D, Boulos A, Turk AS, et al. The safety and effectiveness of the LVIS stent system for the treatment of wide-necked cerebral aneurysms: final results of the pivotal US LVIS trial. J Neurointerv Surg 2019. Available at: https://jnis.bmj.com/content/11/4/357. Accessed November 17, 2021.

17. Jankowitz BT, Hanel R, Jadhav AP, et al. Neuroform Atlas Stent system for the treatment of intracranial aneurysm: primary results of the ATLAS Humanitarian Device Exemption Cohort. J Neurointerv Surg 2019. Available at: https://jnis.bmj.com/content/11/8/801. Accessed November 17, 2021.

18. Burkhardt J-K, Srinivasan V, Srivatsan A, et al. Multi-center postmarket analysis of the Neuroform Atlas Stent for stent-assisted coil embolization of intracranial aneurysms. Am J Neuroradiol 2020. https://doi.org/10.3174/ajnr.A6581. https://pubmed.ncbi.nlm.nih.gov/32467183/. Accessed December 6, 2021.

19. Santillan A, Greenberg E, Patsalides A, et al. Long-term clinical and angiographic results of Neuroform stent-assisted coil embolization in wide-necked intracranial aneurysms. Neurosurgery 2012. Available at: https://www.ncbi.nlm.nih.gov/pubmed/22095221 Lawson. Accessed November 17, 2021.

20. Lawson MF, Newman WC, Chi YY, et al. Stent-associated flow remodeling causes further occlusion of incompletely coiled aneurysms. Neurosurgery 2011;69(3):598–604.

21. De Leacy RA, Fargen KM, Mascitelli JR. Wide-neck bifurcation aneurysms of the middle cerebral artery and basilar apex treated by endovascular techniques: a multicentre, core lab adjudicated study evaluating safety and durability of occlusion (BRANCH). J Neurointerv Surg 2019. Available at: https://pubmed.ncbi.nlm.nih.gov/29858397/. Accessed December 14, 2021.

22. Becske T, Kallmes DF, Saatci I. Pipeline for un-coilable or failed aneurysms: results from a multi-center clinical trial. Radiology 2013. Available at: https://pubmed.ncbi.nlm.nih.gov/23418004/. Accessed December 13, 2021.

23. Hanel RA, Kallmes DF, Lopes DK. Prospective study on embolization of intracranial aneurysms with the pipeline device: the premier study 1 year results. J Neurointerv Surg 2020. Available at: https://pubmed.ncbi.nlm.nih.gov/31308197/. Accessed December 13, 2021.

24. Becske T, Brinjikji W, Potts MB. Long-term clinical and angiographic outcomes following pipeline embolization device treatment of complex internal carotid artery aneurysms: five-year results of the pipeline for uncoilable or failed aneurysms trial. Neurosurgery 2017. Available at: https://pubmed.ncbi.nlm.nih.gov/28362885/. Accessed December 13, 2021.

25. Cagnazzo F, Di Carlo DT, Cappucci M. Acutely ruptured intracranial aneurysms treated with flow-diverter stents: a systematic review and meta-analysis. AJNR Am J Neuroradiol 2018. Available at: https://pubmed.ncbi.nlm.nih.gov/30049721/. Accessed December 13, 2021.

26. Cagnazzo F, Di Carlo DT, Petrella G, et al. Ventriculostomy-related hemorrhage in patients on antiplatelet therapy for endovascular treatment of acutely ruptured intracranial aneurysms. A meta-analysis - neurosurgical review. 2018. Available at: https://pubmed.ncbi.nlm.nih.gov/29968172/; https://link.springer.com/article/10.1007/s10143-018-0999-0.

27. Hudson JS, Nagahama Y, Nakagawa D. Hemorrhage associated with ventriculoperitoneal shunt placement in aneurysmal subarachnoid hemorrhage patients on a regimen of dual antiplatelet therapy: a retrospective analysis. J Neurosurg 2018. Available at: https://pubmed.ncbi.nlm.nih.gov/29125410/. Accessed December 13, 2021.

28. Martínez-Galdámez M, Lamin SM, Lagios KG, et al. Treatment of intracranial aneurysms using the pipeline flex embolization device with shield technology: angiographic and safety outcomes at 1-year follow-up. J Neurointerv Surg 2018. Available at: https://www.ncbi.nlm.nih.gov/pmc/articles/PMC6582709/. Accessed December 12, 2021.

29. Yeomans J, Sandu L, Sastry A. Pipeline flex embolisation device with shield technology for the treatment of patients with intracranial aneurysms: Periprocedural and 6 month outcomes - James Yeomans, Lilian Sandu, Anand Sastry, 2020. SAGE Journals 2020. Available at: https://journals.sagepub.com/doi/abs/10.1177/1971400920966749. Accessed December 12, 2021.

30. Spelle L, Herbreteau D, Caroff J, et al. Clinical assessment of web device in ruptured aneurysms (clarys): results of 1-month and 1-year assessment of rebleeding protection and clinical safety in a multicenter study. J Neurointerv Surg 2021. Available at: https://jnis.bmj.com/content/early/2021/09/07/neurintsurg-2021-017416. Accessed November 4, 2021.

31. Pierot L, Moret J, Barreau X, et al. Safety and efficacy of aneurysm treatment with WEB in the cumulative population of three prospective, Multicenter Series. J Neurointerv Surg 2018. Available at: https://www.ncbi.nlm.nih.gov/pmc/articles/PMC5969386/. Accessed November 4, 2021.

32. Pierot L, Moret J, Barreau X, et al. Aneurysm treatment with Woven Endobridge in the cumulative population of 3 prospective, multicenter series: 2-year follow-up. Neurosurgery 2020. Available at: https://www.ncbi.nlm.nih.gov/pmc/articles/PMC7534535/. Accessed November 4, 2021.

33. Cognard C, Januel AC. Remnants and recurrences after the use of the WEB intrasaccular device in large-neck bifurcation aneurysms. Neurosurgery 2015. Available at: https://pubmed.ncbi.nlm.nih.gov/25710103/. Accessed November 4, 2021.

34. Goertz L, Liebig T, Siebert E. Woven Endobridge embolization versus microsurgical clipping for unruptured anterior circulation aneurysms: a propensity score analysis. Neurosurgery 2020. Available at: https://pubmed.ncbi.nlm.nih.gov/33372215/. Accessed November 5, 2021.

35. Thormann M, Mpotsaris A, Behme D. Treatment of a middle cerebral artery bifurcation aneurysm with the novel contour neurovascular system compatible with 0.021″ catheters - Maximilian Thormann, Anastasios Mpotsaris, Daniel Behme, 2021. SAGE Journals 2021. Available at: https://journals.sagepub.com/doi/10.1177/19714009211041523. Accessed November 22, 2021.

36. Akhunbay-Fudge CY, Deniz K, Tyagi AK. Endovascular treatment of wide-necked intracranial aneurysms using the novel contour neurovascular system: a single-center safety and feasibility study. J Neurointerv Surg 2020. Available from: https://pubmed.ncbi.nlm.nih.gov/31974281/. Accessed November 22, 2021.

37. Piotin M, Biondi A, Sourour N, et al. The Luna aneurysm embolization system for intracranial aneurysm treatment: short-term, mid-term and long-term clinical and angiographic results. J Neurointerv Surg 2018. Available at: https://jnis.bmj.com/content/10/12/e34?ijkey=54d35d40ee6f1e44eadd75a4a1763c33f954737a&keytype2=tf_ipsecsha. Accessed November 23, 2021.

38. Frölich AM, Nawka MT, Ernst M, et al. Intra-aneurysmal flow disruption after implantation of the Medina Embolization Device depends on aneurysm neck coverage. PLoS One 2018. Available at: https://doaj.org/article/8a9a292ccc1d4c81a345b2f69a952b0d. Accessed November 23, 2021.

39. Abalia-Didi H. A medical device to treat brain aneurysms [Internet]. ClinicalTrials.gov. 2021. Available at: https://clinicaltrials.gov/ct2/show/NCT04963933.

40. Sirakov A, Matanov S, Bhopal P. Nautilus-assisted coil embolization for a complex Acoma wide-necked aneurysm in the setting of acute subarachnoid hemorrhage. J Neurointerv Surg 2021. Available at: https://pubmed.ncbi.nlm.nih.gov/34140287/. Accessed December 8, 2021.

41. Matanov S, Sirakov A, Sirakova K. Nautilus-assisted coiling of an unruptured wide-necked aneurysm of the posterior communicating artery. World Neurosurg 2021. Available at: https://pubmed.ncbi.nlm.nih.gov/33989820/. Accessed December 8, 2021.

42. Aguilar-Salinas P, Brasiliense LBC, Walter CM. Current status of the Pulserider in the treatment of bifurcation aneurysms: a systematic review. World Neurosurg 2018. Available at: https://pubmed.ncbi.nlm.nih.gov/29698797/. Accessed December 14, 2021.

43. O'Connor KP, Strickland AE, Bohnstedt BN. Pulserider use in ruptured basilar apex aneurysms. World Neurosurg 2019. Available at: https://www.ncbi.nlm.

nih.gov/pubmed/30980983. Accessed December 14, 2021.

44. Folzenlogen Z, Seinfeld J, Kubes S, et al. Use of the Pulserider device in the treatment of ruptured intracranial aneurysms: a case series. World Neurosurg 2019;127:e149–54. https://doi.org/10.1016/j.wneu. 2019.03.003. https://pubmed.ncbi.nlm.nih.gov/ 30862588/. Accessed December 14, 2021.

45. .Narsinh KH, Caton MT, Mahmood NF, et al., Intrasaccular flow disruption (WEB) of a large wide-necked basilar apex aneurysm using PulseRider-assistance, Interdiscip Neurosurg, 24, 2021, 101072, doi:10.1016%2Fj.inat.2020. 101072 https://www.ncbi.nlm.nih.gov/pmc/articles/ PMC8018600/ Accessed December 14, 2021.

46. Sorenson TJ, Iacobucci M, Murad MH, et al. The PCONUS bifurcation aneurysm implants for endovascular treatment of adults with intracranial aneurysms: a systematic review and meta-analysis. Surg Neurol Int 2019. Available at: https://www.ncbi.nlm. nih.gov/pmc/articles/PMC6416758/. Accessed November 17, 2021.

47. Perez MA, AlMatter M, Hellstern V, et al. Use of the PCONUS HPC as an adjunct to coil occlusion of acutely ruptured aneurysms: early clinical experience using single antiplatelet therapy. J NeuroInterv Surg 2020. Available at: https://jnis.bmj.com/ content/12/9/862. Accessed November 17, 2021.

48. Perez MA, Hellstern V, Candel CS, et al. Use of PCONUS HPC for the treatment of unruptured wide-necked bifurcation aneurysms: early clinical experience using single antiplatelet therapy. Stroke Vasc Neurol 2021. Available at: https://svn.bmj.com/ content/6/1/57. Accessed November 17, 2021.

49. Vries JD, Boogaarts HD, Sørensen L, et al. Eclips bifurcation remodeling system for treatment of wide neck bifurcation aneurysms with extremely low dome-to-neck and aspect ratios: a multicenter experience. J NeuroInterv Surg 2021. Available at: https://jnis.bmj.com/content/13/5/438. Accessed December 7, 2021.

50. Scott Wn. Evasc neurovascular announces the new eclips bifurcation flow diverter. Business Wire 2021. Available at: https://www.businesswire.com/news/ home/20211019006102/en/Evasc-Neurovascular-Announces-the-New-eCLIPs-Bifurcation-Flow-Diverter. Accessed December 7, 2021.

51. Molina-Nuevo JD, López-Martínez L, Pedrosa-Jiménez MJ, et al. Comaneci device-assisted embolization of wide-necked carotid aneurysms with an unfavorable ratio. BMC Neurol 2021. Available at: https://pubmed.ncbi.nlm.nih.gov/33092561/. Accessed November 15, 2021.

52. Sirakov A, Minkin K, Penkov M, et al. Comaneci-assisted coiling as a treatment option for acutely ruptured wide neck cerebral aneurysm: case series of 118 patients. Neurosurgery 2020. Available at: https://www.ncbi.nlm.nih.gov/pmc/articles/ PMC7666901/. [Accessed 15 November 2021]. Accessed November 15, 2021.

53. Sirakov S, Sirakov A, Hristov H, et al. Early experience with a temporary bridging device (COMANECI) in the endovascular treatment of ruptured wide neck aneurysms. J NeuroInterv Surg 2018. https://doi.org/10.1136/neurintsurg-2017-013641. Available at: https://pubmed.ncbi.nlm.nih.gov/ 29438035/. Accessed November 15, 2021.

54. Molyneux A, Kerr R. International subarachnoid aneurysm trial (ISAT) of neurosurgical clipping versus endovascular coiling in 2143 patients with ruptured intracranial aneurysms: a randomized trial. J Stroke Cerebrovasc Dis 2003. Available at: https:// www.sciencedirect.com/science/article/abs/pii/ S1052305702000630. Accessed December 9, 2021.

55. McDougall CG, Spetzler RF, Zabramski JM, et al. The barrow ruptured aneurysm trial. 2012. Available at: https://thejns.org/view/journals/j-neurosurg/116/ 1/article-p135.xml.

56. Mascitelli JR, Lawton MT, Hendricks BK. Analysis of wide-neck aneurysms in the Barrow ruptured aneurysm trial. Neurosurgery 2019. Available at: https:// pubmed.ncbi.nlm.nih.gov/30346618/. Accessed December 9, 2021.

57. Mascitelli JR, Lawton MT, Hendricks BK. Endovascular therapy versus microsurgical clipping of ruptured wide neck aneurysms (EVERRUN registry): a multicenter, prospective propensity score analysis. J Neurosurg 2021. Available at: https://pubmed. ncbi.nlm.nih.gov/34740187/. Accessed December 9, 2021.

58. Mascitelli JR, Mocco J, Hardigan T. Endovascular therapy versus microsurgical clipping of unruptured wide-neck aneurysms: a prospective multicenter study with propensity score analysis. J Neurosurg 2021;. https://pubmed.ncbi.nlm.nih.gov/34952522/. Accessed December 28, 2021.

59. Peitz GW, McDermott RA, Baranoski JF, et al. Extended retrosigmoid craniotomy and approach through the glossopharyngeal cochlear triangle for clipping of a high-riding vertebral-posterior inferior cerebellar artery aneurysm: 2-dimensional operative video. Oper Neurosurg 2021;21(3):E270–1. https:// doi.org/10.1093/ons/opab140. https://pubmed.ncbi. nlm.nih.gov/33989426/. Accessed December 9, 2021.

Minimally Invasive and Outpatient Aneurysm Surgery: New Concepts

Spyridon Karadimas, MD, PhD[a,b,1], Husain Shakil, MD, MSc[a,b,1],
João Paulo Almeida, MD, PhD[c], Michael Tymianski, MD, PhD, FRCSC[d],
Ivan Radovanovic, MD, PhD[a,b,d],*

KEYWORDS

- Minimally invasive aneurysm surgery • Key-hole aneurysm surgery • Outpatient aneurysm surgery

KEY POINTS

- The supraorbital, lateral supraorbital (LSO), and mini-pterional (PT) craniotomy are safe alternatives to the PT craniotomy for successful treatment of anterior circulation aneurysm.
- Minimally invasive approaches can be used to safely conduct outpatient aneurysm surgery.
- Minimally invasive approaches offer greater cosmetic results with comparative long-term aneurysm outcomes compared with the classic open approach.

 Video content accompanies this article at http://www.neurosurgery.theclinics.com.

INTRODUCTION

Sir Victor Horsley has been credited as a pioneer in the treatment of intracranial aneurysms.[1] In the late 19th century, he popularized the use of Hunterian ligation for aneurysm treatment. Since then, treatment strategies for intracranial aneurysms have evolved. In 1937 Dandy used a frontotemporal craniotomy to first apply a hemostatic clip on a posterior communicating artery (PCoA). In the 1970s, Yasargil described and popularized the use of the pterional (PT) craniotomy and splitting of the sylvian fissure for microsurgical clipping of aneurysms.[2] With the use of the operating microscope, the PT allowed for open surgical treatment of predominantly anterior circulation aneurysms, with minimal retraction of the frontal and temporal lobes.

The last 2 decades have seen a notable paradigm shift, with minimally invasive surgery (MIS) coming to the forefront.[3] The workhorse of these MIS strategies has been endovascular treatment, which has now been widely adopted. However, there have also been several advancements in open MIS strategies for intracranial aneurysm treatment. Many of these are modifications of the original PT, and function around a smaller bony opening. They were designed to center the craniotomy on the optimal surgical corridor to the desired target structures, and to minimize trauma to surrounding skin, muscle, bone, and most importantly neural structures. The classic PT requires a long incision, with extensive drilling of the sphenoid bone, and dissection of the temporalis muscle.[4] The term keyhole craniotomy was coined to describe the mini-craniotomies used as an alternative to the PT. The use of a keyhole or minicraniotomy widens the intracranial surgical field with increasing distance from the keyhole to

[a] Department of Surgery, Temerty Faculty of Medicine, University of Toronto, Toronto, ON, USA; [b] Division of Neurosurgery, Sprott Department of Surgery, University Health Network, Toronto, ON, USA; [c] Department of Neurosurgery, Mayo Clinic, Jacksonville, FL, USA; [d] Krembil Brain Institute, Toronto, ON, USA
[1] Equal Contribution.
* Corresponding author. Division of Neurosurgery, Toronto Western Hospital, University Health Network, 4W433, 399 Bathurst Street, Toronto, Ontario M5T 2S8, Canada.
E-mail address: ivan.radovanovic@uhn.ca

Neurosurg Clin N Am 33 (2022) 371–382
https://doi.org/10.1016/j.nec.2022.05.005
1042-3680/22/© 2022 Elsevier Inc. All rights reserved.

a point where contralateral structures can be well visualized.

Their advent has allowed for reducing morbidity and improved cosmesis related to open surgical treatment of intracranial aneurysms.[3] In this review we summarize the main minimally invasive surgical treatment options.

SUPRA-ORBITAL
History

The supra-orbital (SO) craniotomy was first described in 1982 by Jane and colleagues as an approach to lesions within the anterior cranial fossa, and for aneurysms of the anterior communicating artery (ACoA) complex.[5] They described the use of a bicoronal incision, with a large anteriorly reflected skin flap to expose the superior orbital ridge. The original craniotomy involves 2 burr holes. One above the superior orbital ridge at the midline, often invading the frontal sinus. The second is in the classic keyhole, or McCarty position, near the lateral extent of the superior orbital ridge, and behind the zygomatic process.

Technique

Perneczky pioneered a modification of this technique to a more minimally invasive that was he used it since the end of 80s and reported it in almost 160 patients.[6,7] In their articles they implemented the now well-known eyebrow incision at the lateral two-thirds of the eyebrow. Typically, this incision beings lateral to the superior orbital notch and supraorbital nerve to the lateral extent of the eyebrow to expose the orbital ridge, the supraorbital frontal bone, the anterior root of the zygoma, and the keyhole region just under the superior temporal line. The incision can be further extended along the anterior root of the zygomatic arch to allow a lateral extension of the craniotomy. However, a shorter version of the classical PT can be used. The incision behind the hairline extends from 2 cm above the zygomatic arch to the midline and allows for exposure of the lateral extent of the superior orbital rim, the anterior portion of the superior temporal line, and the frontal zygomatic process. The skin incision is made superficial to temporalis fascia. The temporalis is then minimally incised with monopolar cautery off the anterior portion of the superior temporal line for 2 to 3 cm and reflected posteriorly.

Head positioning for this procedure is supine with an approximately 20° head rotation to the contralateral side. The rotation of the head can be adjusted to the location of the aneurysm, for example, and anterior communicating aneurysm may require more rotation, to assist in the alignment of the operative corridor to the target aneurysm. Additionally, the extension of the head by 10 to 15° allows for the frontal lobe to fall away from the anterior cranial fossa, assisting in a subfrontal approach to midline structures. Finally, slight lateral flexion of the head to the contralateral side provides additional comfort to the primary operator.

The MIS SO is made with a single burr hole immediately behind the superior temporal line of the frontal bone. The size, shape, and positioning of the mini-craniotomy can be tailored to the lesion of target, however, are typically 2.5 cm × 1.5 cm in width and height. The medio-lateral limits of the craniotomy usually extend between the supraorbital notch and the frontozygomatic suture. The inner orbital rim is then drilled for a linear view over the orbital roof toward midline and paramedian structures and facilitates the introduction of microinstruments.

Indications

The SO craniotomy typically allows for microsurgical clipping of the internal carotid artery (ICA), ACoA projecting anterior and inferior, proximal middle cerebral artery (MCA), and PCoA aneurysms. The use of extradural drilling of bony prominences of the frontal floor further optimizes the working corridor for subfrontal access in cases of ICA and ACoA aneurysms. For microsurgical clipping of MCA aneurysms, the proximal part of the sylvian fissure coursing medio-laterally can be easily opened through a subfrontal route allowed by the SO approach. However, in cases of a long M1 segment whereby M1-M2 bifurcation aneurysm is located in the distal sylvian fissure over the insula, an SO is less practical.

The SO can also be used for different vascular pathologies in the anterior cranial fossa or inferior frontal lobes using either the eyebrow, supra-eyebrow, or transpalpebral incision. In our institution we also use the eyebrow incision for SO regularly for microsurgical management of ethmoidal dural arteriovenous fistula (dAVF). In **Fig. 1**, the use of an SO through a supra-eyebrow incision for surgical disconnection of an ethmoidal dAVF is depicted. The patient had presented with subarachnoid hemorrhage (SAH) and small intraparenchymal component in the left frontal lobe. Extradural drilling of the internal bone edge of the medial end of craniotomy allows access to the anterior midline skull base such as the olfactory groove region. This optimizes the working corridor and opens the view above the orbital roof eminence for microsurgical treatment of ethmoidal dAVF and other lesions.

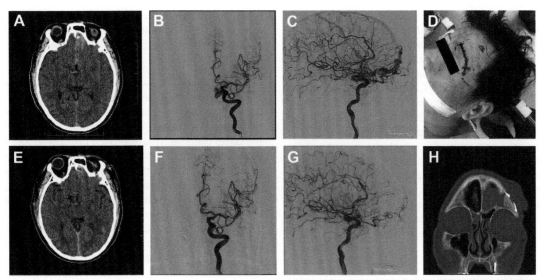

Fig. 1. Left supraorbital approach for microsurgical disconnection of ethmoidal arteriovenous fistula (dAVF). (*A*) Plain axial CT head shows subarachnoid blood in the anterior interhemispheric fissure and small parenchymal hematoma anteriorly within the parasagittal inferior left frontal region. AP (*B*) and lateral (*C*) views following left ICA injection demonstrate an anterior ethmoidal fistula. (*D*) Planned eyebrow incision just above the hairline. (*E–G*) Plain axial CT head and DSA confirm the evacuation of SAH and complete the disconnection of the ethmoidal dAVF. (*H*) Bone window CT head demonstrates the location and size of the bone flap.

Disadvantages/considerations

Microsurgical expertise along with careful patient selection allows minimally invasive aneurysmal obliteration without neurologic complications and with excellent cosmetic results. The SO allows an essential a subfrontal approach with more limited variations in angles of attack for a defined target. While a keyhole opening allows a wide-angle and panoramic view of deep structures, the maneuverability around a selected surgical target is more limited and therefore necessitates a more coaxial work with surgical instruments. The use of various angled aneurysms clips, single, or malleable shafted low profile clip appliers allowing rotational adjustment of the loaded clips and meticulous microsurgical technique can overcome the challenges posed by the coaxial instrument maneuverability for noncomplicated saccular aneurysms. Another important consideration during the SO is the possible breach of the frontal sinus and the subsequent cerebrospinal fluid (CSF) rhinorrhea. The incidence of CSF rhinorrhea after SO ranges between 0% and 9.1%.[8] In a retrospective study of 350 participants who underwent SO craniotomy for different pathologies, Thaher and colleagues reported a 25.1% rate a radiographic invasion of the frontal sinus.[8] However, only 2.3% of these patients developed. Associated meningitis was developed in only one of the patients with CSF rhinorrhea. Frontalis or supraorbital nerve palsies have also been described related to this approach.

SPHENOID RIDGE AND MINI-PTERIONAL
History

In his 1975 article, Yasargil described the versatile use of the PT for access to a wide variety of aneurysms in the circle of Willis.[2] The PT provides good access to the sylvian fissure, allowing for a wide split between the frontal and temporal lobes, and access to midline structures with minimal brain retraction. A key step in the original approach is drilling of the sphenoid ridge to the base of the anterior clinoid. It allows wide access to many of the midline structures, including anterior and posterior circulation aneurysms, lesion within the sellar and parasellar regions, cavernous sinus, sphenoid wing, and midbrain. One of the drawbacks of the PT is the need for the dissection of the temporalis. This results in atrophy of the muscle, and possible unfavorable cosmesis for patients. Further, there is a risk of injury to the frontal branch of the facial nerve resulting in frontalis palsy.

In 2005 Nathal and colleagues first described the use of a smaller keyhole craniotomy centered around the sylvian fissure.[9] This technique uses a smaller 3 × 3 cm focal craniotomy encompassing a frontozygomatic point, the sylvian line, and the pterion. The frontozygomatic point is located just below the lateral and superior edge of the orbital rim, and roughly 2.5 cm above whereby the frontal zygomatic arch joins the orbital rim. The key step to the sphenoid ridge craniotomy is drilling of the sphenoid ridge to the base of the anterior clinoid, similar to the original PT, which provides adequate access to the proximal sylvian for standard microsurgical dissection. This thereby provides a corridor to the basal cisterns for an approach to the sella and parasellar structures comparable to the PT. The authors were able to use this modification to treat aneurysms of the ICA, PCoA, anterior choroidal (AChor), MCA, and ACoA. In 2007, Figueiredo and colleagues described a similar approach, with a focal craniotomy at the proximal sylvian fissure, and coined the term mPT.[9]

Technique

Patient positioning principles for the mPT are similar to that described in the SO craniotomy section. However, the rotation to the contralateral side extends to 40°. An arcuate scalp incision is used. The incision starts 1 cm above the base of the zygomatic arch and at the anterior border of the hairline. It extends cranially 4 to 5 cm toward the ipsilateral superior temporal line. The scalp flap is reflected anteriorly in a routine fashion. The temporalis is elevated subperiostally and then retracted caudally and posterior, until the pterion is exposed. The temporalis has to be disinserted from the superior temporal line over about 2 to 3 cm to allow a good exposure of the pterions.

The craniotomy is positioned with a burr hole just above the frontozygomatic suture, and below the superior temporal line. The craniotomy cuts are then made such that the superior cut follows the superior temporal line until the stephanion, then curving sharply down to make a posterior cut to include the pterion, a second cut from the initial burr hole is taken inferiorly and then anteriorly until the sphenoid ridge is reached from later in discussion. The 2 cuts can be connected with a high-speed drill. The mPT is thereby designed to include the lateral portion of the sphenoid bone. The sphenoid ridge is then drilled down and flattened. The medial extent of this drilling is the meningo-orbital band at the lateral extent of the superior orbital fissure. The dura is typically opened in a curvilinear fashion and flapped toward the skull base.

Esposito and colleagues recently described their modification to the mPT and their experience. In their approach, there is no need for interfascial dissection, and the temporalis muscle is split in a T-shaped fashion with a vertical incision 1 cm anteriorly to the skin incision.[10] Forward retraction of the temporalis sufficiently exposes the pterion but covers the keyhole and the orbitozygomatic process of the frontal bone.

Indications

The mPT is centered on the sphenoid wing and exposes both the frontal and temporal lobe. This allows an optimal access to the sylvian fissure and the basal cisterns. This approach provides access to the proximal sylvian fissure, typically until the anterior ascending ramus. Standard microsurgical dissection of the sylvian fissure, with the opening of the optico-carotid, chiasmatic, and crural cisternal allows for access to the microsurgical clipping of typically MCA, PCoA, and AChor aneurysms. With regards to MCA aneurysms, the depth of aneurysm within the sylvian fissure helps determine the suitability of mPT. The more superficial (as indicated by the distance of the aneurysm from the M1 origin) the more suitable the mPT.[10]

Disadvantages

A disadvantage of the mPT is the limited access to the distal end of the sylvian fissure, making this approach suboptimal in cases of ruptured aneurysms whereby hemorrhage or brain swelling can be encountered. The frontal limit of the craniotomy may significantly restrict dynamic or static retraction of the frontal lobe during sylvian fissure dissection and exposure. While the exposure of the proximal sylvian fissure and M1 segment is adequate, it is achieved from behind and tangentially. For short M1 segments with a bifurcation occurring before the limen insulae, a more subfrontal angle may be useful as provided by the lateral supraorbital (LSO) approach (discussed later in discussion). The limitation of the subfrontal route as used in the SO, LSO, and regular PT, results in a more lateral approach to the midline structures such as the chiasm and ACoA complex. Finally, the temporalis dissection is more extensive than in other keyhole approaches. This may result in more postoperative mastication pain and muscle atrophy. Moreover, it may put the frontal branch of the facial nerve at risk of injury.[11]

LATERAL SUPRAORBITAL
History

In 2005, Hernesniemi published his description and experience with the LSO craniotomy.[12] The approach was designed to be an alternative to the PT. The LSO incorporates a smaller version of the frontal aspect of the classic PT, coming to the sphenoid ridge laterally with no drilling of the sphenoid wing and no temporal bone exposure.

The LSO focuses on the subfrontal approach to the midline and sellar structures, but allows relatively easy access to the sylvian fissure as well. The approach has been used to access numerous aneurysms of the anterior circulation, and for tumors in the anterior skull base, parasellar, and sphenoid wing region.

Technique

Principles of patient positioning are similar to those that which has been described in the SO craniotomy section. A short curvilinear scalp incision is placed at the edge of the hairline. The incision starts 3 cm above the zygoma and curved gently toward the midline. A myocutaneous skin flap is reflected anteriorly after subperiosteal dissection. This helps prevent injury to the frontal branch of the facial nerve. In this approach, only the superior and anterior portion of the temporalis is split, which minimizes atrophy of the muscle. The flap is dissected anteriorly until the lateral two-thirds of the superior orbital rim is exposed, along with the superior portion of the frontal zygomatic process. The craniotomy centered around the intersection of the superior temporal line with the superior orbital rim. It is typically conducted with a single burr hole 2.5 cm posterior to the keyhole on the superior temporal line or just below it. This helps maintain cosmesis, as the burr hole is tucked under the muscle. The craniotomy is usually placed one-half above and one-half below the superior temporal line. The inferior part of the craniotomy should be flush with the sphenoid wing and the orbital roof. The superior part of the craniotomy is cut in the frontal bone superior to the temporal line and curves back inferiorly along the anterior skull base. It can be tailored to the lesion and can be extended in the direction of the midline if necessary.

After the flap is raised on the medial side of the sphenoid ridge, the orbital rim and orbital roof are drilled to maintain an even subfrontal view of the parasellar structures. The use of "hot" drilling with less irrigation with a diamond burr can be used to maintain bone hemostasis. Dura is opened with a curvilinear incision flapped toward the skull base. The sylvian fissure is located at the temporal edge of the craniotomy. It can be split from the frontal side. A standard subfrontal microsurgical approach can be used to access the midline structures. The approach has been used by our group to treat ruptured and unruptured MCA aneurysms (**Figs. 2** and **3**, Video 1). The deepest and more proximal the MCA aneurysm locates in the sylvian fissure the more suitable the LSO is to approach the lesion. In general, and in line with Esposito

and colleagues we think the LSO is optimal to approach MCA aneurysms with a short M1 segment located in the proximal sylvian fissure up to the limen insulae, while more distal aneurysms over the insula may be better approached with a sylvian centered approach such as the mPT as discussed above. We also use this approach for ruptured and unruptured ACoA (**Fig. 4**), PCoA, and Anchor aneurysm.

Our group has described a modification to this technique, which we refer to as the extended lateral supraorbital approach (ELSO).[13] In this technique we describe a method for performing an extradural anterior clinoidectomy through an LSO craniotomy with no extension of the craniotomy over the temporal bone. This allows the operator to reach not only the anterior clinoid extradurally but the entire extradural antero lateral skull base, including the cavernous sinus, the lateral orbit, and the middle fossa. The extradural anterior clinoidectomy was first described by Dolenc, to provide better access and safer management of ophthalmic and paraclinoid aneurysms.[14,15] When described, it was used in combination with a PT, or orbitozygomatic craniotomy. In the ELSO, the standard LSO craniotomy is performed, followed by the dissection of the dura off the orbital roof and sphenoid wing. These two bony surfaces are then thinned down with a 5 mm diamond drill under microscopic vision, until the lateral extent of the superior orbital fissure, meningo-orbital fold, lateral temporal dura, medial temporal dura, and anterior temporal dura are exposed. This drilling provides a fronto-pterional-orbital window to the extradural skull base through a purely frontal (LSO) keyhole craniotomy. The superior orbital fissure is unroofed, and the meningo-orbital fold cut, to separate the temporal dura from the anterior clinoid process. The ACP is then resected extradurally. The optic canal is opened with a 2 mm diamond drill, with subsequent resection of the anterior clinoid process. This technique provides better visualization of critical paraclinoid neurovascular structures and provides access to surgical clip ligation of paraclinoid aneurysms. Intradurally, it allows a wider exposure of the sylvian fissure, and access to temporomesial structures that are less accessible with the SO or the LSO keyhole approaches.

Disadvantages

The LSO is positioned primarily for a subfrontal approach with lateral reach of the mid and proximal sylvian fissure but has limited access to the temporal lobe and distal sylvian fissure. This approach is, therefore, limited to cases with a

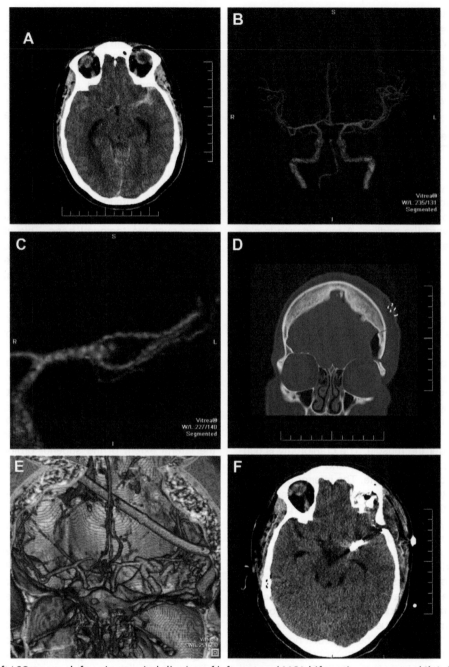

Fig. 2. Left LSO approach for microsurgical clipping of left ruptured MCA bifurcation aneurysm. (*A*) Axial section of CT head shows SAH in sylvian fissures greater on the left and acute hydrocephalus. (*B, C*) 3D reconstructions of coronal CT angiogram show a 3 mm left MCA bifurcation aneurysm. (*D–F*) Left LSO was used to obliterate this aneurysm using microsurgical clips. No postoperative venous or arterial infarct were identified.

large temporal clot, or brain swelling, that can be encountered in cases of ruptured aneurysms. Despite these limitations, the LSO may be the more versatile, "in-between" minimally invasive version of the PT, compared with the more medial, purely subfrontal SO and the more lateral mPT.

MINIMALLY INVASIVE SURGERY INTERHEMISPHERIC
History

In 1936, Wilhelm Tonnis first introduced the frontal interhemispheric approach for surgical treatment of ACoA aneurysm.[16] In the initial description, a

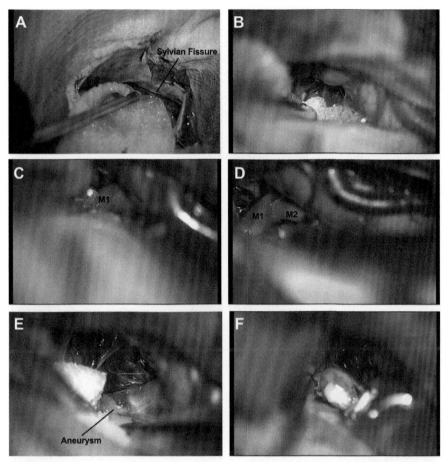

Fig. 3. Right LSO for microsurgical clipping of a right unruptured M1 aneurysm. (*A, B*) The craniotomy resides two-thirds above and one-third below the superior temporal line. In the LSO approach, the sylvian fissure lies just below the postero-inferior edge of the craniotomy. The intact sphenoid ridge, main point of LSO, serves as natural fixed retractor between the frontal and temporal lobes. Gentle retraction on the frontal lobe brings the sylvian fissure into view and allows fissure dissection. (*C–F*) Sylvian fissure dissection reveals the aneurysm in the M1 and its microsurgical clipping.

bifrontal craniotomy and midline subfrontal exposure was used. The bifrontal basal anterior interhemispheric approach provides faster proximal control and access to the basal cisterns, however, includes more soft tissue and bony exposure.[17] In 1991 Fukushima described a keyhole anterior interhemispheric approach for distal ACA and ACoA aneurysms.[18] This was further refined by Zheng and colleagues who introduce a hairline incision for this approach.[19] In our institution, the minimal invasive anterior interhemispheric approach is used for both ruptured and unruptured distal ACA aneurysms requiring surgical treatment.

Technique

Patient is placed supine on the surgical table and the head fixed on the head frame in a neutral and flexed position. A right-side incision, asymmetric to the side of craniotomy, across the midline is placed behind the hairline according to the location of the aneurysm along the ACA. The location of the aneurysm in relationship with the genu of corpus callosum guides the extent of flexion of the head and subsequently the location of craniotomy and working angle. Neuronavigation can be used to further verify the craniotomy site, the angle of trajectory, and the presence of parasagittal veins. The right side is usually chosen to minimize the risk of injury on the dominant hemisphere. For the craniotomy one burr hole is made on the superior sagittal sinus and a 2.5 × 3 cm right median/paramedian craniotomy is performed. The dura is incised with care not to injure any of the bridging veins and then it is pediculated over the midline. Under microscopic vision, an interhemispheric approach is carried out along the falx and then the dissection of the

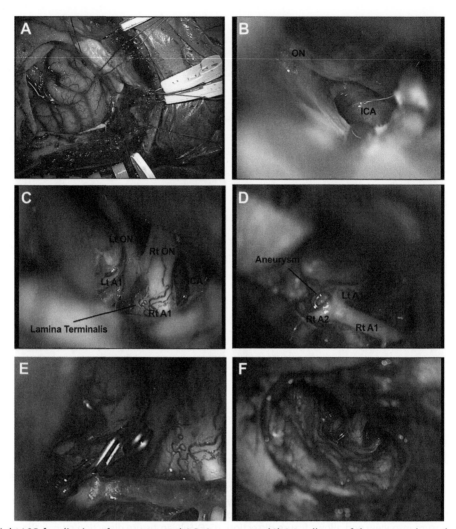

Fig. 4. Right LSO for clipping of an unruptured ACoA aneurysm. (*A*) A small part of the temporal muscle has been detached from the temporal line and retracted anteriorly along with the soft tissue. Following a single burr hole in the posterior end of the superior temporal line, a 3 × 3cm craniotomy ending at the sphenoid wing and orbital rim is made. The dura is flap is retracted anteriorly and the frontal lobe is revealed. The sylvian fissure locates just below the postero-inferior edge of the craniotomy. (*B*) Using dynamic retraction the optic nerve (ON) and internal carotid artery (ICA) are identified. (*C*) Under dynamic retractions, opening of the basal cisterns is performed and the bilateral ONs, the optic chiasm, the lamina terminalis, bilateral A1s, and right A2 are identified. (*D*) At this stage, a fixed retractor is placed gently on the frontal lobe and the aneurysm is dissected. (*E*) Single straight clip excluded the aneurysm from the circulation. (*F*) Low magnification image reveals the operative window.

interhemispheric fissure and between the 2 cingulate gyri is performed. In our experience, the intraoperative corridor for microsurgical clipping of unruptured aneurysms via anterior interhemispheric keyhole approach is sufficient. For ruptured cases, an external ventricular drain can be inserted in the lateral edge of craniotomy allowing CSF release and subsequent brain relaxation. **Fig. 5** depicts the use of MIS interhemispheric craniotomy for microsurgical clipping of a ruptured saccular aneurysm at the junction of the right A2-A3 segments.

ENDOSCOPIC TRANSPTERIONAL PORT APPROACH
History

The endoscope has served as a useful adjunct for keyhole approaches by bringing areas hidden "around the corner" into view and providing illumination to these areas. However, purely endoscopic approaches have also been described as a method of aneurysm treatment. For example, Perneczky and colleagues performed microsurgical clipping of 7 aneurysms using exclusively an endoscope through a PT.[20]

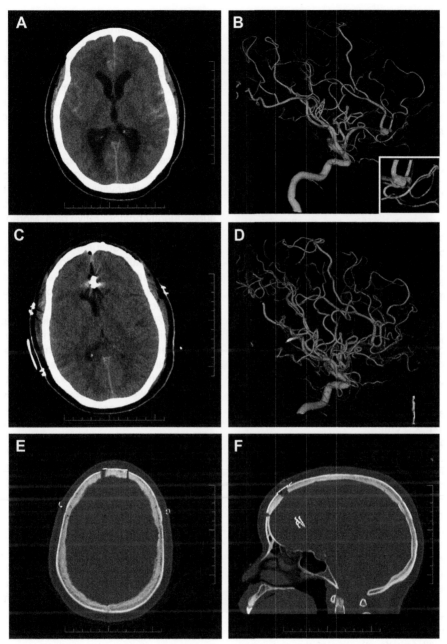

Fig. 5. Anterior interhemispheric keyhole approach for microsurgical clipping of right ACA aneurysm. (*A*) Plain axial CT head demonstrates thick SAH in bilateral sylvian fissures and in the anterior interhemispheric fissure as well as acute hydrocephalus (*B*) 3D reconstruction image from a right ICA injection demonstrates a wide-neck, lobulated saccular aneurysm arising from the junction of the A2-A3 segments of the right ACA and directed anteriorly. The aneurysm measures 5.1 × 7.7 mm and has a 3.3 mm neck. (*C*) Postoperative plain CT head shows aneurysm clips in the interhemispheric fissure, no new arterial or venous infarct, and stable SAH. (*D*) Postoperative 3D reconstruction image from a right ICA injection confirms complete obliteration of the aneurysm. (*E, F*) Axial and sagittal cuts show the extent of bone window (2.5 cm anteroposterior x 3 cm medial to lateral).

As a refinement of both minimally invasive microscopic keyhole approaches and the use of endoscopy in transcranial approaches, our group has developed a port-based endoscopic trans-pterional (ETPA) approach for clip ligation of unruptured anterior circulation aneurysms and other lesions of the antero-lateral skull base.[21] We have published the results from our experience with ETPA, which includes 13 aneurysms treated using this method. Twelve were MCA aneurysms, and one was a PcoA aneurysm. In all patients treated with this technique, complete obliteration of the aneurysm was achieved without intraoperative complications. In long-term follow-up for these patients, there was no change in their modified ranking score. All patients also reported a good cosmetic satisfaction level in long-term follow-up.

Technique

Patients are positioned supine with their heads rotated 20 to 30° toward the contralateral side. The ETPA approach involves two small incisions. The first one measures 3.5 to 4 cm with the epicenter on the lateral projection of the sphenoid wing. It is placed behind the hairline and below the superior temporal line. The second incision is smaller measures 0.5 to 1 cm and is placed just above the fronto-zygomatic suture. The second incision is optional, however, its use as a second port for the endoscope provides an orthogonal view of the sylvian fissure. The craniotomy is designed by placing a burr-hole at the posterior end of pterion and centering the bone flap over the lateral projection of the sphenoid wing. The craniotome is used to drill to a bone window of 1.5 × 1.5 to 2 × 3 cm.

The dura is opened over the sylvian fissure in a curvilinear fashion and flapped toward the skull base. The dural flap can be secured in place using an aneurysmal clip. The sylvian fissure, and basal cisterns are opened using the standard endoscopic technique, similar to endonasal skull base surgery, with the use of single shafted instruments with bimanual microneurosurgical technique. The endoscope is maneuvered by the assistant surgeon through the small port skin incision or through the main posterior incision depending on the angle of view needed. This allows exposure of the ipsilateral optic nerve (ON), supraclinoid ICA, and the proximal segments of the MCA and ACA, to facilitate safe clipping of the aneurysm (Video 2). Wide sylvian fissure and a relatively simple aneurysms configuration with no major branches adherent to the aneurysm dome and a well-defined neck on preoperative imaging are for now elements required to choose this approach in our practice.

OUTPATIENT ANEURYSM SURGERY

Day surgery is well implemented in many different aspects of surgical care. Day surgery decreases dramatically the length of hospital stay and thus the risk of perioperative complications. Day

surgery has a significant impact on global health and on health care budgets. Day surgery has been well described in the neurosurgical practice. Our institution has established the outpatient surgery for brain tumor resection with great outcomes.[22–24] Stepping on this tradition, in 2009 the first outpatient clipping of an unruptured cerebral aneurysm was established by one of the senior authors (M.T.) at the Toronto Western Hospital, University Health Network.

Outpatient surgery for microsurgical clipping of unruptured aneurysms requires the implementation of minimally invasive craniotomies that minimize bone and soft tissue injury and subsequently postoperative pain. Moreover, great collaboration with anesthesiology team is necessary to ensure adequate preoperative assessment, optimization of perioperative quality of care and anesthetic safety as well as management and of postoperative nausea, vomiting, and pain.

Retrospective analysis of our data between 2009 and 2012 identified 25 patients that met the neurosurgical and anesthetic criteria to undergo day surgery for one or more aneurysms of the anterior circulation.[25] Seventeen patients successfully completed the day surgery. Of the 17 patients that were successfully treated in an outpatient manner only one required readmission for a minor cerebral ischemic event. However, 32% of the participants failed to be discharged the same day secondary to perioperative complications (decreased level of consciousness, bradycardia, fever, severe postoperative nausea, severe postoperative pain, generalized motor weakness, and seizures).[25]

The implementation of the careful selection neurosurgical and medical criteria along with minimally invasive surgical techniques and excellent perioperative anesthetic management may make day surgery a viable option for the treatment of unruptured anterior circulation aneurysms.

DISCUSSION

Our group has primary experience in keyhole approaches for anterior circulation aneurysms. These include the SO craniotomy, mPT, LSO craniotomy, and keyhole interhemispheric craniotomy. In 2014 we completed a comparative analysis of safety and cost of MIS and outpatient approaches relative to classic open surgery for aneurysms.[26] In this retrospective cohort study, MIS and standard open strategies were comparable in surgical complications, aneurysm obliteration, and patient outcome measured by the modified Rankin Scale (mRS). MIS strategies were found to result in significantly shorter operative time relative to standard open approaches. Finally, in the treatment of unruptured aneurysms, MIS strategies resulted in a significantly shorter length of hospital stay, and reduced treatment costs. These results highlight the benefit of MIS approaches to the health care system and patient experience.

Jagersberg and colleagues conducted a study comparing the various MIS approaches with respect to maneuverability and working volumes in relation to different aneurysm targets.[27] The authors used the SO craniotomy, mPT, and LSO and perform anatomic dissection on cadavers. Using image guidance, 3D CT reconstructions, and image analysis software they calculate the surface area, distance to specific anatomic targets, and working volume for each keyhole approach to derive a target-specific maneuverability index. In their study, the different MIS approaches provided comparable deep surface exposure relative to the standard PT, despite using a smaller superficial surface area, thereby validating the keyhole concept. The 3 keyhole approaches did not differ significantly with respect to deep surface area exposed, or surgical corridor volume. The authors also quantified maneuverability around specific deep anatomic targets to compare the different keyhole approaches. They defined a maneuverability index that factors in the distance to target, the presence of bony obstacles or critical neurovascular structures, and the presence of a target within the surgical working corridor. Based on this maneuverability index the mPT had the best maneuverability for ophthalmic, PCoA, and MCA, and PCA aneurysms. The LSO had the best maneuverability for basilar tip aneurysms. The SO, mPT, and LSO had comparable maneuverability for ICA bifurcation and ACoA aneurysms.

In 2021, Mandel and colleagues published results from a prospective randomized controlled study comparing MIS and standard PT for the treatment of unruptured intracranial aneurysms.[3] In their study, they noted significantly better cosmetic results from MIS strategies as evaluated by 2 independent observers. They also reported significantly less temporalis muscle atrophy. Additionally, patients scored significantly higher on satisfaction and quality of life measures when undergoing MIS aneurysm procedures. They also noted comparable functional outcomes in the mRS scores at an 8 to 12 month follow-up in patients undergoing both MIS and standard open treatment of aneurysms.

Disadvantages of the keyhole approach include narrow working space, reduced light intensity, and limited space for instruments. Even though the reduced light intensity is of less worry with the most advanced microscopes, efficient movement and positioning of the operative microscope, and the use of endoscope can overcome this barrier.

Finally, it is important to remember that all main keyhole approaches, the SO, the mPT, and the LSO are smaller variants that have primarily evolved from the classic PT craniotomy. They exploit the same optimal antero-lateral routes along the MCA, ICA, and ACA axes and toward the skull base. They require the same microsurgical techniques and aneurysm surgery concepts that those used for many decades to treat anterior circulation aneurysms. In essences, they are relatively small variations, adaptations, and refinements on a standard long-standing, and conserved theme that has not changed as Dandy clipped the first PCoA aneurysm through a fronto-temporal craniotomy in 1938. Yasargil has revolutionized modern neurosurgery by the introduction of the microscope, understanding and exploiting cisternal anatomy and expanded surgical corridors by removing bone (sphenoid ridge) while still using, like Dandy, a fronto-temporal route to the anterior circulations. Current day keyhole approaches likewise conserve the main gains of previous advances while introducing nuances along the same evolutionary force toward reduced invasiveness which from Dandy to Yasargil to modern-day endoscopic approaches has been the main impetus and driver of progress in neurosurgery.

CLINICS CARE POINTS

- Minimally invasive approaches for anterior circulation aneurysms offer great outcomes with appropriate patient selection and higly trained cerebrovascular team.

SUPPLEMENTARY DATA

Supplementary data related to this article can be found online at https://doi.org/10.1016/j.nec.2022.05.005.

REFERENCES

1. Polevaya NV, Kalani MY, Steinberg GK, et al. The transition from hunterian ligation to intracranial aneurysm clips: a historical perspective. Neurosurg Focus 2006;20(6):E3.

2. Yasargil MG, Fox JL. The microsurgical approach to intracranial aneurysms. Surg Neurol 1975;3(1):7–14.

3. Mandel M, Tutihashi R, Li Y, et al. MISIAN (Minimally Invasive Surgery for Treatment of Unruptured Intracranial Aneurysms): A Prospective Randomized Single-Center Clinical Trial With Long-Term Follow-Up Comparing Different Minimally Invasive Surgery Techniques with Standard Open Surgery. World Neurosurg 2021;151:e533–44.

4. Wong JH, Tymianski R, Radovanovic I, et al. Minimally Invasive Microsurgery for Cerebral Aneurysms. Stroke 2015;46(9):2699–706.

5. Jane JA, Park TS, Pobereskin LH, et al. The supraorbital approach: technical note. Neurosurgery 1982; 11(4):537–42.

6. Paladino J, Pirker N, Stimac D, et al. Eyebrow keyhole approach in vascular neurosurgery. Minim Invasive Neurosurg 1998;41(4):200–3.

7. van Lindert E, Perneczky A, Fries G, et al. The supraorbital keyhole approach to supratentorial aneurysms: concept and technique. Surg Neurol 1998; 49(5):481–9 [discussion: 489–90].

8. Thaher F, Hopf N, Hickmann AK, et al. Supraorbital Keyhole Approach to the Skull Base: Evaluation of Complications Related to CSF Fistulas and Opened Frontal Sinus. J Neurol Surg A Cent Eur Neurosurg 2015;76(6):433–7.

9. Nathal E, Gomez-Amador JL. Anatomic and surgical basis of the sphenoid ridge keyhole approach for cerebral aneurysms. Neurosurgery 2005;56(1 Suppl):178–85 [discussion: 178–85].

10. Esposito G, Dias SF, Burkhardt JK, et al. Selection Strategy for Optimal Keyhole Approaches for Middle Cerebral Artery Aneurysms: Lateral Supraorbital Versus Minipterional Craniotomy. World Neurosurg 2019;122:e349–57.

11. Rychen J, Croci D, Roethlisberger M, et al. Minimally Invasive Alternative Approaches to Pterional Craniotomy: A Systematic Review of the Literature. World Neurosurg 2018;113:163–79.

12. Hernesniemi J, Ishii K, Niemela M, et al. Lateral supraorbital approach as an alternative to the classical pterional approach. Acta Neurochir Suppl 2005;94: 17–21.

13. Andrade-Barazarte H, Jagersberg M, Belkhair S, et al. The Extended Lateral Supraorbital Approach and Extradural Anterior Clinoidectomy Through a Frontopterio-Orbital Window: Technical Note and Pilot Surgical Series. World Neurosurg 2017;100: 159–66.

14. Dolenc VV. A combined epi- and subdural direct approach to carotid-ophthalmic artery aneurysms. J Neurosurg 1985;62(5):667–72.

15. Dolenc VV. Extradural approach to intracavernous ICA aneurysms. Acta Neurochir Suppl 1999;72: 99–106.

16. Buchfelder M. From trephination to tailored resection: neurosurgery in Germany before World War II. Neurosurgery 2005;56(3):605–13 [discussion: 605–13].

17. Chhabra R, Gupta SK, Mohindra S, et al. Distal anterior cerebral artery aneurysms: bifrontal basal anterior interhemispheric approach. Surg Neurol 2005; 64(4):315–9 [discussion: 320].

18. Fukushima T, Miyazaki S, Takusagawa Y, et al. Unilateral interhemispheric keyhole approach for anterior cerebral artery aneurysms. Acta Neurochir Suppl (Wien) 1991;53:42–7.

19. Zheng SF, Yao PS, Yu LH, et al. Surgical Technique for Aneurysms at the A3 Segment of Anterior Cerebral Artery Via Anterior Interhemispheric Keyhole Approach. Turk Neurosurg 2017;27(1):22–30.

20. Perneczky A, Boecher-Schwarz HG. Endoscope-assisted microsurgery for cerebral aneurysms. Neurol Med Chir (Tokyo) 1998;38(Suppl):33–4.

21. Andrade-Barazarte H, Patel K, Turel MK, et al. The endoscopic transpterional port approach: anatomy, technique, and initial clinical experience. J Neurosurg 2019;132(3):884–94.

22. Boulton M, Bernstein M. Outpatient brain tumor surgery: innovation in surgical neurooncology. J Neurosurg 2008;108(4):649–54.

23. Carrabba G, Venkatraghavan L, Bernstein M. Day surgery awake craniotomy for removing brain tumours: technical note describing a simple protocol. Minim Invasive Neurosurg 2008;51(4):208–10.

24. Grundy PL, Weidmann C, Bernstein M. Day-case neurosurgery for brain tumours: the early United Kingdom experience. Br J Neurosurg 2008;22(3): 360–7.

25. Goettel N, Chui J, Venkatraghavan L, et al. Day surgery craniotomy for unruptured cerebral aneurysms: a single center experience. J Neurosurg Anesthesiol 2014;26(1):60–4.

26. Radovanovic I, Abou-Hamden A, Bacigaluppi S, et al. A safety, length of stay, and cost analysis of minimally invasive microsurgery for anterior circulation aneurysms. Acta Neurochir (Wien) 2014; 156(3):493–503.

27. Jagersberg M, Brodard J, Qiu J, et al. Quantification of Working Volumes, Exposure, and Target-Specific Maneuverability of the Pterional Craniotomy and Its Minimally Invasive Variants. World Neurosurg 2017; 101:710–7.e2.

Evolution in Cerebrovascular Bypass
Conceptual Framework, Technical Nuances, and Initial Clinical Experience with Fourth-Generation Bypass

Visish M. Srinivasan, MD[a,1], Redi Rahmani, MD[a,1],
Mohamed A. Labib, MD, CM[a], Michael J. Lang, MD[b],
Joshua S. Catapano, MD[a], Christopher S. Graffeo, MD, MS[a],
Michael T. Lawton, MD[a,*]

KEYWORDS

- Aneurysm • Bypass • Cerebral • Cerebrovascular • Fourth generation • Intracranial
- Moyamoya disease

KEY POINTS

- There have been three generations of cerebrovascular bypass: direct extracranial-intracranial (first generation), extracranial-intracranial with interposition graft (second generation), and intracranial-intracranial (third generation).
- Fourth-generation bypasses include constructs that use an atypical anastomotic technique (type 4A) or an atypical vascular orientation (type 4B).
- The fourth-generation bypass concept deepens the armamentarium of options available to cerebrovascular surgeons for treating complex aneurysms, ischemic disease, and other conditions.

INTRODUCTION

Cerebrovascular bypass was first described by Donaghy and Yaşargil in 1967; it was initially conceptualized as a flow augmentation technique for ischemic indications[1] and was later expanded to encompass flow replacement in the setting of complex aneurysms or skull base tumors.[2–4] Cerebrovascular bypass for complex cerebral aneurysms has evolved over the years, influenced heavily by the changes in endovascular technology. At present, routine indications for open cerebrovascular bypass in the treatment of intracranial aneurysms are limited to complex and challenging lesions, including lesions characterized by a wide neck, large size, dolichoectatic morphology, intraluminal thrombus, recurrent or residual aneurysm after endovascular therapy, or severe atherosclerosis.[5–7] Although numerous stepwise technical advances have been reported over time, the major innovations in cerebrovascular bypass are readily grouped into three well-described generations: direct extracranial-intracranial (EC–IC, first generation), interposition

Financial support: None.

Submission category: original article.

[a] Department of Neurosurgery, Barrow Neurological Institute, St. Joseph's Hospital and Medical Center, Phoenix, AZ, USA; [b] Department of Neurosurgery, University of Pittsburgh Medical Center, Pittsburgh, PA, USA

[1] Denotes equal contribution to the manuscript.

* Corresponding author. Neuroscience Publications, Barrow Neurological Institute, St. Joseph's Hospital and Medical Center, 350 West Thomas Road, Phoenix, AZ 85013.

E-mail address: Neuropub@barrowneuro.org

Neurosurg Clin N Am 33 (2022) 383–402
https://doi.org/10.1016/j.nec.2022.06.004

EC–IC (second generation), and intracranial-intracranial (IC–IC, third generation).

The first generation of superficial temporal artery to M4 middle cerebral artery (MCA) operations established and popularized the technique, with many surgeons achieving proficiency and favorable patency outcomes.[8] Indications proliferated, ranging from flow augmentation in the setting of ischemic disease to flow replacement or revascularization for the treatment of intracranial aneurysms.[9–12] These early successes laid the foundation for innovative approaches to more complex lesions, such as paraclinoid and cavernous segment aneurysms, that required high-flow bypass and gave rise to the second generation of cerebrovascular bypass operations. Novel techniques pioneered by Dr Thoralf Sundt and others included several variations on the EC–IC interposition graft, in which a saphenous vein or radial artery is sutured to the external carotid or vertebral artery (VA) extracranially and a large circle of Willis vessel intracranially.[13] Although such bypasses are still applicable to certain unusual cases of ischemic disease or failed endovascular treatment, indications for second-generation bypass have become less prominent since the introduction of flow diversion.[14]

Third-generation bypass evolved in response to the major limitations of second-generation techniques, including donor site complications, tunneling, multiple anastomoses, and recipient-graft mismatch.[15,16] The first reported IC–IC anastomoses were the side-to-side in situ bypasses (p3 posterior inferior cerebellar artery [PICA] to p3 PICA and A3 anterior cerebral artery [ACA] to A3 ACA bypasses), with subsequent expansion to include reanastomosis, reimplantation, and IC–IC interposition.[5,15,17,18] These operations represent the contemporary workhorses of cerebrovascular bypass and the putative limit of innovation that is accessible by the selection of new vessels for rearrangement. The utility of third-generation bypass nonetheless remains limited for treating certain highly complicated aneurysms, motivating further innovations at a higher level of resolution. Specifically, technical variations incorporating novel suturing techniques or vessel orientations have been described, yielding a fourth generation of cerebrovascular bypasses.[5,19]

The designation "fourth generation" is arrived at by two avenues, classified as type 4A and 4B operations (Fig. 1). Although most conventional bypass procedures involve manipulation of the donor vessel in three-dimensional space to complete the backside suture line, the mobility of certain vessels is highly restricted due to the presence of tethering branches, perforators, or neural structures, which renders them poor candidates for third-generation constructs. The innovative solution to this obstacle is to adapt the intraluminal suturing technique from classical side-to-side anastomoses into more advanced constructs, resulting in the type 4A bypass.

In parallel, certain configurations of aneurysm and branch vessels are poorly suited to conventional bypass constructs (eg, the double reimplantation construct for a large MCA bifurcation aneurysm). In a more typical construct, the two efferent MCA branches would require separate end-to-side reanastomosis into either an EC–IC donor or the interposition graft, a rearrangement that may be complicated by the number and configuration of MCA perforators, the aneurysm dome, or other features. In this scenario, replacement of one end-to-end anastomosis with an end-to-side reconstruction between the two M2 vessels or one M2 and the donor graft may offer a more advantageous rearrangement. Still other variations combine multiple third-generation techniques. Put more generally, although type 4A bypasses are defined by the use of unconventional suturing techniques, type 4B bypasses involve the unconventional arrangement and anastomosis of the involved vessels, collectively resulting in at least 15 novel fourth-generation bypass possibilities (Table 1),[5,20–32] 9 of which are illustrated in Fig. 2.

METHODS
Patient Source, Outcomes, and Data Collection

A cohort study design was selected to capture all patients treated with cerebrovascular bypass by the senior author (MTL) during the study period (November 1, 1997 to November 30, 2021). A prospectively maintained neurosurgical registry was used. Age, sex, diagnosis, and all pertinent procedural details, including bypass type and generation, were captured for patients included in the study. Fourth-generation bypasses were identified by retrospective review of the operative report and patient registry, using a classification scheme described elsewhere.[5] All available postoperative cerebrovascular imaging studies and associated reports were reviewed by the study staff to define bypass patency. The study was approved by the St. Joseph's Hospital and Medical Center Institutional Review Board, and the need for patient consent was waived because of the retrospective nature of the study.

Data Management and Statistical Analysis

Data aggregation and exploratory analysis were performed in Microsoft Excel (version 16, Microsoft Corp). Descriptive statistics include

Type 4A

Type 4B

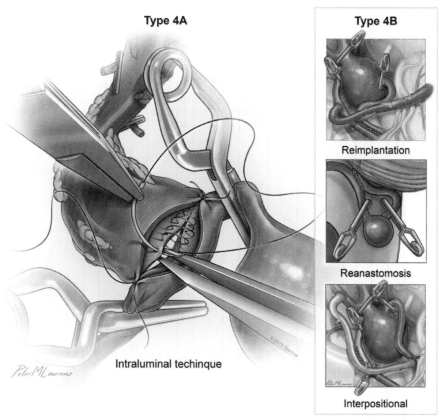

Reimplantation

Reanastomosis

Intraluminal techinque

Interpositional

Fig. 1. Illustration of the fourth-generation bypass subtypes, 4A and 4B. Type 4A bypasses (*left*) are conventional constructs but are created with an unconventional technique (ie, intraluminal technique on an end-to-end [E–E] or end-to-side [E–S] anastomosis). In this example, an intraluminal technique is used on an E–S anastomosis, which is atypical. Type 4B bypasses are unconventional constructs, created with conventional or unconventional suturing techniques. The three panels show reimplantation (*top right*; typically E–S, but here side-to-side [S–S]), reanastomosis (*middle right*; typically E–E, but here S–S), or intracranial-intracranial interpositional bypass (*bottom right*; typically E–S or E–E, but here S–S). (*Courtesy of* Barrow Neurological Institute, Phoenix, Arizona, USA.)

percentages and proportions for categorical variables and means with standard deviations for continuous variables. Categorical variables were assessed for associations using the χ^2 or Fisher exact tests as indicated by expected cell counts using GraphPad Prism 9 (GraphPad, San Diego, CA). Statistical significance was defined using the 0.05 alpha threshold.

RESULTS

Of 750 cerebrovascular bypass operations performed by the senior author (MTL), 44 (5.9%) were classified as fourth generation. The index fourth-generation bypass was a type 4A double reimplantation, completed in 2005. The index type 4B bypass, performed in 2007, was a double reimplantation with side-to-side reimplantation of the first recipient.

Indications included aneurysm ($n = 39$), moyamoya disease ($n = 2$), carotid circulation ischemia

($n = 2$), and compressive VA dolichoectasia ($n = 1$). Aneurysms predominantly involved the anterior circulation ($n = 22$), but there was a marked proportional representation in the posterior circulation ($n = 17$).

Revision or repair of the anastomosis was performed intraoperatively in 12 of 44 cases (27%). Troubleshooting took on various forms, including anastomosis revision ($n = 5$), excision of redundant or diseased artery ($n = 2$), thrombectomy with Fogarty balloon ($n = 2$), anastomosis cutdown ($n = 1$), "nursing" of a white plug along the suture line ($n = 1$), and papaverine treatment ($n = 1$). All repairs were made during the index operation.

Patency was determined by intraoperative indocyanine green videoangiography in 41 cases and postoperative angiography or computed tomography angiography in all 44 cases. The three earliest bypasses predated the availability of

Table 1
Generations of bypasses and comparative characteristics of fourth-generation bypasses

Bypass, Coding Example[a]	Reference	Seven Bypasses No.[b]	Bypass Generation	No. of Anastomoses	Anastomosis Orientation	Suturing Technique
EC–IC bypass		1				
STA (E–S) M4	Bot et al.[20]		1	1	E–S	Conventional
STA (E–S*) M4[c]			4A	1	E–S	Intraluminal
STA (S–S*) M4	Lang et al.[21]		4B	1	S–S	Intraluminal
EC–IC interpositional bypass		2				
ECA (S–E) RAG (E–S) M2	Tayebi Meybodi et al.[22]	2	2	2	E–S, E–E	Conventional
ECA (S–E*) RAG (E–S*) M2[c]			4A	2	E–S, E–E	Intraluminal
ECA (S–E) SVG (S–S*) M2 + A2 (E–S)[c]			4B	3	S–E, S–S, E–S	Conventional or intraluminal
Reimplantation		3				
L p3 PICA (S–E) R p3 PICA	Benet and Lawton[23]	3	3	1	E–S	Conventional
V4 (S–E*) p3 PICA[c]			4A	1	E–S	Intraluminal
M2 (E–E*) M2'			4B	1	E–E	Conventional or intraluminal
V4 (S–S*) a3	Baranoski et al.[24]		4B	1	S–S	Intraluminal
In situ bypass		4				
R A3 (S–S) L A3	Benet et al.[25]	3	3	1	S–S	Intraluminal
Reanastomosis		5				
R a2 (E–E) a2	Baranoski et al.[24]		3	1	E–E	Conventional
L V4 (E–E*) V4	Srinivasan et al.[26]		4A	1	E–E	Intraluminal
R p2 (S–E^i) p3[c]	Lazaro et al.[27]		4B	1	E–S	Conventional or intraluminal
L p2 (S–S*) L p3	Lee and Choi[28]		4B	1	S–S	Conventional or intraluminal

Example bypass	Reference	[b]	[a]	No.	Type	Technique
IC–IC interpositional bypass		6				
V3 (S–E) SVG (E–S) a3	Baranoski et al.[24]		3	2	E-S, E-E	Conventional
M2 (E–S*) RAG (E–S) P2	Lawton et al.[29]		4A	2	E-S, E-E	Intraluminal
R A1 (S–E) RAG [(S–S*) M2 + (E–S*) M2']	Lawton and Lang[5]		4B	2	S-S	Intraluminal
Combination bypass		7				
R A3 (S–S) L A3 + R A2 (S–E) RAG (E–S) ATA	Srinivasan et al.[30]		3	≥2	E-S, S-S, E-S	Conventional or intraluminal
L CmaA (S–E) RAG [(S–E*) R CmaA + (E–S) PcaA]	Mirzadeh et al.[31]		4A	3	E-S	Intraluminal
R STA (E–E) RAFF (E–S) [R A3 + (½S–½S*) L A3]	Ravina et al.[32]		4B	1 (three suture lines)	E-S	Conventional or intraluminal
R M1 (½ E) + R M2 (½E) + R M2'(½Eⁱ)			4B	1 (three suture lines)	E-E	Conventional or in situ

Example bypasses are coded using the schema described by Tayebi Meybodi et al.[45] The examples given are completed bypasses in the surgical series unless denoted as a "dream bypass." Since the publication of the initial version of this table, a new example of fourth-generation bypass has been described, the side-to-side STA-MCA bypass. The term "intraluminal" has been used to clarify the suturing technique, as opposed to the term "in situ technique," which has been previously used. Asterisk (*) indicates use of intraluminal suturing technique. Superscript "i" indicates use of interrupted suturing technique.

Abbreviations: a2, lateral pontine segment of anterior inferior cerebellar artery (AICA); a3, flocculopeduncular segment of AICA; A2, postcommunicating segment of anterior cerebral artery (ACA); A3, precallosal segment of ACA; ATA, anterior temporal artery; CmaA, callosomarginal artery; ECA, external carotid artery; EC-IC, extracranial-intracranial; E-E, end-to-end; E-S, end-to-side; L, left; M2, insular segment of middle cerebral artery (MCA); M4, cortical segment of MCA; p2, lateral medullary segment of posterior inferior cerebellar artery (PICA); p3, tonsillomedullary segment of PICA; PcaA, pericallosal artery; PICA, posterior inferior cerebellar artery; R, right; RAFF, radial artery fascial flow-through free flap; RAG, radial artery graft; S-S, side-to-side; STA, superficial temporal artery; SVG, saphenous vein graft; V3, extradural segment of vertebral artery; V4, intradural segment of vertebral artery.

a Coded according to the schema outlined in Tayebi Meybodi et al.[45]

b Designated according to the schema outlined in Lawton.[15] 1 = EC–IC bypass, 2 = EC–IC interposition bypass, 3 = reimplantation, 4 = in situ bypass, 5 = reanastomosis, 6 = IC–IC interposition bypass, 7 = combination bypass.

c "Dream bypass," which has not been performed.

Adapted from Lawton MT, Lang MJ. The future of open vascular neurosurgery: perspectives on cavernous malformations, AVMs, and bypasses for complex aneurysms. J Neurosurg. May 1 2019;130(5):1409-1425.

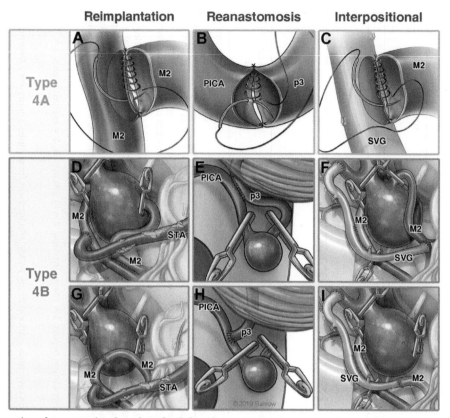

Fig. 2. Examples of type 4A (*A–C*) and 4B (*D–I*) fourth-generation bypasses, adapted from Lawton and Lang.[5] When conventional combinations of anastomoses and techniques are reshuffled, a fourth generation of bypasses results in 15 new types of bypasses, of which 9 are shown here. For example, the two efferent trunks of a complex right middle cerebral artery (MCA) aneurysm can be treated with trapping and bypass of the efferent trunks. Options include end-to-side reimplantation with the intraluminal technique (type 4A; *A*) or either side-to-side reimplantation or end-to-end reimplantation (type 4B; *D* and *G*, respectively). A fusiform posterior inferior cerebellar artery (PICA) aneurysm can be treated with excision and end-to-end reanastomosis; the construction can use the intraluminal technique (type 4A; *B*). Alternatively, the efferent and afferent PICA may be brought together in side-to-side reanastomosis or end-to-side reanastomosis (type 4B; *E* and *H*, respectively). Finally, the two efferent trunks of a complex right MCA aneurysm can be treated with trapping and interpositional bypass. When mobility is limited, one may use the intraluminal technique (type 4A; *C*) or either side-to-side reimplantation or end-to-end reimplantation (type 4B; *F* and *I*, respectively). M2, insular segment of MCA; p3, tonsillomedullary segment of PICA; STA, superficial temporal artery; SVG, saphenous vein graft. (*Used with permission from* Barrow Neurological Institute, Phoenix, Arizona, USA.)

indocyanine green videoangiography at our center. Postoperative imaging findings indicated that 39 (89%) of the bypasses were patent and 5 (11%) were occluded.

Postoperative neurologic examination findings (*n* = 20) were improved in 4 patients, were unchanged in 11 patients, and worsened in 5 patients. In the five patients whose neurologic examination findings were worse after the operation, the neurologic decline was attributable to the bypass or ischemia and correlated with the five cases of angiographic occlusion.

Data on discharge disposition were available for the 16 most recent consecutive patients. Discharge destinations included home (*n* = 7),

acute inpatient rehabilitation (*n* = 2), and skilled nursing (*n* = 4); 3 patients died during hospitalization.

Follow-up neurologic status was available for 17 patients, at a mean 6 months of total follow-up (median [range] 2 [0–20] months). Late imaging findings were available for 12 patients; construct patency was confirmed in all 12 patients. All-cause mortality as of the last follow-up was 11% (5 of 44 patients).

A literature review identified eight cases of fourth-generation bypass reported by surgeons other than the senior author (**Table 2**),[20,22,25–28,32–37] including 2 novel bypass configurations classifiable within the fourth-generation framework. The distribution

Table 2
Fourth-generation bypasses in the literature excluding those reported in the present series

Reference	Seven Bypasses No.[a]	Bypass Type	Bypass Coding[b]	Bypass Generation
Benes et al.[33]	3	Reimplantation	L V4 (E–E) L p1	4B
Matsushima et al.[34]	3	Reimplantation	L PcaA (E–E) L CmaA	4B
Lee and Choi[28]	5	Reanastomosis	L p2 (S–S) L p3	4B
Lazaro et al.[27]	5	Reanastomosis	R p2 (S–E) p3	4B
Sekhar et al. [35]	7	Combination (IC–IC interposition and reimplantation)	R M2 (S–E) SthG [(S–E) M3 + (E–E) M3']c	4B
Nakajima et al.[36]	7	Combination (EC–IC interposition and double reimplantation)	R STA (E–S) R M2 + R STA' [(S–S) M2' + (E–S) M2"] + R M2' (E–E) Perf + M1 (E–E) M2	4B
Arnone et al.[37]	7	Combination (EC–IC and reimplantation)	L STA [(S–S) L M4 + (E–S) L M4']d	4A and 4B
Ravina et al.[32]	7	Combination (EC–IC and in situ)	R STA (E–E) RAFF (E–S) [R A3 + (½S-½S*) L A3]	4B

Combination bypasses consist of multiple component bypasses. Please note the update to the earlier version of the table published in Lawton and Lang,[5] with the exclusion of cases by Kato et al.[49] and Lee et al.[50] After additional review, these cases were determined to not use 4B atypical construction. Asterisk (*) indicates use of intraluminal suturing technique.

Abbreviations: A3, precallosal segment of ACA; CmaA, callosomarginal artery; E–E, end-to-end; E–S, end-to-side; L, left; M1, sphenoidal segment of middle cerebral artery (MCA); M2, insular segment of MCA; M3, opercular segment of MCA; M4, cortical segment of MCA; p1, anterior medullary segment of posterior inferior cerebellar artery (PICA); p2, lateral medullary segment of PICA; p3, tonsillomedullary segment of PICA; PcaA, pericallosal artery; Perf, perforating artery; R, right; RAFF, radial artery fascial flow-through free flap; S–E, side-to-end; S–S, side-to-side; STA, superficial temporal artery; SthG, superior thyroid artery graft; V4, intradural segment of vertebral artery.

[a] Designated according to the schema outlined in Lawton.[15] 1 = EC–IC bypass, 2 = EC–IC interposition bypass, 3 = reimplantation, 4 = in situ bypass, 5 = reanastomosis, 6 = IC–IC interposition bypass, 7 = combination bypass.
[b] Coded according to the schema outlined in Tayebi Meybodi et al.[45]
c M2, M2', and M2" signify different middle cerebral artery trunks. Similarly, STA and STA' denote different postbifurcation superficial temporal artery trunks.
d The L STA (E–S) L M4'-MCA anastomosis was done with an intraluminal technique and therefore is considered both type 4A and type 4B.
Adapted with permission from Lawton and Lang.[5]

of fourth-generation bypass subtypes is shown in **Table 3**. Combination bypasses, which included type 4A and 4B bypasses, were the most common (*n* = 12), followed by the use of an intraluminal technique (type 4A) in IC–IC interposition bypass (*n* = 10) or in reanastomosis (*n* = 8). Several bypass subtypes have been conceived that have not yet been performed, adding to the list of "dream bypasses."[15]

Many of these complex bypasses preceded the development of the bypass coding nomenclature. Based on imaging, operative notes, and assessment of intraoperative photographs, bypass codes were assigned to all 44 bypasses (**Table 4**). The use of these codes both highlights the unique nature of these fourth-generation bypasses and shows the value of the code in conveying atypical constructs.

The use of these techniques was also assessed in the progression of the senior author's career. The senior author completed 148 first-generation bypasses before performing the first fourth-generation bypass in 2005; overall, first-generation operations account for 59% of all bypasses in the sample, a proportion that has remained relatively stable since the advent of fourth-generation procedures.[15] Overall, approximately 8% of aneurysms treated required bypass (254 bypasses among 4479 aneurysms in 3313 patients), of which 181 were performed using IC–IC techniques (71%).

DISCUSSION

We report the first cohort study of fourth-generation bypass operations, with particular attention to the distinguishing features of these novel techniques, and the preliminary experiences reported by our center and others in the contemporary literature. These new bypasses reflect the

Table 3
Distribution of fourth-generation bypass types

Bypass	Seven Bypasses No.[a]	Bypass Generation	No. of Anastomoses	Anastomosis Orientation	Suture Technique	No. of Cases
EC–IC	1	4B	1	S–S	Intraluminal	3
		4B	1	E–E	Conventional	1
EC–IC interpositional bypass	2	4A	2	E–S, E–E	Conventional	2
Reimplantation	3	4A	1	E–S	Intraluminal	4
		4B	1	E–E	Conventional or intraluminal	1
		4B	1	S–S	Intraluminal	1
Reanastomosis	5	4A	1	E–E	Intraluminal	8
		4B	1	E–S	Conventional or intraluminal	1
		4B	1	S–S	Conventional or intraluminal	0
IC–IC interpositional bypass	6	4A	2	E–S, E–E	Intraluminal	10
		4B	2	E–S, E–E	Conventional or intraluminal	0
		4B	2	S–S	Intraluminal	0
Combination bypass	7	4A, 4B	≥2	E–S, S–S, E–S	Conventional or intraluminal	12
EC–EC bypass	N/A	4A	2	E–S	Intraluminal	1
Total						44
All IC–IC bypasses						181

Combination bypasses consist of component bypasses and can be either 4A or 4B and were counted as such if any of the component bypasses were fourth generation. Double reimplantation bypasses accounted for several of the fourth-generation combination bypasses. The total number of all IC–IC bypasses is provided as a comparison only. Because fourth-generation bypasses are defined by the technique used rather than which vessels are brought together, this classification applies to EC–IC bypasses as well as EC–EC bypass.

Abbreviations: EC–EC, extracranial to extracranial; EC–IC, extracranial to intracranial; E–E, end-to-end; E–S, end-to-side; IC–IC, intracranial to intracranial; N/A, not applicable; S–S, side-to-side; 1, EC–IC bypass; 2, EC–IC interposition bypass; 3, reimplantation; 4, in situ bypass; 5, reanastomosis; 6, IC–IC interposition bypass; 7, combination bypass.

[a] Designated according to the schema outlined in Lawton.[15]

importance of evolution and innovation in the open cerebrovascular space as well as the need to maintain proficiency in microsurgical skills to provide care to a wide range of patients, however rare the pathology.

Fourth-Generation Bypass: Evolution of Practice

A large body of preceding literature has defined the indications for and outcomes associated with cerebrovascular bypass, in particular first-generation EC–IC operations, which have been widely validated as improving outcomes across a range of disease.[38] More contemporary evidence has expanded support for revascularization in the treatment of complex aneurysms.[39–41] Increasingly, patients with

aneurysms presenting for microsurgical treatment have required bypass; this change is likely attributable to the increasing portion of routine cases that are managed with endovascular techniques.

Long-term patency in the senior author's bypass series was recently assessed, with a very high overall percentage of patent bypasses (97%).[42] The percentage of bypasses with long-term patency was marginally lower among constructs involving high-flow grafts or multiple anastomotic sites.[42] Historical data reported by Sundt and coworkers confirmed a reproducible association between clinical volume and patency outcome in high-flow bypass operations, indicating that experience with at least 20 high-flow bypasses

Table 4
Coding system applied to 44 fourth-generation bypasses

Case No.	Bypass Generation[a]	Seven Bypasses No.[b]	Operative Title	Standard Naming	Full Bypass Code[c]
1	4A	7 (3, 6)	Anterior cerebral artery to pericallosal artery bypass with reimplantation of callosomarginal artery	R A1-RAG R CmaA-R PcaA	R A1 (S–E) RAG [(S–E*) CmaA + (E–S) PcaA]
2	4A	3	Reimplantation of pericallosal artery onto callosomarginal artery (end-to-side in situ bypass)	PcaA-CmaA	PcaA (E–S*ᶜ) CmaA
3	4B	7 (3, 6)	A1 anterior cerebral artery to middle cerebral artery bypass (double reimplantation)	R A1-RAG R M2+R M2'	R A1(S–E) RAG [(S–S) M2 + (E–S) M2']
4	4A, 4B	7 (3, 6)	R A2 anterior cerebral artery to L pericallosal artery and L callosomarginal artery bypass with radial artery graft (R ACA-L PcaA-L CmaA bypass, double reimplantation)	R A2-RAG-L CmaA + L PcaA	R A1 (S–E) RAG [(E–S*ᶜ) L CmaA + (S–S) L PcaA]
5	4B	3	Trapping of vertebral artery dissecting aneurysm, posterior inferior cerebellar artery reimplantation (bypass, × 2)	L PICA-VA	L PICA (E–Eᶜ) V3
6	4A	6	Middle cerebral artery to posterior cerebral artery bypass with radial artery graft	R M2-RAG-PCA	R M2 (S–E) RAG (E–S*ᶜ) P2
7	4A	7 (2, 6)	Common carotid artery to middle cerebral artery bypass, M2 middle cerebral artery to middle cerebral artery in situ bypass (reimplantation)	R CCA-RAG-MCA, MCA'-MCA'	R CCA (S–E*ᶜ) RAG (S–E) M2 + M2' (E–S) M2''
8	4A	2	Common carotid artery to middle cerebral artery bypass, M2 middle cerebral artery to middle cerebral artery in situ bypass (reimplantation)	L CCA-RAG-MCA	L CCA (S–E*) RAG (E–S) L MCA
9	4A	5	Middle cerebral artery to middle cerebral artery reanastomosis (bypass)	L M1-M2	L M1 (E–E*ᶜ) M2

(continued on next page)

Table 4
(continued)

Case No.	Bypass Generation[a]	Seven Bypasses No.[b]	Operative Title	Standard Naming	Full Bypass Code[c]
10	4A	5	Excision-reanastomosis of fusiform distal L posterior inferior cerebellar artery aneurysm (bypass)	L PICA-PICA	L p3 PICA (E–E*[c]) p3
11	4A, 4B	6	Middle cerebral artery to A1 anterior cerebral artery bypass with saphenous vein graft	R MCA-SVG-A1	R M2 (S–E) SVG (E–E*[c]) A1
12	4A	7 (3, 5)	M2-M2 reanastomosis, M2-M2 reimplantation	M2-M2'	R STA (E–S) M2' (failed intraoperatively) R M2' (E–E) M2' + M2" (E–S*) M2'
13	4A	6	Middle cerebral artery to posterior cerebral artery bypass, harvest of saphenous vein graft	R M2-SVG-PCA	R M2 (S–E) SVG (E–S) P2
14	4A	5	Excision of distal fusiform R middle cerebral artery aneurysm, reanastomosis of middle cerebral artery (bypass)	R M2-M3	R M2 (E–E*) M3
15	4A	6	Middle cerebral artery to posterior cerebral artery bypass with saphenous vein graft	R M2-SVG-PCA	R M2 (S–E) SVG (E–S) P2
16	4A	5	Vertebral artery to anterior inferior cerebellar artery bypass, anterior inferior cerebellar artery to anterior inferior cerebellar artery reanastomosis	L VA-AICA-AICA	L V4 (S–S*) a3 AICA (failed intraoperatively) L a3 (E–E*) a3
17	4A	2	External carotid artery to middle cerebral artery bypass, harvest of radial artery graft	R ECA-RAG-MCA	R ECA (S–E) RAG (E–S) M2
18	4A	6	Middle cerebral artery to posterior cerebral artery bypass, endoscopic harvest of saphenous vein graft	R M2-SVG-PCA	R M2 (S–E) SVG (E–S*) P2
19	4A	3	Middle cerebral artery to anterior temporal artery reimplantation (bypass)	R MCA'-ATA	R ATA (S–E) M2'
20	4A	3	R posterior inferior cerebellar artery to L posterior inferior cerebellar artery reimplantation (bypass)	R PICA-L PICA	R p3 (E–S*) L p3

21	4A	6	M1 middle cerebral artery to M2 middle cerebral artery bypass, harvest of radial artery graft	R M1-RAG-M2	R M1 (E–E) RAG (E–E) M2
22	4A, 4B	7 (3, 6)	A1 anterior cerebral artery to M2 middle cerebral artery double reimplantation bypass, harvest of radial artery graft	R A1-RAG-M2+M2'	R A1 (S–E) RAG [(S–S*) M2 + (E–S*) M2']
23	4A	5	R distal posterior inferior cerebellar artery aneurysm, end-to-end reanastomosis (bypass)	R PICA-PICA	R p3 (E–E*ᶜ) p3
24	4A, 4B	7 (4, 6)	A1 anterior cerebral artery to middle cerebral artery bypass (double reimplantation)	R A1-SVG-M2+M2'	R A1 (S–E) SVG [(S–S) M2 + (E–S*ᶜ) M2']
25	4A	7 (1, 6)	Superficial temporal artery to middle cerebral artery bypass, A1 anterior cerebral artery to M2 middle cerebral artery bypass with radial artery graft	L A1-RAG L M2	L A1 (S–E) RAG (E–S) M2
26	4A, 4B	7 (3, 6)	Anterior cerebral artery to M2 middle cerebral artery + M2 middle cerebral artery double reimplantation bypass	R A1-RAG R M2+M2'	R A1 (S–E) RAG [(S–S) M2 + (E–S*ᶜ) M2']
27	4A	6	M2 middle cerebral artery to P2 posterior cerebral artery bypass	L P2-RAG-L M2	L M2 (S–E) RAG (E–S) P2
28	4A	5	Anterior inferior cerebellar artery reanastomosis (bypass)	L AICA-AICA'	L a2 (E–E) a3
29	4A	3	L pericallosal artery-R pericallosal artery reimplantation (bypass)	R A3-L A3	R A3 (E–S*ᶜ) L A3
30	4A	6	M2 middle cerebral artery to P2 posterior cerebral artery interpositional bypass with radial artery graft	R M2-RAG-P2	R M2 (E–S*ᶜ) RAG (E–Sᶜ) R P2
31	4A	6	M2 middle cerebral artery to P2 posterior cerebral artery bypass	R M2-RAG-P2	R M2 (E–S*ᶜ) RAG (E–Sᶜ) R P2
32	4A	7(2, 3)	External carotid artery to M2 middle cerebral artery interpositional bypass with radial artery graft, reimplantation of temporal M2 middle cerebral artery onto frontal M2 middle cerebral artery (bypass)	L ECA-RAG-M2 (MCoA case 2)	L ECA (S–E) RAG (E–S) M2' + M2' (E–S*) M2

(continued on next page)

Table 4
(continued)

Case No.	Bypass Generation[a]	Seven Bypasses No.[b]	Operative Title	Standard Naming	Full Bypass Code[c]
33	4A	5	Excision of dolichoectatic, distal R middle cerebral artery aneurysm, reanastomosis of middle cerebral artery (type 4A)	R M3-M3	R M3 (E-E*^{c}) M3
34	4A	1	Superficial temporal artery to middle cerebral artery bypass (side-to-side) for moyamoya disease	R STA-M4	R STA (S-S^c) M4
35	4A	1	Superficial temporal artery to middle cerebral artery bypass (side-to-side) for moyamoya disease	R STA-M4	R STA (S-S^c) M4
36	4A	1	Superficial temporal artery to middle cerebral artery bypass (side-to-side) for moyamoya disease	R STA-M4	R STA (S-S^c) M4
37	4B	5	Posterior inferior cerebellar artery reanastomosis (end-to-side bypass, type 4B)	L p2-p3	L p2 (E-S^c) p3
38	4B	1	Occipital artery-to-anterior inferior cerebellar artery bypass (type 4B, end-to-end anastomosis)	L OA-a1	L OA (E-E^c) a1
39	4A, 4B	7 (3, 6)	A1 anterior cerebral artery to M2 middle cerebral artery interpositional bypass, M2 middle cerebral artery–M2 middle cerebral artery reimplantation (middle communicating artery)	L A1-RAG-L M2+M2	L A1 (S-S^c) RAG (E-S^c) M2' + M2' (E-E*^{c}) M2
40	4A, 4B	7 (1, 3)	Double-barrel superficial temporal artery to middle cerebral artery bypass, end-to-end reimplantation of middle cerebral artery	L STA-M2 double barrel + M2-M2	L STA (E-S^c) M2' + L STA' (E-S^c) M2" + M2' (E-E*^{c}) M2''

41	4A		Subclavian artery to internal carotid artery bypass with radial artery graft	L SclA-RAG-L C1 ICA		L Scl (S–Eᶜ) RAG (E–S*ᶜ) C1 ICA
42	4A	5	Left V4-V4 reanastomosis for dolichoectatic vertebral artery	L V4-V4		L V4 (E–E*ᶜ) V4 VA
43	4B	3	R M2-M2 reimplantation for recurrent MCA aneurysm	R M2-M2		R M2 (E–S*) M2" (failed intraoperatively) R M2' (S–S) M2"
44	4A	6	Left M2-RAG-s2 interposition bypass with proximal occlusion of giant vertebrobasilar dolichoectatic aneurysm	L M2-RAG-s2		L M2 (E–S*) RAG (S–E*) s2

A comparison of the baseline description of the bypass, with various levels of detail, is shown. The rightmost column, using the recently described coding scheme from Tayebi Meybodi et al.,[45] captures the full essence of these complex bypasses. Even the surgeon's own operative description of the bypass (operative title) may not accurately convey the details of the bypass. Operative reports and intraoperative photographs were evaluated to accurately code these bypasses. The details of whether an intraluminal technique or continuous suturing was used were noted in superscript only when it could be confirmed, although use of the continuous technique is the senior author's typical practice, and the continuous technique was certainly used for intraluminal suturing. The portion of the operative title in the database that described the bypass is displayed. Combination bypasses consist of multiple component bypasses, which each have their own *Seven Bypasses* type (1–6), as described in Lawton.[15] Attempted bypasses are also included to demonstrate the troubleshooting value of fourth-generation techniques. Asterisk (*) indicates use of intraluminal suturing technique. Superscript "c" indicates use of continuous suturing technique.

Abbreviations: a1, anterior pontine segment of anterior inferior cerebellar artery (AICA); a2, lateral pontine segment of AICA; a3, flocculopeduncular segment of AICA; A1, precommunicating segment of anterior cerebral artery; A3, precallosal segment of anterior cerebral artery; ACA, anterior cerebral artery; AICA, anterior inferior cerebellar artery; ATA, anterior temporal artery; CCA, common carotid artery; CmaA, callosomarginal artery; ECA, external carotid artery; E–E, end-to-end; E–S, end-to-side; ICA, internal carotid artery; L, left; M1, sphenoidal segment of MCA; M2, insular segment of MCA; M3, opercular segment of MCA; M4, cortical segment of MCA; MCA, middle cerebral artery; MCoA, middle communicating artery; OA, occipital artery; p2, lateral medullary segment of posterior inferior cerebellar artery (PICA); p3, tonsillomedullary segment of PICA; P2, postcommunicating segment of PCA; PCA, posterior cerebral artery; PcaA, pericallosal artery; PICA, posterior inferior cerebellar artery; R, right; RAG, radial artery graft; s2, lateral pontomesencephalic segment of superior cerebellar artery; S–E, side-to-end; S–S, side-to-side; STA, superficial temporal artery; SclA, subclavian artery; SVG, saphenous vein graft; V3, extradural segment of VA; V4, intradural segment of VA; VA, vertebral artery; 1, EC–IC bypass; 2, EC–IC interposition bypass; 3, reimplantation; 4, in situ bypass; 5, reanastomosis; 6, IC–IC interposition bypass; 7, combination bypass.

[a] The cited bypass generation type reflects only the successfully completed bypass.

[b] Designated according to the schema outlined in Lawton.[15]

[c] Coded according to the schema outlined in Tayebi Meybodi et al.[45]

was mandatory to maintain a patency percentage of more than 90%.[13,43]

In the current study, we observed graft patency in 89% of fourth-generation bypasses (39 of 44 cases). This difference most likely reflects the marked increase in case complexity and diversity. The Sundt experience was restricted to a narrow range of second-generation procedures, whereas the study cohort includes 14 distinct fourth-generation subtypes, only one of which accumulated more than 20 cases, namely, the type 4A end-to-side reimplantation with intraluminal suturing. This subset had a patency rate of 91% (21 of 23 cases). Considered within that context, and in light of the numerous instances of intraoperative troubleshooting required (unpublished data), we consider the study outcomes to be very reassuring, and they are likely to improve further with additional cases.

Mandate to Innovate

Type 4A fourth-generation bypass was developed in response to the need to perform anastomoses in very narrow operative corridors or between vessels with relatively fixed positions, restricting visualization of one side of the suture line. As the intraluminal suturing technique was adapted to these cases, it became increasingly apparent that certain anastomoses would benefit substantially if intraluminal suturing was elevated to the default technique (eg, the MCA component of an M2 MCA end-to-side radial artery graft [RAG] side-to-end P2 bypass). Thus, in the most recent such case (case 44, see **Table 4**), both end-to-side anastomoses were performed with an intraluminal technique on the back wall (ie, to anastomose RAG to M2 and s2).[44] This 4A bypass, using either an RAG or a saphenous vein graft as an interposition graft, was used to treat a total of 10 patients (**Fig. 3**). With still further experience, the intraluminal suturing technique has been adapted across a diverse range of bypass operations, including unusual circumstances such as treatment for a compressive dolichoectatic VA (coded as L V4 VA (E–E*c) V4 VA, using the coding schema discussed below and described elsewhere[45]) or extracranial vascular reconstruction, coded as L SclA (S–Ec) RAG (E–S*c) C1 internal carotid artery (ICA).

The type 4B bypass emerged from the need to optimize double reimplantation operations. The first such procedure was an early double

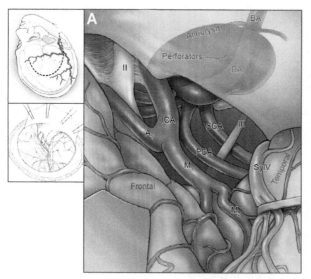
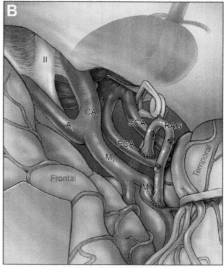

Fig. 3. M2 to radial artery graft (RAG) to postcommunicating (P2) segment of posterior cerebral artery (PCA) bypass. This bypass is one of the most common 4A bypasses.[29] (A) The senior author (MTL) has developed this bypass to function as a high-flow alternative to the posterior communicating artery for treatment of a dolichoectatic basilar trunk aneurysm. This bypass enables flow reversal. (B) The deep anastomosis, RAG side-to-end P2, is performed in the narrow corridor of the oculomotor-tentorial triangle. The RAG may obscure visualization within the field during the bypass and may be relatively immobile. Thus, use of the intraluminal suturing technique on the first (deep) suture line facilitates performance of the bypass while keeping the RAG in a favorable position.[44] Insets show the incision (*top*) and an overview of the surgical exposure (*bottom*). II, optic nerve; III, oculomotor nerve; A1, precommunicating segment of anterior cerebral artery; BA, basilar artery; ICA, internal carotid artery; M1, sphenoidal segment of middle cerebral artery (MCA); M2, insular segment of MCA; PCA, posterior cerebral artery; SCA, superior cerebellar artery; SylV, sylvian vein. *Used with permission from Lawton MT. Seven Bypasses, Tenets and Techniques for Revascularization; New York, Thieme; 2018.*

reimplantation bypass, coded as R A1 (S–E) RAG [(S–E) CmaA + (E–S) PcaA], during which it was discovered that the second reimplantation could more easily be performed using the side-to-side technique rather than the end-to-side technique. This discovery yielded the construct coded as R A2 (S–E) RAG [(E–S*c) L CmaA + (S–S) L PcaA] for ACA double reimplantation. Still further evolution of the double reimplantation techniques yielded additional type 4B operations, such as the "middle communicating artery" reconstruction.[46] Similarly, type 4B approaches were identified as the safest and most efficient options for atypical reanastomoses (eg, end-to-side reanastomosis with a p2 PICA that could not be mobilized because of perforators), reimplantations (eg, side-to-side reimplantation of a3 anterior inferior cerebellar artery [AICA] due to immobility of perforators), and other unusual circumstances. Rarely, single operations may incorporate indications for both type 4A and type 4B bypasses, as we have described for the treatment of particularly challenging M2 or AICA reimplantations (see **Table 4**) (reimplantation video [unpublished data]) or AICA[24] reimplantations. An example of such a case is shown in **Fig. 4**, and an example of type 4A bypass is shown in **Fig. 5**.

Scope of Practice and Generalizability

Critical reading of clinical research, such as the present work (a relatively small single-surgeon cohort study describing a rarified practice) invites important questions regarding the generalizability of the findings. In our view, the mandate for detailed reporting of these uncommon operations and their outcomes serves at least 4 critical functions, each of which has a major positive influence on the care of critical cerebrovascular patients.

Perhaps most obviously, the existence of patients who will require similar operations in the future highlights the need for objective data describing outcomes, such that patients can be educated and counseled with respect to the range of possible interventions, risks, benefits, and alternatives. In this same vein, although our experience with fourth-generation bypass is the most robust, at least 8 other similar cases have been reported by other cerebrovascular neurosurgeons (see **Table 2**). The limits of publication bias are such that these numbers likely underrepresent the true scope of practice, and a commitment to sharing outcomes after these uncommon and challenging procedures will hopefully encourage others to similarly describe their experiences, such that the literature overall will more accurately reflect the contemporary state of practice for fourth-generation bypass.

Two other key arguments are forward-looking in terms of the importance of describing advanced bypass techniques. As endovascular strategies proliferate and become safer, more effective, and better able to encompass broader indications, open cerebrovascular neurosurgery will continue to shift toward a smaller number of more difficult cases, many of which will require bypass techniques for optimal treatment. Practices will simultaneously shift toward consolidation in environments where a small number of bypass subspecialists are able to take on these challenging operations. This cadre of subspecialists will benefit from a robust literature describing this focused but highly granular clinical niche. Finally, the very existence of fourth-generation bypass is a testament to the potential for creativity and innovation within the open cerebrovascular space, and the yet-to-be-imagined fifth generation of bypass operations depends on the next generation of cerebrovascular neurosurgeons being invested with a strong foundation in the accomplishments and experiences of their predecessors.

Cerebrovascular Bypass Nomenclature

Envisioning new bypasses and communicating the thought process behind those bypasses is only possible with a common language. This bypass description enables communication of even these complex fourth-generation bypasses, including potential new bypasses that are listed as "dream bypasses" in **Table 1**.

In a recent series of studies co-authored by the senior author, a coding schema[45] has been used to accurately convey the true construction of these unique bypasses.[5,26,46] This coding schema adds a sense of the basic architecture and "math" of a bypass, using simple arithmetical operators and the distributive property. However, bypass surgery is also an art; it is the most creative expression in cerebrovascular surgery. Thus, neurosurgeons have applied creative names to help describe the unique nature of their bypasses and provide a colorful metaphor for the function and shape of a bypass. Examples include Spetzler's bonnet bypass[47] and Russin's arborization bypass.[48] In this series, we have included the "azygos bypass,"[31] the "middle communicating artery,"[46] and the "binder ring bypass"[26] as examples of fourth-generation bypasses. Other surgeons have conjured interesting names, such as Lee and Choi's "closing omega" bypass for L p2 (S–S) L p3.[28] We encourage those that create new bypasses to continue to put forth these artfully descriptive names, but we ask them to also consider communicating their novel bypasses with the coding schema for clarity and consistency.

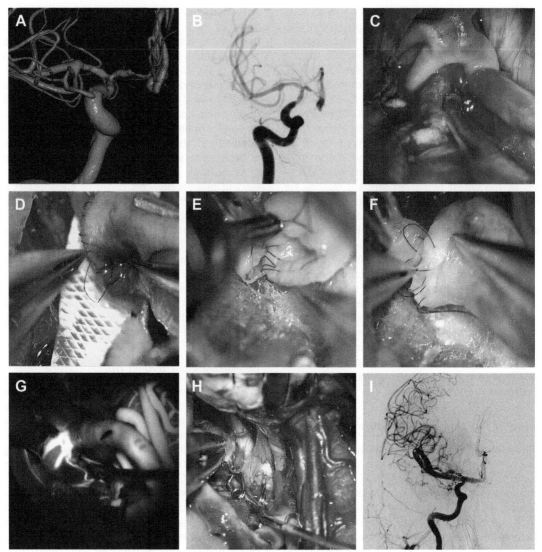

Fig. 4. Example of type 4A and 4B bypasses. A woman in her mid-70s presented with Hunt-Hess grade 2 and Fisher grade 4 subarachnoid hemorrhage from a right A1 dissecting aneurysm (case 11 in **Table 4**). The aneurysm was not amenable to the available endovascular techniques at that time. (*A*) Preoperative 3D rotational angiogram shows the small dissecting aneurysm at the mid-A1. (*B*) Digital subtraction angiography with posterior-anterior projection shows a robust M2 donor and diminutive postdissection A1. (*C*) Intraoperative photograph from a right orbitopterional approach shows the diseased A1 segment. (*D*) Completion of the saphenous vein graft (SVG) end-to-side M2 anastomosis. Because of the patient's atherosclerosis, the radial artery graft was unfavorable. (*E*) Intraluminal suturing of the A1 end-to-end (E–E) SVG anastomosis. (*F*) Completion of the E–E anastomosis with extraluminal suturing on the other side. (*G*) Indocyanine green videoangiography confirmed patency of the bypass and flow into the bilateral A2s. (*H*) Overview of the bypass shows the resected and absent A1, lamina terminalis fenestration, and clip assistance to adjust for SVG-A1 mismatch. This bypass was both type 4A (because intraluminal suturing was used) and type 4B (because of the atypical use of E–E anastomosis). The combined code is thus R M2 (S–E) SVG (E–E*^c^) A1.[45] (*I*) Postoperative posterior-anterior projection digital subtraction angiography shows patent bypass and excision of the aneurysm. (*Courtesy of* Barrow Neurological Institute, Phoenix, Arizona, USA.)

Limitations

This study is subject to the typical limitations of all retrospective, observational, single-surgeon studies, including selection bias, confounding factors, small sample size, and limited generalizability. A limitation that is more specific to this project is that the intended audience and associated patient population are

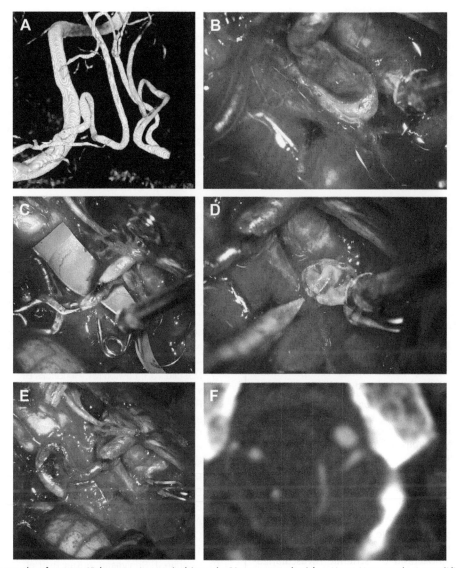

Fig. 5. Example of a type 4B bypass. A man in his early 60s presented with a Hunt-Hess grade 4, modified Fisher grade 4 rupture of a dissecting, fusiform left posterior inferior cerebellar artery (PICA) aneurysm (case 37 in **Table 4**). (*A*) Preoperative 3D rotational angiogram shows the dissecting aneurysm involving the p2 PICA. (*B*) Intraoperative photograph, seen via a left far lateral approach, shows the aneurysm. Note the proximity of the healthy p2 just proximal to the aneurysm and the p3 distal to the aneurysm. Perforating arteries along the p2 segmented and at the distal aneurysm prevented donor and recipient mobilization for end-to-end reanastomosis, but in their native position they were favorable for end-to-side reanastomosis (type 4B). (*C*) Intraoperative photograph showing that the bypass, coded as L p2 (E–S^c) p3,[44] has been completed. (*D*) The interior of the arterial dissection is explored. (*E*) Overview of the field, with the left p2 donor now supplying the distal PICA (p3 and beyond) with exclusion of the aneurysmal segment with a clip on the inflow. (*F*) Postoperative computed tomography angiogram shows patency of the bypass and distal PICA, with the end-to-side orientation seen here. (*Courtesy of Barrow Neurological Institute, Phoenix, Arizona, USA.*)

relatively few in number. Despite these considerations, this study describes a unique, important, and illuminating clinical experience with a novel subset of cerebrovascular techniques that will be critically important to that audience and their patients, as we have discussed in detail.

SUMMARY

Fourth-generation bypass represents the contemporary frontier of open cerebrovascular microsurgery. By evolving past novel vessel configurations to incorporate novel suturing techniques or vascular orientations, type 4A and 4B bypasses are expanding the treatment capacity of open cerebrovascular neurosurgery, rendering the treatment of these highly unusual and challenging cases safer and more efficient. We anticipate that this study will empower the treatment of complex pathologies, helpfully inform patient counseling, and provide a foundation for creative innovation among future generations of cerebrovascular neurosurgeons.

CLINICS CARE POINTS

- Fourth-generation bypass techniques build on the previous generations and are characterized by the use of atypical (ie, intraluminal) suture techniques or unconventional arterial orientation.

- Type 4A bypasses use atypical suturing techniques (ie, intraluminal suturing in an end-to-side or end-to-end anastomosis).

- Type 4B bypasses are characterized by atypical arterial configuration (eg, end-to-end reimplantation, when typical reimplantation would be performed end to side).

- Fourth-generation bypasses are not commonly required, but the techniques can be applied to challenging situations to simplify a bypass or make it more technically feasible.

- Several other studies have independently described unique bypass constructs performed using fourth-generation techniques.

- Fourth-generation techniques are most commonly applicable to bypasses for complex aneurysms but may be used in the treatment of dolichoectasia or ischemic revascularization.

ACKNOWLEDGMENTS

The current affiliation of Redi Rahmani, MD, is Department of Neurosurgery, University of Rochester, Rochester, New York. The authors thank the staff of Neuroscience Publications at Barrow Neurological Institute for assistance with article preparation.

DISCLOSURE

The authors have no personal, financial, or institutional interest in any of the drugs, materials, or devices described in this manuscript. No prior submissions or presentations.

REFERENCES

1. Donaghy RM, Yaşargil MG. Micro-vascular surgery. Report of first conference, October 6-7, 1966, Mary Fletscher Hospital. Burlington, Vermont. Stuttgart: Thieme; 1967.

2. Esposito G, Amin-Hanjani S, Regli L. Role of and Indications for Bypass Surgery After Carotid Occlusion Surgery Study (COSS)? Stroke 2016;47(1): 282–90.

3. Lawton MT, Spetzler RF. Internal carotid artery sacrifice for radical resection of skull base tumors. Skull Base Surg 1996;6(2):119–23.

4. Walcott BP, Lawton MT. Carotid artery occlusion and revascularization in the management of meningioma. Handb Clin Neurol 2020;170:209–16.

5. Lawton MT, Lang MJ. The future of open vascular neurosurgery: perspectives on cavernous malformations, AVMs, and bypasses for complex aneurysms. J Neurosurg 2019;130(5):1409–25.

6. Lawton MT, Quinones-Hinojosa A, Chang EF, et al. Thrombotic intracranial aneurysms: classification scheme and management strategies in 68 patients. Neurosurgery 2005;56(3):441–54; discussion 441-454.

7. Mascitelli JR, Lawton MT, Hendricks BK, et al. Analysis of Wide-Neck Aneurysms in the Barrow Ruptured Aneurysm Trial. Neurosurgery 2019; 85(5):622–31.

8. Group EIBS. Failure of extracranial-intracranial arterial bypass to reduce the risk of ischemic stroke. Results of an international randomized trial. N Engl J Med 1985;313(19):1191–200.

9. Burkhardt JK, Winkler EA, Gandhi S, et al. Single-Barrel Versus Double-Barrel Superficial Temporal Artery to Middle Cerebral Artery Bypass: A Comparative Analysis. World Neurosurg 2019; 125:e408–15.

10. Cherian J, Srinivasan V, Kan P, et al. Double-Barrel Superficial Temporal Artery-Middle Cerebral Artery Bypass: Can It Be Considered "High-Flow? Oper Neurosurg (Hagerstown) 2018;14(3): 288–94.

11. Duckworth EA, Rao VY, Patel AJ. Double-barrel bypass for cerebral ischemia: technique, rationale, and preliminary experience with 10 consecutive cases. Neurosurgery 2013;73(1 Suppl Operative): 30–8; discussion ons37-38.

12. Gandhi S, Rodriguez RL, Tabani H, et al. Double-Barrel Extracranial-Intracranial Bypass and Trapping of Dolichoectatic Middle Cerebral Artery Aneurysms: 3-Dimensional Operative Video. Oper Neurosurg (Hagerstown) 2019;17(1):E14–5.

13. Sundt TM Jr, Piepgras DG, Marsh WR, et al. Saphenous vein bypass grafts for giant aneurysms and intracranial occlusive disease. J Neurosurg 1986; 65(4):439–50.

14. Sharma M, Ugiliweneza B, Fortuny EM, et al. National trends in cerebral bypass for unruptured intracranial aneurysms: a National (Nationwide) Inpatient Sample analysis of 1998-2015. Neurosurg Focus 2019;46(2):E15.

15. Lawton MT. Seven bypasses: Tenets and Techniques for Revascularization. New York: Thieme; 2018.

16. Sanai N, Zador Z, Lawton MT. Bypass surgery for complex brain aneurysms: an assessment of intracranial-intracranial bypass. Neurosurgery 2009;65(4):670–83; discussion 683.

17. Abla AA, Lawton MT. Anterior cerebral artery bypass for complex aneurysms: an experience with intracranial-intracranial reconstruction and review of bypass options. J Neurosurg 2014;120(6): 1364–77.

18. Abla AA, McDougall CM, Breshears JD, et al. Intracranial-to-intracranial bypass for posterior inferior cerebellar artery aneurysms: options, technical challenges, and results in 35 patients. J Neurosurg 2016; 124(5):1275–86.

19. Lawton MT, Quinones-Hinojosa A. Double reimplantation technique to reconstruct arterial bifurcations with giant aneurysms. Neurosurgery 2006;58(4 Suppl 2):347–53; discussion ONS-353-354.

20. Bot GM, Gandhi S, Tabani H, et al. Superficial Temporal Artery to Middle Cerebral Artery Bypass in a 1-Year-Old Moyamoya Patient: 2-Dimensional Operative Video. Oper Neurosurg (Hagerstown) 2018; 15(5):E60.

21. Lang MJ, Kan P, Baranoski JF, et al. Side-to-Side Superficial Temporal Artery to Middle Cerebral Artery Bypass Technique: Application of Fourth Generation Bypass in a Case of Adult Moyamoya Disease. Oper Neurosurg (Hagerstown) 2020;18(5):480–6.

22. Tayebi Meybodi A, Huang W, Benet A, et al. Bypass surgery for complex middle cerebral artery aneurysms: an algorithmic approach to revascularization. J Neurosurg 2017;127(3):463–79.

23. Benet A, Lawton MT. Revascularization of the Posterior Inferior Cerebellar Artery With Contralateral Reimplantation of Right Posterior Inferior Cerebellar Artery to Left Posterior Inferior Cerebellar Artery: 3-Dimensional Operative Video. Oper Neurosurg (Hagerstown) 2016;12(3):305.

24. Baranoski JF, Przybylowski CJ, Mascitelli JR, et al. Anterior Inferior Cerebellar Artery Bypasses: The 7-Bypass Framework Applied to Ischemia and Aneurysms in the Cerebellopontine Angle. Oper Neurosurg (Hagerstown) 2020;19(2):165–74.

25. Benet A, Bang JS, Lawton MT. A3-A3 In Situ Bypass and Distal Clip Occlusion of Giant Serpentine Anterior Communicating Artery Aneurysm: 3-Dimensional Operative Video. Oper Neurosurg (Hagerstown) 2017;13(6):755.

26. Srinivasan VM, Labib MA, Furey CG, Catapano JS, Lawton MT. The "binder ring" bypass: transection, rerouting, and reanastomosis as an alternative to macrovascular decompression of a dolichoectatic vertebral artery. Oper Neurosurg (Hagerstown) 2022;22(4):224–30.

27. Lazaro TT, Srinivasan VM, Cotton PC, et al. Trapping and P2-P3 Posterior Inferior Cerebellar Artery Reanastomosis for Treatment of a Ruptured Fusiform Aneurysm: Application of Fourth-Generation Technique: 2-Dimensional Operative Video. Oper Neurosurg (Hagerstown) 2021;21(6):E539–40.

28. Lee SH, Choi SK. In Situ Intersegmental Anastomosis within a Single Artery for Treatment of an Aneurysm at the Posterior Inferior Cerebellar Artery: Closing Omega Bypass. J Korean Neurosurg Soc 2015;58(5):467–70.

29. Lawton MT, Abla AA, Rutledge WC, et al. Bypass Surgery for the Treatment of Dolichoectatic Basilar Trunk Aneurysms: A Work in Progress. Neurosurgery 2016;79(1):83–99.

30. Srinivasan VM, Labib MA, Catapano JS, et al. Combination A3-A3 In Situ Bypass and ATA-RAG-A2 Interpositional Bypas with Partial Trapping of Giant Anterior Communicating Artery Aneurysm. Covideos Available at: https://www.barrowneuro.org/for-physicians-researchers/education/grand-rounds-publications-media/covideos-19/. Accessed January 18, 2021.

31. Mirzadeh Z, Sanai N, Lawton MT. The azygos anterior cerebral artery bypass: double reimplantation technique for giant anterior communicating artery aneurysms. J Neurosurg 2011;114(4):1154–8.

32. Ravina K, Yim B, Lam J, et al. Three-Vessel Anastomosis for Direct Bihemispheric Cerebral Revascularization. Oper Neurosurg (Hagerstown) 2020;19(3): 313–8.

33. Benes L, Kappus C, Sure U, et al. Treatment of a partially thrombosed giant aneurysm of the vertebral artery by aneurysm trapping and direct vertebral artery-posterior inferior cerebellar artery end-to-end anastomosis: technical case report. Neurosurgery 2006;59(1 Suppl 1). ONSE166–167; discussion ONSE166-167.

34. Matsushima K, Kawashima M, Suzuyama K, et al. Thrombosed giant aneurysm of the distal anterior cerebral artery treated with aneurysm resection and proximal pericallosal artery-callosomarginal artery end-to-end anastomosis: Case report and review of the literature. Surg Neurol Int 2011;2:135.

35. Sekhar LN, Stimac D, Bakir A, et al. Reconstruction options for complex middle cerebral artery aneurysms. Neurosurgery 2005;56(1 Suppl):66–74; discussion 66-74.

36. Nakajima H, Kamiyama H, Nakamura T, et al. Direct surgical treatment of giant middle cerebral artery

aneurysms using microvascular reconstruction techniques. Neurol Med Chir (Tokyo) 2012;52:56–61.

37. Arnone GD, Hage ZA, Charbel FT. Side-to-side and end-to-side double anastomosis using the parietal-branch of the superficial temporal artery—a novel technique for extracranial to intracranial bypass surgery: 3-dimensional operative video. Oper Neurosurg (Hagerstown) 2019;16:112–4.

38. Rumalla K, Srinivasan VM, Gaddis M, et al. Readmission following extracranial-intracranial bypass surgery in the United States: nationwide rates, causes, risk factors, and volume-driven outcomes. J Neurosurg 2020;1–9.

39. Bardach NS, Olson SJ, Elkins JS, et al. Regionalization of treatment for subarachnoid hemorrhage: a cost-utility analysis. Circulation 2004;109(18):2207–12.

40. Sughrue ME, Saloner D, Rayz VL, et al. Giant intracranial aneurysms: evolution of management in a contemporary surgical series. Neurosurgery 2011;69(6):1261–70; discussion 1270-1271.

41. Davies JM, Lawton MT. Advances in open microsurgery for cerebral aneurysms. Neurosurgery 2014;74(Suppl 1):S7–16.

42. Yoon S, Burkhardt JK, Lawton MT. Long-term patency in cerebral revascularization surgery: an analysis of a consecutive series of 430 bypasses. J Neurosurg 2018;131(1):80–7.

43. Sundt TM 3rd, Sundt TM Jr. Principles of preparation of vein bypass grafts to maximize patency. J Neurosurg 1987;66(2):172–80.

44. Graffeo CS, Srinivasan VM, Manjila S, Lawton MT. Fourth-generation bypass and flow reversal to treat a symptomatic giant dolichoectatic basilar trunk aneurysm [published online ahead of print, 2022 Jul 1]. Acta Neurochir (Wien). 2022; https://doi.org/10.1007/s00701-022-05292-w.

45. Tayebi Meybodi A, Gadhiya A, Borba Moreira L, et al. Coding cerebral bypasses: a proposed nomenclature to better describe bypass constructs and revascularization techniques. J Neurosurg 2022;136(1):163–74.

46. Frisoli FA, Catapano JS, Baranoski JF, et al. The middle communicating artery: a novel fourth-generation bypass for revascularizing trapped middle cerebral artery bifurcation aneurysms in 2 cases. J Neurosurg 2020;134(6):1879–86.

47. Spetzler RF, Roski RA, Rhodes RS, et al. The "bonnet bypass". Case report. J Neurosurg 1980;53(5):707–9.

48. Russin JJ. The arborization bypass: Sequential intracranial-intracranial bypasses for an unruptured fusiform MCA aneurysm. J Clin Neurosci 2017;39:209–11.

49. Kato N, Prinz V, Finger T, et al. Multiple reimplantation technique for treatment of complex giant aneurysms of the middle cerebral artery: technical note. Acta Neurochir (Wien) 2013;155(2):261–9.

50. Lee SH, Chung Y, Ryu JW, et al. Rescue bypass for the treatment of pseudoaneurysm on the distal anterior cerebral artery: a case report of vertical side-to-side anastomosis of the distal callosomarginal artery-pericallosal artery. Acta Neurochir (Wien) 2017;159(9):1687–91.

Rethinking Cerebral Bypass Surgery

Robert C. Rennert, MD[a], Jonathan J. Russin, MD[b],*

KEYWORDS

• Cerebral bypass • Revascularization • Innovation • Vasospasm • Ischemia

KEY POINTS

- Cerebral bypass remains an important treatment for selected patients with moyamoya disease, steno-occlusive cerebrovascular disease, complex aneurysms, and tumors.
- Cerebral bypass has evolved from first-generation superficial temporal artery-to-middle cerebral artery constructs to complex fourth-generation bypasses using unconventional suturing techniques and/or unconventional bypass structures.
- Ongoing advances across all generations have focused on developing more personalized bypass strategies.
- Technical and technological innovations have continued to address challenges in the field to increase the safety of cerebral bypass.

INTRODUCTION

Following the first successful superficial temporal artery (STA)–middle cerebral artery (MCA) bypass by Yaşargil in 1967,[1] cerebral bypass was increasingly used in the treatment of a variety of pathologies, including moyamoya disease (MMD), steno-occlusive cerebrovascular disease (SOCD), complex aneurysms, and tumors. However, after 2 large randomized trials (the Extracranial-to-Intracranial [EC-IC] Bypass Study in 1985 and the Carotid Occlusion Surgery Study [COSS] in 2011) failed to demonstrate a benefit of cerebral bypass for stenosis or occlusion of either the internal carotid artery (ICA) or MCA,[2,3] bypass rates for SOCD in the United States decreased dramatically.[4–6] Although the rates of cerebral bypass increased during this time for MMD,[6] and were largely stable for intracranial aneurysms despite the rise of endovascular therapies,[7] there is an ongoing evolution in the indications and clinical application of this procedure.

As highlighted by the reactions to the EC-IC and COSS trials, which were criticized for their exclusion of dynamically ischemic patients, relatively short follow-up period, and a lack of standardized neuroanesthesia and postoperative care protocols,[8] it remains an open question whether a subset of patients with progressive or refractory symptomatic SOCD may still benefit from cerebral bypass. Across all indications, the continued development of tailored revascularization constructs to match a patient's individual needs and technical and technological innovations to decrease complication rates will be critical to the success of cerebral bypass moving forward. This review summarizes ongoing refinements in patient selection criteria, recent creative innovations, and future challenges in the field.

DISCUSSION

Precisely identifying the patients who will benefit from cerebral revascularization and improving the technical and perioperative safety of the procedure are ongoing goals of cerebral bypass research.

a Department of Neurological Surgery, Center for Neurorestoration, Keck School of Medicine, University of Southern California, 1200 North State Street # 4250 Los Angeles, CA 90033, USA; b Department of Neurological Surgery, Center for Neurorestoration, Keck School of Medicine, University of Southern California, 1200 North State Street # 4250 Los Angeles, CA 90033, USA
* Corresponding author.
E-mail address: jonathan.russin@med.usc.edu

Neurosurg Clin N Am 33 (2022) 403–417
https://doi.org/10.1016/j.nec.2022.05.004
1042-3680/22/© 2022 Elsevier Inc. All rights reserved.

Indications for Cerebral Bypass

Flow preservation

Broadly speaking, bypass can be performed for flow preservation (ie, aneurysms, tumors) or flow augmentation (ie, MMD, SOCD). The goal of flow preservation surgery is to replace the blood flow sacrificed during treatment of an aneurysm or tumor, or as a rescue procedure in the event of a vascular injury.

Bypass for cerebral aneurysms is rare (roughly 0.4% of unruptured aneurysms), and typically reserved for complex lesions. Although the overall rate of bypass for unruptured aneurysms was not affected by the initial rise of flow diversion in the early 2010s, its practice is now limited to a small cohort of surgeons in tertiary care centers.[7] Flow diversion is likely to increasingly affect the indications for cerebral bypass, especially for proximal, fusiform ICA aneurysms, a subset of patients historically treated with revascularization but who are increasingly being managed with flow diversion.[9] The recent advent of flow diverters with reduced thrombogenicity requiring only single agent antiplatelet therapies (Pipeline Embolisation Device with Shield technology [PED-Shield], Medtronic Neurovascular, Irvine, CA) may also impact the indications for bypass in the setting of aneurysmal subarachnoid hemorrhage,[10] although additional data on rehemorrhage rates owing to the often-delayed securement of the hemorrhage source are needed. The influence of intrasaccular devices such as the Woven EndoBridge device (Sequent Medical, Aliso Viejo, CA)[11] on bypass remains to be seen, although the relatively simple wide-necked bifurcation aneurysms amenable to this treatment are less likely to require revascularization if treated with open surgery as compared with fusiform or more complex bifurcation aneurysms involving parent vessels.

The net effect of these endovascular advancements will likely be a decreased number but increased complexity of aneurysms requiring bypass as part of their treatment algorithm. The variety of EC–IC and intracranial-to-intracranial (IC–IC) bypass constructs that have been described for the treatment of both ruptured and unruptured complex saccular, fusiform, and blister aneurysms will be important to meet this need.[12–16] Modern outcomes data for patients treated with bypass for ruptured aneurysms are also promising. Although all-cause complication rates in these patients are as high as 70%, surgical complication rates are more acceptable at approximately 20%, and a majority of patients can achieve good functional outcomes.[13] Traditionally not performed in patients with higher Hunt and Hess grades after aneurysmal subarachnoid hemorrhage owing to the complexity and additional length of surgery, risk of vasospasm, and overall poor prognosis of this patient subset, it has recently been shown that the functional outcomes with revascularization can be comparable with open clipping in this high-risk patient cohort for aneurysms not amenable to stand-alone endovascular therapy.[17]

Although well-described and still an important skill for skull base surgeons,[18,19] the use of planned bypass for complex skull base tumors involving the cerebrovasculature has decreased as practice patterns have increasingly favored subtotal tumor resections and adjuvant radiation or chemotherapy, thereby avoiding the potentially high morbidity associated with aggressive resections and revascularization.[20–22] Rescue bypass for flow preservation after iatrogenic vessel injury remains an important but relatively rare indication in tumor surgery.

Flow augmentation

The goal of flow augmentation surgery is to provide additional perfusion to an risk territory, most often in patients with MMD or SOCD.

The benefit of EC–IC bypass for MMD is well-established for hemorrhagic MMD, with rebleeding rates in this population decreased from as high as 44% to as low as 7.7% with revascularization,[23–25] and future ischemic events reduced by nearly 80% on a recent meta-analysis.[26] Although there are mixed aggregate data on the benefit of bypass for secondary stroke prevention in patients with ischemic MMD,[26,27] individual analyses provide compelling supporting evidence and suggest that the benefit from revascularization may not be realized for a decade or more.[28,29] For example, in one of the larger studies on the topic analyzing more than 400 patients presenting with ischemic MMD, the 10-year rate of ischemic stroke was decreased from 13.3% in the nonsurgical group to 3.9% in the revascularization group (3.9%) ($P = 0.019$), equating to a 70.7% relative risk reduction.[28] In selecting a bypass technique, data from meta-analyses suggests that direct or combined revascularization is more effective than indirect bypass for secondary stroke prevention in adult MMD, without increased perioperative risk,[26,27,30] although a consensus on technique has not been reached.[31–34] Despite ongoing debate, in pediatric patients with MMD, there is likely equipoise in the relative efficacy of indirect versus direct bypass.[35–38] The role of prophylactic bypass for asymptomatic MMD is also controversial, despite an annual stroke risk of more than 3% in this population.[39] Explorations of the neurocognitive effects of revascularization for MMD have thus far demonstrated the potential to restore cerebral connectivity to normal levels,[40] with mixed data on functional changes in IQ, processing speed, and attention.[41,42]

Despite the null results of the EC-IC and COSS trials, cerebral bypass is likely still beneficial for a subset of patients with symptomatic SOCD refractory to medical management.[43,44] Limiting perioperative stroke risk and identifying those patients at highest risk for future stroke without surgical intervention is nonetheless critical and challenging.[8] Performance at high-volume bypass centers and the use of dedicated neuroanesthesia and formal perioperative and postoperative treatment protocols are some of the proposed methods to limit perioperative stroke risk in this fragile population. Patient selection is an ongoing question. Addressing a criticism of the EC-IC trial, COSS used positron emission tomography scans to identify hemodynamic impairment from SOCD via elevated oxygen extraction fraction ratios.[3] However, patients with dynamic symptoms were excluded in both trials, with COSS requiring neurologic stability for at least 72 hours before an enrollment scan,[3] and the EC-IC trial requiring 8 weeks between the last ischemic event and enrollment.[2]

The revascularization of patients with acute, progressive symptoms refractory to maximal medical management owing to SOCD in either the anterior or posterior circulation (the latter a population not assessed in EC-IC or COSS) with a corresponding significant perfusion core/penumbra mismatch and not amenable to endovascular treatment has accordingly shown promise in recent series.[43,44] A 2019 systematic review comparing medical management to bypass for symptomatic intracranial atherosclerotic disease also demonstrated reductions in the rates of ischemic stroke and cerebrovascular death from 16.0% and 4.5% in the medical cohort, respectively, to 7.0% and 1.9% with direct bypass.[45] Although this study represents a heterogenous dataset that includes data predating the EC-IC and COSS trials, the performance of selected revascularization surgery for SOCD is in line with American Heart Association guidelines, with bypass considered investigational for patients with recurrent or progressive ischemic symptoms from surgically inaccessible stenoses or occlusions of the ICA refractory to medical therapy.[46] Current American Heart Association guidelines nonetheless do not address the usefulness of bypass in patients with medically refractory vertebrobasilar or more distal anterior circulation intracranial stenosis and actively progressing symptoms, likely owing to a paucity of relevant data. Similar to the evolution rather than complete abandonment of intracranial stenting after the Stenting versus Aggressive Medical Therapy for Intracranial Arterial Stenosis trial,[47] ongoing technological advancements and refinements in patient selection will likely continue to elucidate those SOCD patients most likely to benefit from cerebral revascularization.

Innovations in Cerebral Bypass

In response to this smaller but increasingly complex cohort of patients, multiple strategic, technical, and technological innovations in cerebral bypass surgery have occurred in recent years with the goal of providing increasingly tailored revascularization constructs and improving the surgical and perioperative safety of bypass.

Strategic innovations

Strategic innovations in cerebral bypass have centered on the development of new as well as the refinement of existing revascularization strategies. Using the evolutionary view of cerebral bypass as described by Lawton and Lang,[48] advancements are ongoing across all 4 generations of constructs.

First-generation bypasses involve the anastomosis of scalp arteries and cortical recipients (ie, STA-MCA, occipital artery–posterior inferior cerebellar artery [PICA]).[48] Considered low flow (distal STA flow rates range from 10 to 40 mL/min),[49,50] first-generation bypasses are most commonly used for flow augmentation as they generally do not provide enough flow to completely replace an occluded ICA (flow rates of >250 mL/min) or proximal MCA (flow rates of >150 mL/min)[51] without significant assistance from collateral circulation. The progressive nature of both MMD and SOCD allows for the development of collateral flow over time, however, making these pathologies well-suited for first-generation bypass.

Given the ongoing debate on the superiority of direct versus indirect bypass for MMD,[26,27,30–34] combined approaches represent an early iteration of first-generation bypass advancements that appealingly provide immediate flow with the direct component, and allow for secondary maturation of the indirect component over time.[52,53] The indirect component can also function as a backup source of flow if the direct bypass decreases,[54] and, regardless of the source after combined bypass, it has been shown that any resulting collateralization correlates with regression of the hemorrhage-prone abnormal collateral channels that are the hallmark of MMD.[55] Building on this concept, a pedicled temporoparietal fascial flap for combined revascularization in MMD has been

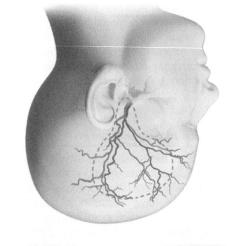

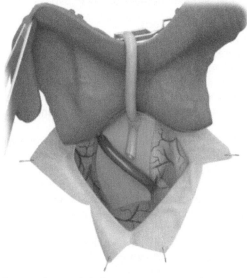

Fig. 1. The pedicled temporoparietal fascial flap (TPFF) has been described for combined revascularization in MMD, where the temporoparietal fascial flap surface area is maximized for indirect revascularization. Importantly, the venous drainage of this tissue is preserved to prevent venous engorgement and mass effect. (© Jonathan J. Russin. Published with permission.)

recently described, maximizing the surface area of the indirect component with a highly vascular pedicled temporoparietal fascial flap, while also importantly maintaining venous drainage to minimize the risk of venous engorgement and mass effect (**Fig. 1**).[56,57]

Other advancements in first-generation bypass include the double-barrel STA–MCA bypass, wherein both the frontal and parietal branches of the STA are anastomosed to cerebral vessels in order to target multiple at-risk territories based on preoperative imaging.[58,59] The addition of the

second distal STA anastomosis site increases overall flow (on average up to 65 mL/min in total),[50] and provides additional versatility to STA-MCA bypass for indications with medium flow needs. In a recent series of 44 patients with a range of indications including MMD, SOCD, and complex aneurysms, this technique demonstrated efficacy for targeted revascularization of multiple territories without affecting bypass patency or complication rates.[60]

Second-generation bypasses were developed to provide increased flow as compared with first-generation constructs, and use interposition grafts and higher caliber donor and recipient vessels. Accordingly, second-generation bypasses are the historic workhorses for large vessel reconstructions in cases of carotid sacrifice for skull base tumors or proximal aneurysms, and most commonly involve external carotid artery-to-M2 or -M3 bypass (medium to high flow based on graft and recipient vessels, 40–140 mL/min).[48,61] Iterations of second generation constructs include use of the proximal STA as a donor vessel with short segment interposition grafts to the M2/M3 or PCA, resulting in a medium flow construct (54–100 mL/min) that avoids the need for a neck incision and graft tunneling.[49] The internal maxillary artery as a donor for EC–IC bypass with a short segment interposition graft similarly avoids a neck incision and tunneling, with access to the infratemporal fossa gained via a lateral subtemporal craniectomy.[62–65] Flow rates of up to 60 mL/min with this technique have been reported,[62] with a versatility to revascularize the M2, proximal ICA, and A2 with relatively short interposition graft lengths ranging from 4.2 cm for the MCA to 6.8 cm for the ACA territories.[65] Other donor vessels for medium to high flow bypass outside of the external carotid artery, STA, and internal maxillary artery include the vertebral artery and occipital artery.[66,67]

In conjunction with donor vessel exploration, the expansion of available interposition grafts has enabled increased customization of second-generation bypasses to more precisely meet flow needs and approximate recipient and donor vessel calibers. Aside from the most commonly used radial artery and saphenous vein interposition grafts,[68] the occipital artery, STA, epigastric artery, thoracodorsal artery, anterior and posterior tibial arteries, and the descending branch of the lateral circumflex femoral artery (DLCFA) have all been developed as viable interposition vessels with a ranges of calibers and lengths.[63,69–75] The most recently reported of these, the DLCFA is a reliable graft (2–3 mm in diameter for up to 15 cm) that has a successful history within the

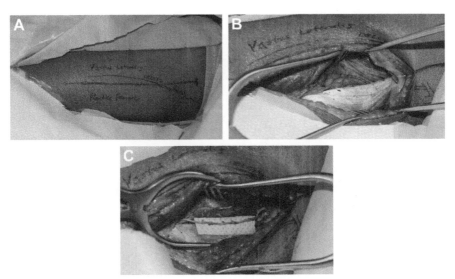

Fig. 2. The DLCFA has been developed as an appealing interposition graft with a cosmetic harvest site and a consistent 2 to 3 mm diameter for up to 15 cm. Used with permission from, [101] *Operative Neurosurgery.*

cardiac and plastic surgery fields and a cosmetically appealing harvest site (**Fig. 2**).[75–79] In comparison with other donor grafts such as the radial artery, the DLCFA may also be less affected by systemic atherosclerosis,[80–82] a potential advantage for long-term patency. The distant harvest site of the DLCFA also enables simultaneous, multiteam surgery to maximize operative efficiency, and has demonstrated efficacy for size- and flow-matched revascularization of the PICA and MCA territories.[13,17,71,75,83,84]

Graft harvest can also be incorporated into the operation (ie, with use of an STA interposition graft for internal maxillary artery–MCA bypass), avoiding the need for a second harvest site and eliminating an additional source of morbidity in cases where a relatively short and small caliber graft is sufficient.[63] Similarly, creative use of the all of the vessels available at the operative site can limit the need for additional graft harvest, as with use of the parietal branch of the STA as an interposition graft extending from the distal frontal STA to the ACA for low-flow revascularization of this territory.[85]

The neurosurgical application of flow-through free flaps has also been described as a customizable solution for patients with pathologies requiring complex cerebral revascularizations (**Fig. 3**).[86] In a recent small series, a radial artery fascial flow-through free flap (RAFF) and radial artery fasciocutaneous flow-through free flap was successfully used in 4 challenging cases.[86] The first 2 patients underwent combined direct STA–ACA and indirect STA–MCA RAFF bypass for

progressive multiterritory MMD with ACA symptom predominance, and the third patient underwent direct STA–ACA and indirect MCA revascularizations with a RAFF, combined with a facial artery–MCA direct bypass with a posterior tibial artery graft for concomitant MMD and a fusiform ICA aneurysm requiring sacrifice. The final patient underwent direct facial artery–MCA bypass (end-to-side anastomosis to a temporal M2 and side-to-side anastomosis to a frontal M3) and scalp reconstruction using a radial artery fasciocutaneous flow-through free flap for a recurrent complex MCA bifurcation aneurysm with an overlying nonhealing wound. The technical nuance of using a single donor graft to revascularize multiple cerebral territories with direct anastomoses as seen in the last patient is an additional innovation to second generation bypasses that enables tailored reperfusion constructs.

Third-generation bypasses are IC–IC constructs that include reanastomosis or reimplantation of disrupted vessels, revascularization with in situ donors (ie, PICA–PICA or A3–A3 bypass), or the use of short intracranial interposition grafts.[48] Despite these constructs often placing a nonaffected territory at risk, they have demonstrated safety and efficacy particularly in complex aneurysm surgery.[12,15,87–90] In the anterior circulation IC–IC constructs include side-to-side A3–A3 bypass for proximal ACA aneurysms. This strategy facilitates surgical or minimally invasive endovascular aneurysm treatment with decreased ischemic risk from parent vessel occlusion.[87,88] Single, or serial IC–IC side-to-side, bypasses

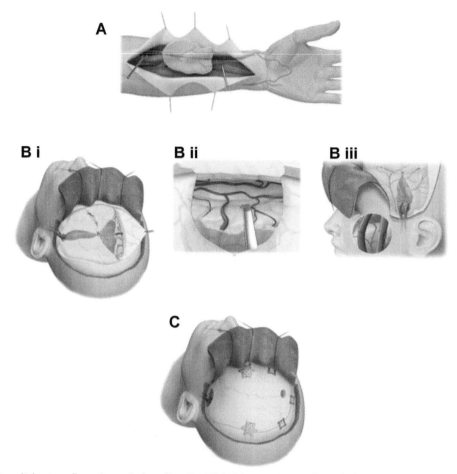

Fig. 3. A radial artery flow through free flap (RAFF) (with a variation if needed to include a fasciocutaneous component [radial artery fasciocutaneous flow-through free flap] for wound coverage) was recently described. In this work, the RAFF was used mainly for direct ACA revascularization with indirect revascularization for the MCA distribution for patients with MMD affecting the MCA and ACA territories with predominantly ACA symptoms. Connection of the venous outflow of this flap promoted normal tissue microcirculation within the flap and prevented venous congestion. © 2017 Center for Neurorestoration, University of Southern California Neurorestoration Center. Used with permission.

have also been described for the treatment of complex MCA aneurysms to revascularize beyond a proximal lesion,[91,92] with the relatively superficial anatomy of the MCA candelabra allowing for keyhole surgical techniques aimed at reducing hospitalization time and surgical morbidity.[91] Similar to A3–A3 constructs, PICA–PICA bypass for proximal PICA/vertebral artery aneurysms allow for the combination of open revascularization with endovascular aneurysm occlusion, thereby limiting deep dissection around the PICA origin and lower cranial nerves.[89,90] Knowledge of the anterior spinal artery is nonetheless critical when considering treatment strategies for such lesions to avoid ischemic spinal cord injury.[93] Proposed advantages of IC–IC noninterposition revascularization include the avoidance of graft

harvest–related morbidity and a single anastomosis site, both of which can limit operative time. In a recent series of 41 bypass patients with complex intracranial aneurysms, IC–IC constructs demonstrated a favorable technical and safety profile when compared directly to EC–IC revascularizations.[12] Although IC–IC bypass with an interposition graft likely has related advantages by limiting surgical exposure and tunneling risks, as well as avoiding the possibility of graft injury with extracranial trauma,[48] the second anastomosis site may theoretically impact long-term patency.[16]

Finally, fourth-generation bypasses as described within the evolutionary construct either (a) maintain the bypass structure of third-generation approaches but use an unconventional suturing technique (ie, intraluminal suturing for

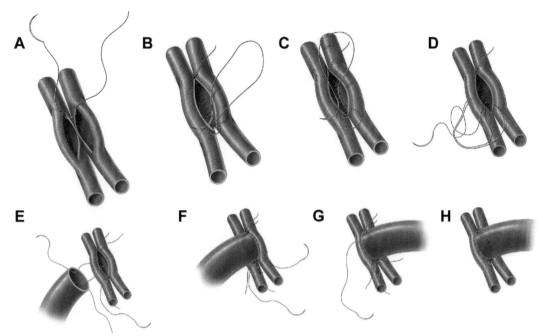

Fig. 4. Three-vessel anastomosis technique as an example of a fourth-generation bypass. (*A*) The back walls of a side-to-side anastomosis are anastomosed in standard fashion. (*B*) After the needle is transitioned from the inside to the outside of the vessels, and reversed, a knot is tied between the free end of the suture and a newly created loop following out-to-in and in-to-out throws (*C, D*). (*E–H*) The donor vessel is then sewn in an end-to-side fashion to the open face of the side-to-side construct. Copyright © Ikumi Kayama/Studio Kayama LLC. Used with permission from Jonathan J. Russin, MD.

back wall end-to-side or end-to-end anastomosis), or (b) use an unconventional bypass structure while using either a conventional or unconventional suturing technique.[48] Recent examples of fourth-generation constructs include the construction of a middle communicating artery for revascularization of the MCA candelabra during treatment of complex MCA bifurcation aneurysms.[94] Specifically, these cases included a double barrel STA–MCA end-to-side bypass to the 2 M2s combined with a proximal M2–M2 end-to-end anastomosis (to connect the flow of the 2 STA donor sites and ensure adequate perfusion of the entire MCA tree), and use of a standard ECA-M2 bypass with a RAG interposition graft combined with an end-to-side anastomosis of the temporal and frontal M2s (to revascularize the entire isolated MCA distribution from the single EC–IC graft).[94] Another novel fourth-generation bypass example is the creation of a 3-vessel anastomosis between 2 recipients and one donor vessel.[95] In this application, a proximal STA to bilateral A3 bypass was performed to revascularize the bilateral ACA territories with a RAFF interposition graft (while simultaneously indirectly bypassing the right MCA territory) in a patient with MMD predominately affecting the right M1

and the bilateral A1s, who had a recent MCA stroke. Avoiding the need for multiple grafts or anastomotic sites, the 3-vessel anastomosis was performed by first completing the back wall of a side-to-side A3–A3 anastomosis, then suturing the radial artery graft in an end-to-side fashion to the open front wall of the A3–A3 construct (**Fig. 4**).

Technical innovation

Recent technical innovations in cerebral bypass surgery have targeted ongoing challenges in the field. For example, interposition graft spasm is a risk with the use of any arterial graft and can result in ischemic complications by decreasing flow through the bypass. Prevention strategies include pharmacologic agents (ex vivo calcium channel blocker and nitroglycerin),[96] pressure–distension manipulation,[61] and preservation of the vena comitantes during arterial graft harvest combined with dual (arterial/venous) anastomosis.[97] Despite these interventions, vasospasm can occur in up to 10% of RAGs.[97] Traditional treatment options for graft spasm once it occurs are limited and include systemic anticoagulation, intra-arterial injections of calcium channel blockers or antispasmodics, and angioplasty.[98,99] In this setting, the *ex vivo* use of botulinum toxin has demonstrated

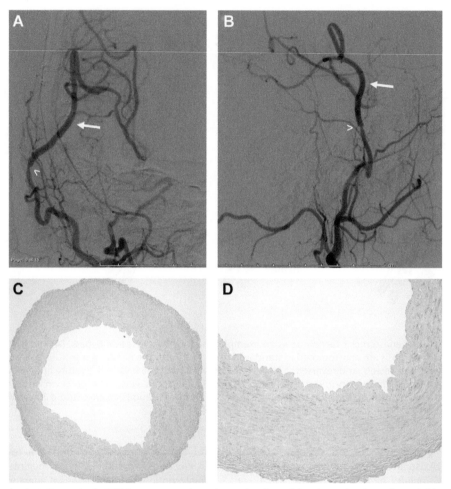

Fig. 5. *Ex vivo* botulinum toxin (BTX) treatments have been developed for the reduction of arterial interposition graft spasm, acting likely through pleotropic effects to reduce vasoconstriction and promote vasodilation. In the reporting series, BTX treated DLCFA grafts demonstrated no spasm, and histologic evaluation showed no endothelial or vascular injury after BTX treatment. (Used with permission from,[100] *JNS.*)

safety and early efficacy in a small series with DLCFA interposition grafts (**Fig. 5**), acting likely through pleotropic effects to reduce the release of vasoconstricting catecholamines and increase the concentration of vasodilating local peptides.[101,102]

Nuances in suturing technique have also been described with the goal of increasing microsuturing efficiency and decreasing clamp time. Recent examples include descriptions of the running-to-interrupted, single loop interrupted, and needle-parking techniques that seek to combine the efficiency of a running stitch with the higher patency rates of interrupted sutures.[103–105] A modification in the initial stay stitch that allows an expedited transition to back-wall suturing for side-to-side anastomosis has also been described (**Fig. 6**).[106] Similarly, use of a half-tied second stay suture technique can limit the obstruction of thick and/ or larger caliber donor vessels during end-to-side anastomosis.[107]

Technological innovations

A variety of technological innovations in the last 2 decades have increased the preoperative, intraoperative, and postoperative information available to bypass surgeons. Regarding patient selection, in addition to advancements in perfusion imaging and analysis that are helping to more clearly define SOCD patients with at risk penumbral tissue,[108,109] large-vessel quantitative magnetic resonance angiography has also shown promise as a tool to identify patients with high stroke risk from SOCD most likely to benefit from revascularization. For example, the Vertebrobasilar Flow Evaluation and Risk of Transient Ischemic Attack and Stroke (VERiTAS) study group has demonstrated that in patients with

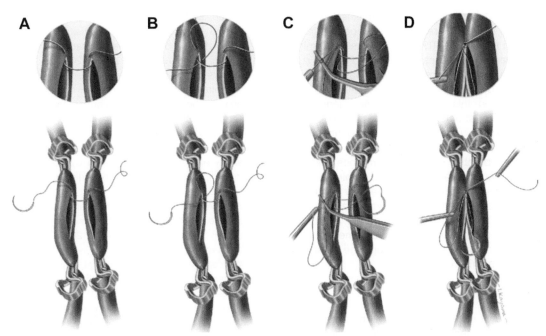

Fig. 6. The expedited transition to back wall suturing for side-to-side anastomosis is one of the many described technical nuances in microsuturing. This technique leaves the apical knot untied during the intraluminal transition, removing the need for a blind needle pass. (© Ikumi Kayama/Studio Kayama LLC. Used with permission from Jonathan J. Russin, MD.)

symptomatic vertebrobasilar disease, impaired quantitative magnetic resonance angiography posterior circulation distal flow (while not well-predicted by the extent of vertebrobasilar disease) was strongly correlated with prospective stroke risk (28% vs 9% in those with normal distal flow over a median of 23 months; hazard ratio, 11.55 [95% confidence interval, 1.88–71.00; $P = .008$]).[110,111] On longer follow-up of this patient cohort, although flow status had the potential to either improve or worsen with medical management alone, the presence of impaired distal flow at any point remained a strong predictor of increased stroke risk.[112] This noninvasive data provides important information for practicing surgeons, while also laying the groundwork for future revascularization clinical trials.

Intraoperatively, to verify bypass patency early advancements beyond the invasive and time-consuming gold standard of intraoperative digital subtraction angiography include the use of Doppler ultrasonography to determine flow velocity and directionality,[113] and microscope-integrated indocyanine green videoangiography.[114] The cut flow index (a ratio of bypass flow [determined by quantitative Doppler imaging]/flow in the cut donor vessel before bypass), has also been described as a simple intraoperative tool, with CFIs of 0.5 or greater shown to have significantly higher long-term patency rates.[115,116]

More recently, microscope-integrated software (Flow 800, Carl Zeiss, Oberkochen, Germany) has been used to provide intraoperative, temporal indocyanine green–based flow information.[117] This technology can semi-quantitatively assess microcirculatory hemodynamic changes in cortical tissue before versus after bypass, and potentially predict the risk of postbypass complications such as hyperperfusion syndrome or a stroke in real time.[117–120] Automated analyses building on this technology and independent of commercial software have also recently been developed adding data on flow directionality.[121] Fluorescein videoangiography is a similar technique that has enhanced visualization of cortical vascular networks as compared with indocyanine green videoangiography, but currently lacks integration into standard imaging platforms for flow-based analyses.[122] Recent advancements in postbypass, longitudinal assessments beyond digital subtraction angiography and computed tomography angiography have also been made, including the use of 4-dimensional flow MRI for the quantitative reconstruction of flow dynamics within the bypass and downstream vasculature.[123]

Future Directions

Despite ongoing advancements in the field of cerebral bypass surgery, data from an international survey of 51 bypass surgeons published in 2020 highlights the relative rarity of this procedure globally, with more than 80% of surgeons performing fewer than 20 bypasses annually and only 3 surgeons performing more than 50 bypasses annually.[124] Additionally, nearly 94% of all bypasses performed in this survey were first-generation STA-MCA constructs. Although the future of cerebral bypass will undoubtedly rely on continued refinements in patient selection and innovations to decrease operative risk, its performance will also likely continue to be concentrated within a select few centers and surgeons, especially for more complex revascularizations. Current and future limitations in trainee exposure during neurosurgical residency will need to be overcome by those interested in this niche field through the pursuit of advanced training opportunities.

SUMMARY

The future of cerebral bypass will be shaped by ongoing refinements in patient selection and creative innovations to continue to improve clinical outcomes. The technical demands of this increasingly complex field will likely result in its continued consolidation to specialized centers.

CLINICS CARE POINTS

- The indications for cerebral bypass have generally decreased in number and increased in complexity over time.

- Strategic innovations in bypass construction have enabled increasingly tailored revascularization solutions.

- Ongoing technical and technological innovations have targeted the operative and perioperative risks of bypass.

- The future of cerebral bypass will rely on refinements in patient selection and continued innovations, likely by a small cohort of specialized surgeons.

DISCLOSURES

The authors have no financial interest to declare in relation to the content of this article.

REFERENCES

1. Hayden MG, Lee M, Guzman R, et al. The evolution of cerebral revascularization surgery. Neurosurg Focus 2009;26(5):E17.

2. Group EIBS. Failure of extracranial-intracranial arterial bypass to reduce the risk of ischemic stroke. Results of an international randomized trial. N Engl J Med 1985;313(19):1191–200.

3. Powers WJ, Clarke WR, Grubb RL, et al. Extracranial-intracranial bypass surgery for stroke prevention in hemodynamic cerebral ischemia: the Carotid Occlusion Surgery Study randomized trial. JAMA 2011;306(18):1983–92.

4. Saber H, Rajah G, Palla M, et al. Utilization and safety of extracranial-intracranial bypass surgery in symptomatic steno-occlusive disorders. Brain Circ 2019;5(1):32–5.

5. Alvi MA, Rinaldo L, Kerezoudis P, et al. Contemporary trends in extracranial-intracranial bypass utilization: analysis of data from 2008 to 2016. J Neurosurg 2019;1–9.

6. Winkler EA, Yue JK, Deng H, et al. National trends in cerebral bypass surgery in the United States, 2002-2014. Neurosurg Focus 2019;46(2):E4.

7. Sharma M, Ugiliweneza B, Fortuny EM, et al. National trends in cerebral bypass for unruptured intracranial aneurysms: a National (Nationwide) Inpatient Sample analysis of 1998-2015. Neurosurg Focus 2019;46(2):E15.

8. Esposito G, Amin-Hanjani S, Regli L. Role of and indications for bypass surgery after carotid occlusion surgery study (COSS)? Stroke 2016;47(1):282–90.

9. Guo Y, Song Y, Hou K, et al. Intracranial fusiform and circumferential aneurysms of the main trunk: therapeutic dilemmas and prospects. Front Neurol 2021;12:679134.

10. Manning NW, Cheung A, Phillips TJ, et al. Pipeline shield with single antiplatelet therapy in aneurysmal subarachnoid haemorrhage: multicentre experience. J Neurointerv Surg 2019;11(7):694–8.

11. Fujimoto M, Lylyk I, Bleise C, et al. Long-term outcomes of the WEB device for treatment of wide-neck bifurcation aneurysms. AJNR Am J Neuroradiol 2020;41(6):1031–6.

12. Ravina K, Rennert RC, Brandel MG, et al. Comparative assessment of extracranial-to-intracranial and intracranial-to-intracranial in situ bypass for complex intracranial aneurysm treatment based on rupture status: a case series. World Neurosurg 2021;146:e122–38.

13. Lam J, Ravina K, Rennert RC, et al. Cerebrovascular bypass for ruptured aneurysms: a case series. J Clin Neurosci 2021;85:106–14.

14. Strickland BA, Rennert RC, Bakhsheshian J, et al. Extracranial-intracranial bypass for treatment of blister aneurysms: efficacy and analysis of complications compared with alternative treatment strategies. World Neurosurg 2018;117:e417–24.

15. Wang L, Cai L, Qian H, et al. Intracranial-intracranial bypass with a graft vessel: a comprehensive

review of technical characteristics and surgical experience. World Neurosurg 2019;125:285–98.

16. Yoon S, Burkhardt JK, Lawton MT. Long-term patency in cerebral revascularization surgery: an analysis of a consecutive series of 430 bypasses. J Neurosurg 2018;131(1):80–7.

17. Lam J, Rennert RC, Ravina K, et al. Bypass and deconstructive technique for Hunt and hess grade 3-5 aneurysmal subarachnoid hemorrhage deemed unfavorable for endovascular treatment: a case series of outcomes and comparison to clipping. World Neurosurg 2020. https://doi.org/10.1016/j.wneu.2020.02.088.

18. Yang T, Tariq F, Chabot J, et al. Cerebral revascularization for difficult skull base tumors: a contemporary series of 18 patients. World Neurosurg 2014;82(5):660–71.

19. Bulsara KR, Patel T, Fukushima T. Cerebral bypass surgery for skull base lesions: technical notes incorporating lessons learned over two decades. Neurosurg Focus 2008;24(2):E11.

20. Kalani MY, Kalb S, Martirosyan NL, et al. Cerebral revascularization and carotid artery resection at the skull base for treatment of advanced head and neck malignancies. J Neurosurg 2013;118(3):637–42.

21. Rennert RC, Ravina K, Strickland BA, et al. Complete cavernous sinus resection: an analysis of complications. World Neurosurg 2018;119:89–96.

22. Couldwell WT, MacDonald JD, Taussky P. Complete resection of the cavernous sinus-indications and technique. World Neurosurg 2014;82(6):1264–70.

23. Miyamoto S, Yoshimoto T, Hashimoto N, et al. Effects of extracranial-intracranial bypass for patients with hemorrhagic moyamoya disease: results of the Japan Adult Moyamoya Trial. Stroke 2014;45(5):1415–21.

24. Choi WS, Lee SB, Kim DS, et al. Thirteen-year experience of 44 patients with adult hemorrhagic moyamoya disease from a single institution: clinical analysis by management modality. J Cerebrovasc Endovasc Neurosurg 2013;15(3):191–9.

25. Abhinav K, Furtado SV, Nielsen TH, et al. Functional outcomes after revascularization procedures in patients with hemorrhagic moyamoya disease. Neurosurgery 2020;86(2):257–65.

26. Li Q, Gao Y, Xin W, et al. Meta-analysis of prognosis of different treatments for symptomatic moyamoya disease. World Neurosurg 2019;127:354–61.

27. Jeon JP, Kim JE, Cho WS, et al. Meta-analysis of the surgical outcomes of symptomatic moyamoya disease in adults. J Neurosurg 2017;1–7.

28. Kim T, Oh CW, Kwon OK, et al. Stroke prevention by direct revascularization for patients with adult-onset moyamoya disease presenting with ischemia. J Neurosurg 2016;124(6):1788–93.

29. Lee SB, Kim DS, Huh PW, et al. Long-term follow-up results in 142 adult patients with moyamoya disease according to management modality. Acta Neurochir (Wien) 2012;154(7):1179–87.

30. Sun H, Wilson C, Ozpinar A, et al. Perioperative complications and long-term outcomes after bypasses in adults with moyamoya disease: a systematic review and meta-analysis. World Neurosurg 2016;92:179–88.

31. Nielsen TH, Abhinav K, Sussman ES, et al. Direct versus indirect bypass procedure for the treatment of ischemic moyamoya disease: results of an individualized selection strategy. J Neurosurg 2020;134(5):1578–89.

32. Macyszyn L, Attiah M, Ma TS, et al. Direct versus indirect revascularization procedures for moyamoya disease: a comparative effectiveness study. J Neurosurg 2017;126(5):1523–9.

33. Park SE, Kim JS, Park EK, et al. Direct versus indirect revascularization in the treatment of moyamoya disease. J Neurosurg 2018;129(2):480–9.

34. Lai PMR, Patel NJ, Frerichs KU, et al. Direct vs indirect revascularization in a North American cohort of moyamoya disease. Neurosurgery 2021;89(2):315–22.

35. Zhao Y, Lu J, Yu S, et al. Comparison of long-term effect between direct and indirect bypass for pediatric ischemic-type moyamoya disease: a propensity score-matched study. Front Neurol 2019;10:795.

36. Ha EJ, Kim KH, Wang KC, et al. Long-term outcomes of indirect bypass for 629 children with moyamoya disease: longitudinal and cross-sectional analysis. Stroke 2019;50(11):3177–83.

37. Rashad S, Fujimura M, Niizuma K, et al. Long-term follow-up of pediatric moyamoya disease treated by combined direct-indirect revascularization surgery: single institute experience with surgical and perioperative management. Neurosurg Rev 2016;39(4):615–23.

38. Ravindran K, Wellons JC, Dewan MC. Surgical outcomes for pediatric moyamoya: a systematic review and meta-analysis. J Neurosurg Pediatr 2019;1–10.

39. Kuroda S, Hashimoto N, Yoshimoto T, et al. Radiological findings, clinical course, and outcome in asymptomatic moyamoya disease: results of multicenter survey in Japan. Stroke 2007;38(5):1430–5.

40. Sakamoto Y, Okamoto S, Maesawa S, et al. Default mode network changes in moyamoya disease before and after bypass surgery: preliminary report. World Neurosurg 2018;112:e652–61.

41. Zeifert PD, Karzmark P, Bell-Stephens TE, et al. Neurocognitive performance after cerebral revascularization in adult moyamoya disease. Stroke 2017;48(6):1514–7.

42. Kazumata K, Tha KK, Tokairin K, et al. Brain structure, connectivity, and cognitive changes following revascularization surgery in adult moyamoya disease. Neurosurgery 2019;85(5):E943–52.

43. Steinberg JA, Rennert RC, Ravina K, et al. Rescue cerebral revascularization in patients with progressive steno-occlusive ischemia of the anterior intracranial circulation. World Neurosurg 2019. https://doi.org/10.1016/j.wneu.2019.09.102.

44. Rennert RC, Steinberg JA, Strickland BA, et al. Extracranial-to-intracranial bypass for refractory vertebrobasilar insufficiency. World Neurosurg 2019;126:552–9.

45. Ilyas A, Chen CJ, Ironside N, et al. Medical management versus surgical bypass for symptomatic intracranial atherosclerotic disease: a systematic review. World Neurosurg 2019;129:62–71.

46. Kernan WN, Ovbiagele B, Black HR, et al. Guidelines for the prevention of stroke in patients with stroke and transient ischemic attack: a guideline for healthcare professionals from the American Heart Association/American Stroke Association. Stroke 2014;45(7):2160–236.

47. Yu Y, Wang T, Yang K, et al. Timing and outcomes of intracranial stenting in the post-SAMMPRIS Era: a systematic review. Front Neurol 2021;12:637632.

48. Lawton MT, Lang MJ. The future of open vascular neurosurgery: perspectives on cavernous malformations, AVMs, and bypasses for complex aneurysms. J Neurosurg 2019;130(5):1409–25.

49. Alaraj A, Ashley WW, Charbel FT, et al. The superficial temporal artery trunk as a donor vessel in cerebral revascularization: benefits and pitfalls. Neurosurg Focus 2008;24(2):E7.

50. Cherian J, Srinivasan V, Kan P, et al. Double-barrel superficial temporal artery-middle cerebral artery bypass: can it be considered "high-flow? Oper Neurosurg (Hagerstown) 2018;14(3):288–94.

51. Zarrinkoob L, Ambarki K, Wåhlin A, et al. Blood flow distribution in cerebral arteries. J Cereb Blood Flow Metab 2015;35(4):648–54.

52. Bang JS, Kwon OK, Kim JE, et al. Quantitative angiographic comparison with the OSIRIS program between the direct and indirect revascularization modalities in adult moyamoya disease. Neurosurgery 2012;70(3):625–32. discussion 632-3.

53. Czabanka M, Peña-Tapia P, Scharf J, et al. Characterization of direct and indirect cerebral revascularization for the treatment of European patients with moyamoya disease. Cerebrovasc Dis 2011;32(4):361–9.

54. Amin-Hanjani S, Singh A, Rifai H, et al. Combined direct and indirect bypass for moyamoya: quantitative assessment of direct bypass flow over time. Neurosurgery 2013;73(6):962–7.

55. Yamamoto S, Kashiwazaki D, Uchino H, et al. Ameliorative effects of combined revascularization surgery on abnormal collateral channels in moyamoya disease. J Stroke Cerebrovasc Dis 2021;30(4):105624.

56. Ravina K, Rennert RC, Strickland BA, et al. Pedicled temporoparietal fascial flap for combined revascularization in adult moyamoya disease. J Neurosurg 2018;1–7. https://doi.org/10.3171/2018.5.JNS18938.

57. Ravina K, Kim PE, Rennert RC, et al. Lessons learned from the initial experience with pedicled temporoparietal fascial flap for combined revascularization in moyamoya angiopathy: a case series. World Neurosurg 2019;132:e259–73.

58. Duckworth EA, Rao VY, Patel AJ. Double-barrel bypass for cerebral ischemia: technique, rationale, and preliminary experience with 10 consecutive cases. Neurosurgery 2013;73(1 Suppl Operative):ons30–8. discussion ons37-38.

59. Burkhardt JK, Winkler EA, Gandhi S, et al. Single-barrel versus double-barrel superficial temporal artery to middle cerebral artery bypass: a comparative analysis. World Neurosurg 2019;125:e408–15.

60. Kan P, Srinivasan VM, Srivatsan A, et al. Double-barrel STA-MCA bypass for cerebral revascularization: lessons learned from a 10-year experience. J Neurosurg 2021;1–9. https://doi.org/10.3171/2020.9.JNS201976.

61. Sekhar LN, Kalavakonda C. Cerebral revascularization for aneurysms and tumors. Neurosurgery 2002;50(2):321–31.

62. Nossek E, Costantino PD, Eisenberg M, et al. Internal maxillary artery-middle cerebral artery bypass: infratemporal approach for subcranial-intracranial (SC-IC) bypass. Neurosurgery 2014;75(1):87–95.

63. Feng X, Meybodi AT, Rincon-Torroella J, et al. Surgical technique for high-flow internal maxillary artery to middle cerebral artery bypass using a superficial temporal artery interposition graft. Oper Neurosurg (Hagerstown) 2017;13(2):246–57.

64. Abdulrauf SI, Sweeney JM, Mohan YS, et al. Short segment internal maxillary artery to middle cerebral artery bypass: a novel technique for extracranial-to-intracranial bypass. Neurosurgery 2011;68(3):804–8. discussion 808-809.

65. Rubio RR, Gandhi S, Benet A, et al. Internal maxillary artery to anterior circulation bypass with local interposition grafts using a minimally invasive approach: surgical anatomy and technical feasibility. World Neurosurg 2018;120:e503–10.

66. Yang T, Tariq F, Duong HT, et al. Bypass using V2-V3 segment of the vertebral artery as donor or recipient: technical nuances and results. World Neurosurg 2014;82(6):1164–70.

67. Benet A, Tabani H, Bang JS, et al. Occipital artery to anterior inferior cerebellar artery bypass with radial artery interposition graft for vertebrobasilar

insufficiency: 3-dimensional operative video. Oper Neurosurg (Hagerstown) 2017;13(5):641.

68. Baaj AA, Agazzi S, van Loveren H. Graft selection in cerebral revascularization. Neurosurg Focus 2009;26(5):E18.

69. Kubota H, Tanikawa R, Katsuno M, et al. Vertebral artery-to-vertebral artery bypass with interposed radial artery or occipital artery grafts: surgical technique and report of three cases. World Neurosurg 2014;81(1):202.e1–8.

70. Liu JK, Kan P, Karwande SV, et al. Conduits for cerebrovascular bypass and lessons learned from the cardiovascular experience. Neurosurg Focus 2003;14(3):e3.

71. Başkaya MK, Kiehn MW, Ahmed AS, et al. Alternative vascular graft for extracranial-intracranial bypass surgery: descending branch of the lateral circumflex femoral artery. Neurosurg Focus 2008; 24(2):E8.

72. Houkin K, Ishikawa T, Kuroda S, et al. Vascular reconstruction using interposed small vessels. Neurosurgery 1998;43(3):501–5.

73. Jain A, O'Neill K, Patel MC, et al. Extracranial-intracranial bypass of the bilateral anterior cerebral circulation using a thoracodorsal axis artery-graft. Asian J Neurosurg 2012;7(4):203–5.

74. Ramanathan D, Starnes B, Hatsukami T, et al. Tibial artery autografts: alternative conduits for high flow cerebral revascularizations. World Neurosurg 2013;80(3–4):322–7.

75. Strickland BA, Bakhsheshian J, Rennert RC, et al. Descending branch of the lateral circumflex femoral artery graft for posterior inferior cerebellar artery revascularization. Oper Neurosurg (Hagerstown) 2018;15(3):285–91.

76. Osman S, Chou S, Rosing J, et al. Total posterior leg open wound management with free anterolateral thigh flap: case and literature review. Eplasty 2013;13:e50.

77. Koshima I, Fukuda H, Yamamoto H, et al. Free anterolateral thigh flaps for reconstruction of head and neck defects. Plast Reconstr Surg 1993; 92(3):421–8. discussion 429-430.

78. Song YG, Chen GZ, Song YL. The free thigh flap: a new free flap concept based on the septocutaneous artery. Br J Plast Surg 1984;37(2):149–59.

79. Gaiotto FA, Vianna CB, Busnardo FF, et al. The descending branch of the lateral femoral circumflex artery is a good option in CABG with arterial grafts. Rev Bras Cir Cardiovasc 2013;28(3):317–24.

80. Zhang Y, Janssen L, Chu FV. Atherosclerosis of radial arterial graft may increase the potential of vessel spasm in coronary bypass surgery. J Thorac Cardiovasc Surg 2005;130(5):1477–8.

81. Lee JH, Choi HJ, Jung KH, et al. Pathologic patency analysis of the descending branch of the lateral femoral circumflex artery in head and neck reconstruction. J Craniofac Surg 2016;27(4): e385–9.

82. Halvorson EG, Taylor HO, Orgill DP. Patency of the descending branch of the lateral circumflex femoral artery in patients with vascular disease. Plast Reconstr Surg 2008;121(1):121–9.

83. Ravina K, Buchanan IA, Rennert RC, et al. Occipital artery to posterior cerebral artery bypass using descending branch of the lateral circumflex femoral artery graft for treatment of fusiform, unruptured posterior cerebral artery aneurysm: 3-dimensional operative video. Oper Neurosurg (Hagerstown) 2018. https://doi.org/10.1093/ons/opy057.

84. Srinivasan VM, Kan P, Huang AT, et al. Occipital artery to middle cerebral artery bypass using the descending branch of the lateral circumflex femoral artery as an interposition graft for blood flow augmentation in progressive moyamoya disease. World Neurosurg 2020;139:208–14.

85. Sudhir BJ, Murali SH, Jamaluddin MA, et al. Superficial temporal artery extended interposition graft to anterior cerebral artery bypass for the treatment of a large fusiform distal anterior cerebral artery aneurysm: 2-dimensional operative video. Oper Neurosurg (Hagerstown) 2021;21(4):E353–4.

86. Rennert RC, Ravina K, Strickland BA, et al. Radial artery fascial flow-through free flap for complex cerebral revascularization: technical notes and long-term neurologic and radiographic outcomes. Oper Neurosurg (Hagerstown) 2018. https://doi.org/10.1093/ons/opy124.

87. Abla AA, Lawton MT. Anterior cerebral artery bypass for complex aneurysms: an experience with intracranial-intracranial reconstruction and review of bypass options. J Neurosurg 2014;120(6): 1364–77.

88. Ravina K, Strickland BA, Rennert RC, et al. A3-A3 anastomosis in the management of complex anterior cerebral artery aneurysms: experience with in situ bypass and lessons learned from pseudoaneurysm cases. Oper Neurosurg (Hagerstown) 2018. https://doi.org/10.1093/ons/opy334.

89. Rennert RC, Strickland BA, Ravina K, et al. Efficacy and outcomes of posterior inferior cerebellar artery (pica) bypass for proximal pica and vertebral artery-pica aneurysms: a case series. Oper Neurosurg (Hagerstown) 2018;15(4):395–403.

90. Abla AA, McDougall CM, Breshears JD, et al. Intracranial-to-intracranial bypass for posterior inferior cerebellar artery aneurysms: options, technical challenges, and results in 35 patients. J Neurosurg 2016;124(5):1275–86.

91. Ravina K, Rennert RC, Kim PE, et al. Orphaned middle cerebral artery side-to-side in situ bypass as a favorable alternative approach for complex middle cerebral artery aneurysm treatment: a case series. World Neurosurg 2019;130:e971–87.

92. Russin JJ. The arborization bypass: Sequential intracranial-intracranial bypasses for an unruptured fusiform MCA aneurysm. J Clin Neurosci 2017;39: 209–11.

93. Ravina K, Strickland BA, Rennert RC, et al. Fusiform vertebral artery aneurysms involving the posterior inferior cerebellar artery origin associated with the sole angiographic anterior spinal artery origin: technical case report and treatment paradigm proposal. J Neurosurg 2018;1–7.

94. Frisoli FA, Catapano JS, Baranoski JF, et al. The middle communicating artery: a novel fourth-generation bypass for revascularizing trapped middle cerebral artery bifurcation aneurysms in 2 cases. J Neurosurg 2020;134(6):1879–86.

95. Ravina K, Yim B, Lam J, et al. Three-vessel anastomosis for direct bihemispheric cerebral revascularization. Oper Neurosurg (Hagerstown) 2020;19(3): 313–8.

96. He GW. Arterial grafts: clinical classification and pharmacological management. Ann Cardiothorac Surg 2013;2(4):507–18.

97. Tecle NEE, Zammar SG, Hamade YJ, et al. Use of a harvested radial artery graft with preservation of the vena comitantes to reduce spasm risk and improve graft patency for extracranial to intracranial bypass: technical note. Clin Neurol Neurosurg 2016;142:65–71.

98. Natarajan SK, Hauck EF, Hopkins LN, et al. Endovascular management of symptomatic spasm of radial artery bypass graft: technical case report. Neurosurgery 2010;67(3):794–8. discussion 798.

99. Liu JK, Couldwell WT. Intra-arterial papaverine infusions for the treatment of cerebral vasospasm induced by aneurysmal subarachnoid hemorrhage. Neurocrit Care 2005;2(2):124–32.

100. Strickland BA, Bakhsheshian J, Rennert RC, et al. Descending Branch of the Lateral Circumflex Femoral Artery Graft for Posterior Inferior Cerebellar Artery Revascularization. Oper Neurosurg (Hagerstown) 2018 Sep 1;15(3):285–91. https://doi.org/10.1093/ons/opx241. PMID: 30125010.

101. Strickland BA, Rennert RC, Bakhsheshian J, et al. Botulinum toxin to improve vessel graft patency in cerebral revascularization surgery: report of 3 cases. J Neurosurg 2018;1–7.

102. Ravina K, Strickland BA, Rennert RC, et al. Role of botulinum neurotoxin-A in cerebral revascularization graft vasospasm prevention: current state of knowledge. Neurosurg Focus 2019;46(2):E13.

103. Rennert RC, Strickland BA, Radwanski RE, et al. Running-to-interrupted microsuture technique for vascular bypass. Oper Neurosurg (Hagerstown) 2018;15(4):412–7.

104. Matsuo S, Amano T, Nakamizo A. Single loop interrupted suture technique for cerebrovascular anastomosis: technical note. J Clin Neurosci 2020;72:434–7.

105. Mehta SH, Belykh E, Farhadi DS, et al. Needle parking interrupted suturing technique for microvascular anastomosis: a technical note. Oper Neurosurg (Hagerstown) 2021;21(5):E414–20.

106. Ravina K, Fredrickson VL, Donoho DA, et al. An expedited transition to the back wall suturing for side-to-side in situ microvascular anastomosis: a technique update. Oper Neurosurg (Hagerstown) 2020;19(6):E583–8.

107. Shimizu S, Osawa S, Kuroda H, et al. Half-tied stay suture technique for cerebrovascular end-to-side anastomosis: a technique to expand the view of the hidden ostium. Neurol Med Chir (Tokyo) 2019; 59(8):326–9.

108. de Havenon A, Khatri P, Prabhakaran S, et al. Hypoperfusion distal to anterior circulation intracranial atherosclerosis is associated with recurrent stroke. J Neuroimaging 2020;30(4):468–70.

109. Yaghi S, Khatri P, Prabhakaran S, et al. What threshold defines penumbral brain tissue in patients with symptomatic anterior circulation intracranial stenosis: an exploratory analysis. J Neuroimaging 2019;29(2):203–5.

110. Amin-Hanjani S, Pandey DK, Rose-Finnell L, et al. Effect of hemodynamics on stroke risk in symptomatic atherosclerotic vertebrobasilar occlusive disease. JAMA Neurol 2016;73(2):178–85.

111. Amin-Hanjani S, Du X, Rose-Finnell L, et al. Hemodynamic features of symptomatic vertebrobasilar disease. Stroke 2015;46(7):1850–6.

112. Amin-Hanjani S, See AP, Du X, et al. Natural history of hemodynamics in vertebrobasilar disease: temporal changes in the veritas study cohort. Stroke 2020;51(11):3295–301.

113. Badie B, Lee FT, Pozniak MA, et al. Intraoperative sonographic assessment of graft patency during extracranial-intracranial bypass. AJNR Am J Neuroradiol 2000;21(8):1457–9.

114. Woitzik J, Horn P, Vajkoczy P, et al. Intraoperative control of extracranial-intracranial bypass patency by near-infrared indocyanine green videoangiography. J Neurosurg 2005;102(4):692–8.

115. Amin-Hanjani S, Du X, Mlinarevich N, et al. The cut flow index: an intraoperative predictor of the success of extracranial-intracranial bypass for occlusive cerebrovascular disease. Neurosurgery 2005;56(1 Suppl):75–85. discussion 75-85.

116. Stapleton CJ, Atwal GS, Hussein AE, et al. The cut flow index revisited: utility of intraoperative blood flow measurements in extracranial-intracranial bypass surgery for ischemic cerebrovascular disease. J Neurosurg 2019;06:1–5.

117. Rennert RC, Strickland BA, Ravina K, et al. Assessment of hemodynamic changes and hyperperfusion risk after extracranial-to-intracranial bypass surgery using intraoperative indocyanine green-based flow analysis. World Neurosurg 2018;114:352–60.

118. Rennert RC, Strickland BA, Ravina K, et al. Intraoperative assessment of cortical perfusion after intracranial-to-intracranial and extracranial-to-intracranial bypass for complex cerebral aneurysms using flow 800. Oper Neurosurg (Hagerstown) 2018. https://doi.org/10.1093/ons/opy154.

119. Yang T, Higashino Y, Kataoka H, et al. Correlation between reduction in microvascular transit time after superficial temporal artery-middle cerebral artery bypass surgery for moyamoya disease and the development of postoperative hyperperfusion syndrome. J Neurosurg 2017;1–7. https://doi.org/10.3171/2016.11.JNS162403.

120. Rennert RC, Strickland BA, Ravina K, et al. Assessment of ischemic risk following intracranial-to-intracranial and extracranial-to-intracranial bypass for complex aneurysms using intraoperative indocyanine green-based flow analysis. J Clin Neurosci 2019. https://doi.org/10.1016/j.jocn.2019.06.036.

121. Jiang Z, Lei Y, Zhang L, et al. Automated quantitative analysis of blood flow in extracranial-intracranial arterial bypass based on indocyanine green angiography. Front Surg 2021;8:649719.

122. Narducci A, Onken J, Czabanka M, et al. Fluorescein videoangiography during extracranial-to-intracranial bypass surgery: preliminary results. Acta Neurochir (Wien) 2018;160(4):767–74.

123. Sekine T, Takagi R, Amano Y, et al. 4D flow MRI assessment of extracranial-intracranial bypass: qualitative and quantitative evaluation of the hemodynamics. Neuroradiology 2016;58(3):237–44.

124. Srinivasan VM, Griessenauer CJ, Rodríguez-Hernández A, et al. A survey of microsurgical technique for extracranial-to-intracranial bypass. World Neurosurg 2020;141:e743–51.

"Dolichoectatic Vertebrobasilar Artery Aneurysms"

Behnam Rezai Jahromi, MD[a,b],*, Mika Niemelä, MD, PhD[a,b]

KEYWORDS

- Dolichoectasia • Fusiform aneurysm • Giant aneurysm • Vertebrobasilar

KEY POINTS

- Vertebrobasilar dolichoectatic artery aneurysms (VBADA) are complex and heterogenous vascular anomalies affecting posterior circulation of the main arteries.
- Natural history of VBADA is poorly understood due to a lack of definition of VBADA.
- The time window to treat patients is narrow, and those VBADAs that show any activity should be controlled closely.
- VBADA lacks an aneurysmatic neck to be excluded from circulation; thus, flow changes are the only available options for treatment. Flow change through VBADA is technically possible via endovascular methods and microneurosurgery but might have catastrophic outcomes.
- Young patients with high vascular plasticity might benefit the most from invasive treatment.

INTRODUCTION

Intracranial artery dolichoectasia (IADE) is a heterogenous arterial disease that is underdiagnosed and identified mainly in stroke patients. The abnormal lengthening (dolicho) and enlargement (ectasia) of intracranial arteries are poorly defined, especially in anterior circulation arteries. IADE of the vertebrobasilar artery was defined by Smoker and colleagues[1] as follows: (1) basilar artery diameter larger than 4.5 mm, (2) tortuous of basilar artery more lies laterally from margin of clivus or dorsum sellae, and (3) basilar artery is above the suprasellar cistern. No definitions or criteria currently exist for anterior circulation dolichoectasia.[2] Accurate natural history and epidemiologic studies are lacking due to an undefined population and cohorts, and also because IADEs are seen as normal anatomic variations.[1–3] Put simply, IADE is excess arterial tissue without malformation.

The lack of classification related to the outcome and progression of IADE, as well as its underdiagnosis by physicians, has resulted in inconsistent studies on its epidemiology, disease progression, definition, and pathophysiology.[4] Most patients are diagnosed after stroke by a neurologist and referred for neurosurgical evaluation when disease progression has reached a level with cranial nerve palsies or other treatments requiring decompression. Most IADE occurs in posterior circulation, making such cases vertebrobasilar dolichoectasia; some develop separate aneurysms, or the whole arterial segment expands aneurysmatically (**Fig. 1**).

IADE is thought to be common among stroke patients (12%), and it has been shown to exist concomitantly with extracranial aneurysm and abdominal artery aneurysm (AAA) in particular.[5–7] Fusiform aneurysms are shown to be more common in AAA patients than in the general population.[7] However, 20% of IADE has been identified without atherosclerosis, which expands the pathophysiological hypothesis behind the entity.

a Department of Neurosurgery, Helsinki University Hospital & University of Helsinki, Helsinki, Finland; b Töölö Hospital, Topeliuksenkatu 5, Helsinki 00260, Finland
* Corresponding author. Department of Neurosurgery, Helsinki University Hospital & University of Helsinki, Helsinki, Finland.
E-mail address: behnam.rezai-jahromi@hus.fi

Neurosurg Clin N Am 33 (2022) 419–429
https://doi.org/10.1016/j.nec.2022.06.003
1042-3680/22/© 2022 Elsevier Inc. All rights reserved.

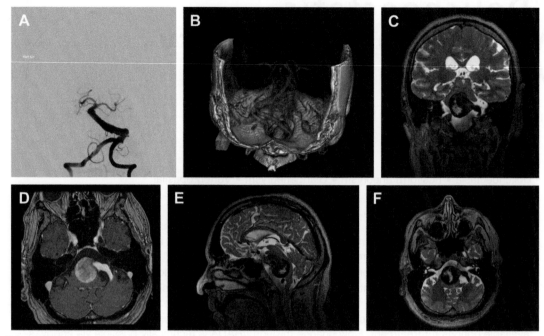

Fig. 1. A 61-year-old man presented with and left side hemiparesis. He had for some time dysphagia. A giant VBADA was seen in imaging. Both VA were feeding the VBADA (*A*, *B*), while dislocating cranial nerves and brainstem (*C–F*). Patient had multiple comorbidities and refused from any treatment.

The terminology of dolichoectatic vertebrobasilar artery aneurysms is heterogeneous. Various terms have been used to describe their features based on anatomic characteristics, including *serpentine, fusiform, megadolichoectasia, aneurysmal malformation, megadolichobasilar anomaly, elongated basilar artery, cirsoid aneurysm, wandering basilar artery,* and *tortous basilar artery.* "*S aneurysms,*" as Dandy referred to this condition, lack a defined neck and are usually segmental, unlike fusiform aneurysms in which some part of the segment can include the intact artery.[8] Often, fusiform and dolichoectatic aneurysms are hard to separate and "translational" terms have been introduced.[9,10] However, there is little evidence of dolichoectasia arising from fusiform formation. In this article, we use vertebrobasilar artery dolichoectatic aneurysms (VBADAs) to define nonsaccular aneurysms in VBA because, in our opinion, they provide a good reflection of the characteristics of this arteriopathy.

Neurosurgeons often encounter a VBADA when the progression of disease has reached the point of inducing compression to the cranial nerves and brainstem or obstructing the third ventricle to induce hydrocephalus (**Fig. 2**). Neurosurgeons see the tip of the iceberg of hemorrhagic cases when the immediate mortality of VBADA is most probably extremely high. Due to the vital perforator being fed through the VBADA and without an obvious neck to be ligated, the microsurgical treatment is challenging with high morbidity and mortality. Unfortunately, advances in an endovascular approach have not provided the needed relief for the progression of VBADAs, despite the application of flow diverters. A correct treatment option in the most fruitful timing is still to be established.

DISCUSSION
Epidemiology

A lack of coherence in the definition of IADE and VBADA has made a precise review of epidemiologic studies difficult. An autopsy study from the United States showed that 0.008% of the population had IADE whereas in a more contemporary study cohort of stroke patients, 12% were analyzed with IADE.[2,11]

In a Japanese selected cohort for patients 60 to 70 years old seeking an annual physical check-up, 1.3% had asymptomatic vertebrobasilar dolichoectasia and the major risk factors, including hypertension, dyslipidemia, smoking, and diabetes mellitus, overlapped with atherosclerosis.[12] On the other hand, a Chinese cohort was used to study the differences between intracranial atherosclerosis stenosis and IADE, and it was found that the only common risk factor was advanced age.[13] There are conflicting results on atherosclerotic involvement in VBADA formation although there are robust data on the involvement of small vessel

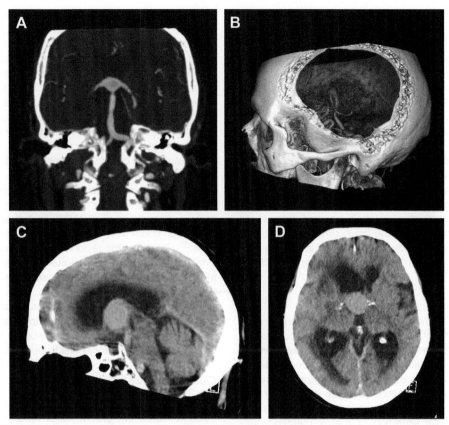

Fig. 2. A 77-year-old woman presented with walking difficulties and memory deficit for 2 years. Symptoms progressed and an elongated BA blocking the CSF pathway was seen in images in computer tomography (CT) [C,D] and in CT-angio [A,B]. Comorbidities were thought to be high risk and patients' symptoms were developed slowly. Family withdrew the support due to risk of hemorrhage after potential shunt placement.

disease and other traditional cardiovascular risk factors. Unlike saccular intracranial aneurysms, there is a predominance of male patients with VBADA.

Although symptomatic VBADAs are more prone to be highlighted, compared with IADE in anterior circulation, there is evidence that the latter is more common in posterior circulation or in both anterior and posterior circulation compared with anterior circulation alone[2,5,6]

Basilar artery (BA) diameter has been shown to be an independent risk factor for mortality of cardiovascular disorders, especially when the diameter is larger than 4.3 mm, and BA height has been shown to be a continuous variable for stroke if the BA is positioned transversely. Coronary artery ectasia and BA ectasia have been shown to be associated.[3] This raises the question of whether systemic pathophysiology is related to some VBADA patients.[2]

In a meta-analysis by Nasr and colleagues,[9] in which only 15 studies were recognized, fusiform and dolichoectatic VBA nonsaccular aneurysms were analyzed. The annual mortality rate of these 827 patients was 13%, making the overall prognosis poor. They found differences between fusiform and dolichoectatic patients, although a heterogenous definition might complicate the setting of the meta-analysis. The growth rates of fusiform and dolichoectatic aneurysms differed (12% vs 3%, respectively).

Most patients in meta-analysis presented with ischemic stroke and compression symptoms. On rare occasions, patients with VBADA are admitted with hemorrhages. This may be due to the high fatality rate of posterior circulation aneurysm ruptures, which prevents them from being admitted to a hospital in time.[14,15] VBADAs that showed growth during follow-up had a high chance of rupture.[14,15]

Pathophysiology

Despite the limited number of pathologic investigations of VBADA, it has been suggested that there are multiple etiologies of the same entity. A small number of VBADAs are related to infections such as human immunodeficiency virus and syphilis whereas other rare forms are related to metabolic disorders such as Fabry's and Pompei diseases.[4] Furthermore, immunologic etiologies such as Ig-4-related diseases have been reported. An embryologic lack of the posterior communicating (Pcom) artery may enforce VBADA formation, and lack of vascular plasticity is among the prognostic factors.[16] The main hypothesis of VBADA formation has been dissection, evolution of fusiform formation, and atherosclerosis as somatic mutations.[17–19] At the point of evolution, the BA diameter increases due to the need for blood flow in vital areas of the brain, such as the pontine region. Some birds, including owls, have fusiformlike dilation in their cervical arteries to allow blood flow to the brain despite being able to turn their head by 270° and disrupting the flow for a short time while using fusiform sacs as reserves.[20]

Hemodynamics and inflammation
The BA's hemodynamic role is noteworthy, as it can be bidirectional depending on the Pcom artery diameter.[21] These changes are dependent on the patient's vascular plasticity, and Pcom arteries and other collaterals can grow or shrink depending on their need. In rabbit models, cervical artery ligation induced BA enlargement and caused a burst of endothelial secretion of matrix metalloproteinases through shear stress.[4] Enlargement of the BA slows the flow in some segments and induces thrombosis. Abnormalities in the hemodynamics of VBADAs are described in computer fluid dynamic modeling.

In saccular intracranial aneurysms, as in AAA, the thrombosis induces inflammation. There are a few anecdotal reports on whether thrombosis formation is a stabilizing factor or whether it accelerates VBADA progression. However, it is noteworthy that an aneurysm is still able to grow despite thrombosis formation, reminding us that there are vasa vasorum that keep the artery functional despite thrombus formation.[20,21] This phenomenon has also been described in saccular aneurysms. There are reports that the thrombus is endothelized toward brainstem perforators in VBADA.

Atherosclerosis and dissection
There are contradictory data regarding the role of atherosclerosis and the formation of VBADAs. This may be caused by the different setups of reported cohorts—20% of VBADAs do not share atherosclerotic plaque, and thus, the term *atherosclerotic aneurysm* is not valid.[4,22] Most of VBADA patients are advanced in age, and many share traditional cardiovascular risk factors. For this reason, atherosclerosis might be a general finding with little significance in the pathophysiology of VBADAs. Nakatomi and colleagues studied the histology of 16 fusiform aneurysms. Of these cases, only five were in posterior circulation and only one affected the BA, indicating that the results were indeed from fusiform lesions rather than dolichoectatic ones. The terminology used during the study period was even more heterogenous despite the finding that "in atherosclerosis, early changes include intimal cell proliferation around lipid deposits and duplication or thinning of IEL, neither of which was observed in our (16) cases."[16]

Mizutani detailed new histologic findings for 3 patients out of a reported 13, showing macroscopic dissection of VBADA and that natural dissection could develop in later stages of the disease.[23] However, the report also demonstrated a similar finding to that of Nakatomi that significant atherosclerotic characteristics were missing in histology.

The expression of rare diseases such as VBADA usually reflects that there are multiple risk factors that must coexist in order for the disease to occur. What is a waving factor is still to be explored.

Clinical Manifestation

VBADA can present incidentally, for example, through routine imaging. Most of VBADA patients present with thromboembolic complications, hemorrhage, mass effects of the brainstem, or stretching of cranial nerves due to the elongation and lateralization of VBADA. When the BA rises sufficiently, it may block the cerebrospinal pathway in the third ventricle and cause hydrocephalus.

Thromboembolic complications
When flow is decreased at certain points of a VBADA and thrombosis formation is induced, it is thought that the aneurysm itself might be stabilized while flow to the brainstem is preserved. It needs to be investigated whether this is caused by collateral formation in the brainstem as thrombosis is formed spontaneously in low shear stress areas, or whether it has to do with inflammation induced to the VBADA's wall from the thrombosis. The embolic material formation in IADE is seen to be high as 12% of stroke patients have been shown to have IADE. In patients with aneurysmatic section of VBADA the thrombosis is more frequent due to the pouch providing a shield for the thrombosis as it is established.[1,9–16] Thrombus in the other hand can force degeneration and thus tip the pathophysiology toward destabilizing nature.

Hemorrhage
Thrombosis in VBADA may induce thrombosis in the vasa vasorum, which may in turn lead to

necrosis of the aneurysm wall and hemorrhage. However, it has been shown that VBADAs that grow during follow-up have the highest risk of rupture, especially after the diameter of the BA increases to 10 mm or more. It can be hypothesized that the VBADA wall is able to grow, permitted by vaso vasorums and collaterals. Degeneration of VBADA, similar to saccular aneurysms, plays a role in the reorganization of the VBADA wall.

Mass effect of brainstem and cranial nerves

It is surprising how long patients can resist and be symptom free when a significant mass stretches the brainstem. This indicates that the development of VBADAs takes place reasonably slowly. Symptoms are related to the part of the brainstem that is under the influence of the mass.

Therapeutic Options

Conservative treatment

Despite the apparently poor prognosis of VBADAs, there have been no randomized clinical trials on this aspect. VBADA patients also have concomitant diseases that force clinicians to treat lesions conservatively.[15] Individual vascular plasticity and collateral formation have brought hope that VBADAs can be treated conservatively: If the patient is lucky, the VBADA may stabilize, and the aneurysm will stop growing while the brain stem perforators are kept intact. After the BA has enlarged by 10 mm or more, the probability of rupture increases whereas enlargement also brings the possibility of the cranial nerve stretching and the brainstem compressing. As mentioned earlier, there are contradictory reports on whether thrombosis formation stabilizes or promotes VBADA's malignant activity. The risk of stroke increases much earlier at 4.5 mm BA diameter, which forces patients to be treated prophylactically with antithrombotic medication (ASA), statins, and hypertension medication. Clinicians should closely follow-up on patients when VBADA shows any signs of activity. **Fig. 2** demonstrates well the conservatively treated patient.

Interventional neuroradiology

The rapid development of endovascular treatments for intracranial procedures initially brought hope that VBADAs could be treated with flow diverters (FD). However, this enthusiasm declined rapidly with the report by Siddiqui and colleagues[24] on their initial experience with FD in nonsaccular VBA aneurysms. The same group reported 12 patients at a later stage who had better outcomes, but none of the cases were of VBADA.[25] The hypothesis was that VBADAs with partial thrombosis have a high risk of perforator occlusion as only channels feeding blood supply to those perforators go through the thrombus itself. The main problem with this is that endothelialization does not start from progenitor cells in the blood but from the intact healthy artery. As VBADA by definition lacks a healthy artery in all parts of the affected segment, the complication and occlusion rates with FD are explainable. In addition, the uneven wall structure of a VBADA causes FDs to be poorly attached to the wall, reducing the regenerative thrombus formation that is seen in saccular aneurysms and FD. Boghal and colleagues[26] reported FD use in 56 patients and 58 nonsaccular VBA aneurysms. The occlusion rate was highly dependent on the definition of aneurysms proposed by Flemming, whereby nonsaccular VBA aneurysms were divided into fusiform (24 aneurysms), translational (28 aneurysms), and dolichoectatic (6 aneurysms). Of the nonfusiform aneurysms in this series (total 34 aneurysms), nine aneurysms were occluded, eight patients died, and two did not have follow-up. Of the fusiform aneurysms that were most successfully treated with FD, 18 achieved occlusion. Wang and colleagues showed that symptomatic VBADA cases had poor outcomes when treated with FD. The findings were similar in other endovascularly treated VBADA cases: Waiting for symptoms or enlargement of the aneurysms increased the risk of complication and decreased the success rate. Wang and colleagues[27] reported 22 VBADA cases treated endovascularly with multiple endovascular tools (coil + stent/multiple stents), but unfortunately, of the 13 patients who were admitted with compressive symptoms, 7 died due to severe compression to the brainstem. Five patients with ischemic symptoms were reported, three of whom benefited, with the modified Rankin scale increasing after treatment; in the other two cases, the neurologic outcome stayed the same. In the same report, three-quarters of patients with hemorrhages achieved good clinical improvement while one patient stayed the same.

Endovascular treatment of VBADA seems to be possible in selected and early treated patients. On the other hand, the impact of thrombus formation seems to be a double-edged sword as it is able to both stabilize aneurysms and induce the progression of VBADA. This is particularly well seen in cases with compression symptoms (**Fig. 3**). The role of the vasa vasorum might be significant in aneurysm behavior and how well FD is able to stabilize them. Dobrocky and colleagues[28] demonstrated the lack of pontine perforators in VBADA cases with the brainstem fed by risen collaterals.

Until now, there have not been endovascular flow reduction devices. Patients may benefit from dynamic and slow changes in VBADAs with the help of computer flow dynamic (CFD) modeling.[29] It has been shown that collateral formation can be formed while stabilizing VBADA if changes are slow enough.[28,30]

Open microneurosurgery

Microneurosurgery has come far since the days of C. G. Drake's first experience with basilar tip aneurysms.[31,32] There have been developments in imaging that have given neurovascular surgeons the option to create new revascularizations while perioperatively checking the patency of bypasses and seeing how neural tissue is affected after closure of the artery via brainstem monitoring.[33–36] Microneurosurgeons have learnt to use CFD modeling before surgery, just like interventionists. When VBADA appears to neurosurgeons in practice, there has been progressive development of one or multiple of the abovementioned clinical manifestations. VBADA admitted with bleeding may not be amenable to treatment. The time window to decompress the mass effect while preserving perfusion to the brainstem might have passed. Many experienced neurosurgeons choose endovascular treatment for small saccular posterior circulation aneurysms, but in selected cases VBADA endovascular treatment is not an option due to the compression of cranial nerves and/or the brainstem or simply because there are no endovascular tools that can be used for enlarged dolichoectasia. Excluding the aneurysmatic part of a VBADA while preserving the vital perforators to the brainstem is the only option, although this task is made particularly challenging because all segments are usually aneurysmatic, and there is no obvious neck to be closed from circulation. Some VBADAs have separate and more active pouches that can be excluded from circulation. This can be achieved both with a straight clip strategy and with a protective bypass. Balloon test occlusion (BTO) should be used before surgery to evaluate the ability of collaterals to fill the reduced flow.[33]

Changing the flow The bypass strategy for complex aneurysms is discussed in another part of this update. Here, we go through the concept of microsurgical treatment of VBADAs.

In a classic and honest bypass surgery series by Lawton and colleagues,[36] 37 patients were reported with true VBADA. Twelve of them were treated microneurosurgically immediately, and the rest of the 25 patients were observed. Four of the patients were selected for surgical treatment due to disease progression from initially conservatively treated cases. Patients underwent different flow alteration surgeries, which were analyzed.

Flow reversal in five patients

Extracranial-to-intracranial (superior temporal artery or graft to posterior cerebral artery (PCA) or superior cerebral artery (SCA)) bypasses were used to revascularize posterior circulation while endovascularly both vertebral arteries were occluded in different sites of posterior inferior artery to reverse the blood flow retrogradely in VBADA. All five patients died, one patient died due to an initial hemorrhage.

Moderate flow reduction in three patients

Intracranial-to-intracranial bypasses were implemented using grafts between the vertebral artery and the superior cerebral artery. Flow to VBADA was reduced by occlusion of the dominant VA, but distally, the flow was established via the created bypass. In one case, VA was already occluded, and the subclavian artery was used as a donor. Two patients had progressive aneurysm growth, and both died—one death was treatment related (VA was sacrificed because of aneurysm growth and suffered from VBADA thrombosis) and the second was due to a progressive deficit (aspiration pneumonia). The third patient—the only survivor in the flow reduction group—went through the same bypass reconstruction, but the bleeding side on the upper basilar trunk was clip reconstructed.

Severe flow reduction in eight cases

Intracranial-to-intracranial bypasses were implemented using grafts between the media cerebral artery (MCA) and the PCA. The aim of the bypass procedures was to create an artificial Pcom artery while occluding VBADA outflow. This strategy significantly reduced VBADA outflow while MCA was feeding the upper half of the posterior circulation, and lower BA flow was feeding the brainstem perforators. The initial four patients were suffering from brainstem infarction; clopidogrel was added immediately after bypass to the next four cases. From this group, one patient tolerated the management well. The remaining patients suffered from brainstem infarction, of which one was related to a clipping technique. Severe flow reduction reduced brainstem perforator inflow in most of the cases and caused brainstem infarction in six patients and SCA territory infarction related to clipping in one patient. Only one patient tolerated the treatment intact.

In a combined cohort from Japan and the United States, Nakatomi and colleagues[37] reported a total of 32 patients with symptomatic large and giant VBADA. From this cohort, 11 patients were conservatively treated and 10 died. Nine of the deaths were caused by VBADA, and one patient's

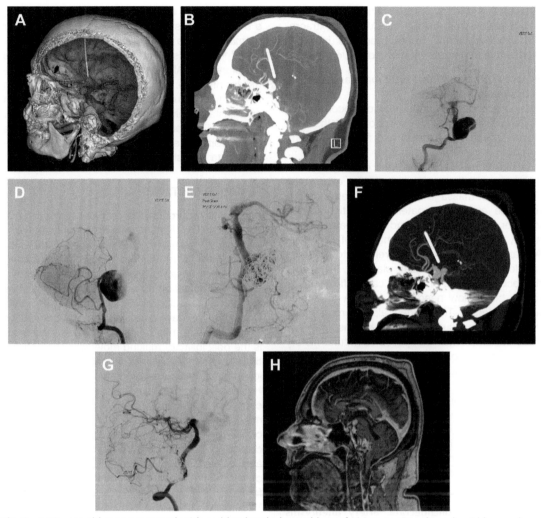

Fig. 3. A 52-year-old man presented with sudden headache and loss of vision. In CT, subarachnoid hemorrhage (SAH) was detected and slowness of VBA perfusion via VBADA (*A, B*). An intraventricular drainage was installed due to acute hydrocephalus related to thrombosis of VBADA and SAH. VBADA had separate aneurysmal sac (*C, D*), which was stent assisted coiled (*E, F*). In short-term follow-up, aneurysmatic sac shrank (*G*) but in the long-term VBADA progressed and enlarged (*H*).

death was associated with atherosclerotic disease.

The treatment methods were divided from the early learning curve of 1980 to the later stages of experience from 2010. Treatment strategies were straight clip construction, proximal parent artery occlusion, remote occlusion of parent artery (endovascular included), and bypass with or without proximal parent artery occlusion.

Straight clip reconstruction in five cases
The same immediate neurologic condition was achieved in two patients; the remaining three patients developed brainstem infarction. Long-term mortality was 80% and morbidity 60% for this group.

Proximal parent artery occlusion in seven cases from which six also received a bypass
Five patients suffered from brainstem infarctions, and two of them died immediately. At the last check, follow-up mortality was 57.1% and morbidity 85.7%. It is noteworthy that in this cohort, one patient had only unilateral VA occlusion because of patient refusal, and this case was lost to follow-up.

Remote occlusion of the parent artery (endovascular included) in six cases from which three also received a bypass
Four patients showed aneurysm shrinkage, with good outcomes. Two patients suffered from brainstem hemorrhage, and one recovered in follow-up.

Interestingly, five out of six patients developed collateral flow from extracranial VA and extracranial external carotid artery branches into BA. Morbidity and mortality in this group were 50%.

Bypass with or without proximal parent artery occlusion in three cases

Two patients suffered from SAH; one occurred the day after surgery and the second 6 months later. Neither of the two patients had favorable Pcom, and both were advanced in age.

In the series of Nakatomi and colleagues, flow attenuation pathway is not clearly expressed. The relevant message of this series relies on patient age and Pcom patency; if patients were younger than 45 year old and had a patent Pcom artery, they had the best chance of surviving. Age and Pcom diameter is in relation to collateral development and vascular plasticity. How well the reconstructions of VBADA can shift in relation to the blood flow need from VBADA to Pcoms and collaterals. This series also demonstrated that microneurosurgical interventions can be more effective when compared to natural history in the selected cohort.

We learned that sudden changes in flow through VBADA are highly thrombogenic (**Fig. 4**). Vascular plasticity and collateral formation might help to stylize VBADA, especially if benign hemodynamic changes happen slowly enough in younger patients.[36–38] There is a possibility that even through thrombus, endothelized pathways to brainstem perforators can develop.

Cranial nerve palsy and microdecompression of vertebrobasilar dolichoectatic artery aneurysms

The tortuous effect of dolichoectasia might lead to cranial nerve palsy. Tortuous BA is more often involved with a single isolated cranial nerve deficit, whereas with an extension of BA diameter multiple cranial nerves can be affected.[1,39] Similar to Janetta's microvascular decompression, there have been reports on macrovascular decompression of the brainstem and cranial nerves while transpositioning the vertebrobasilar artery. If the VBADA has reached a significant mass, its movement is dangerous and can lead to perforator injury and thromboembolic stroke when the hemodynamics are changed. The descriptions are from a small case series and only in a few high-volume cerebrovascular centers with dedicated neurovascular experts who systematically managed VBADA transposition safely. There has been a report on rerouting dolichoectasia via a binder ring bypass for macrovascular decompression.[40]

Hydrocephalus If the VBADA rises high enough, it reaches the third ventricle, inducing disruption in CSF circulation. Some patients might benefit from a shunt whereas others have no changes in their *normal pressure hydrocephalus* statuslike condition.[41,42] There is a fear that a shunt might induce a rupture of VBADA due to a reduction of intraventricular pressure. One common practice has been to insert the shunt before VBADA treatment with an adjustable valve while keeping the valve closed. After VBADA treatment or without treatment, the valve is opened slowly. There is currently no significant data published on the matter.

FUTURE DIRECTIONS

We should approach the problem along several pathways. The first step is to identify patients who are at risk of developing malignant IADE toward VBADA at an early stage. Some fascinating biomarkers have been proposed that require further investigation as does the role of thrombus in the progression and stabilization of VBADAs.[37,43] We have already been introduced to liquid biopsy from intraluminal VBADAs, and there is the possibility of making molecular characteristics to define VBADAs not only based on radiological parameters but also on etiologic background. Heterogenous VBADA still lacks definition, and the course of progression needs to be defined. Treatment options are limited, and the pathophysiology of VBADA should be taken into account when designing treatment both with microneurosurgery and with endovascular procedures. Identification of vascular plasticity and induction of collateral formation might bring hope to VBADA treatment. Perhaps we should ignore the VBADA itself and try to remember the role of the BA. Can we induce the growth of collaterals so that we do not need the diseased segment?

The current state-of-the-art bypasses and flow diverters were not seen as possible in the early days of microneurosurgery and interventional neuroradiology, so there will certainly be more development in both microneurosurgery and endovascular treatments for the treatment of VBADA.

SUMMARY

An aging population may bring with it the evolving problem of intracranial dolichoectasia and its vertebrobasilar dolichoectasia subgroup, which is the most challenging to treat. Little is known about VBADAs, and we continue to lack knowledge of their natural history, prognosis, pathophysiology, and prevalence of disease. Specifically, we are limited by the definition of early-stage VBADA and IADE partially because of interphysician

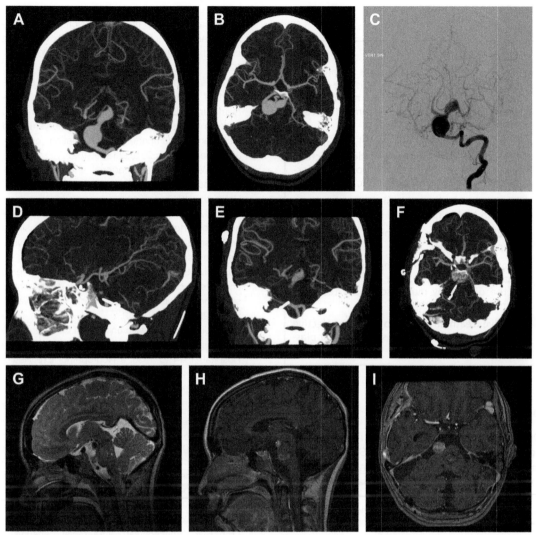

Fig. 4. A 14-year-old patient with previously diagnosed and treated right side internal carotid aneurysm by endovascular closure of ICA and STA-MCA bypass in another center. STA-MCA bypass was not patent after ICA closure and VBA was feeding the anterior circulation in significant amount. In follow-up, the patient presented with VBADA and oculomotor paresis (*A–C*). Symptoms and aneurysm progressed in 3 years of follow-up, and it was decided for microneurosurgical treatment of VBADA. Right side VA-MCA via radial artery graft was performed and STA-MCA was redone. BA was proximally closed (*D–F*). Flow changed happened rapidly and unfortunately BA thrombosed and patient suffered from brainstem infarction (*G–I*).

variability in identifying risk cases that need to be closely monitored. There are methods to reduce stroke risk when a VBADA still has a benign course, but a BA diameter of 4.5 mm is reached, the VBADA becomes risky. Cranial nerve palsy occurs with laterality of dolichoectasia and enlargement of the VBADA will naturally have an impact on the brainstem. The risk of rupture increases with the size of the BA. Endovascular procedures and microneurosurgery can be effective compared with natural history, but case selection should be made carefully. Sudden hemodynamic changes should be avoided, and if needed, complex bypasses should be used for treatment of VBADA. Treatment is most effective when given in the early stages of the disease prognosis and at a younger age when vascular plasticity is still impactful to hemodynamic changes. Therefore, there is a need for new, surgical, endovascular, and biological means to stop this ominous disease.

CLINICS CARE POINTS

- Clinicians should look for signs of high-risk patients in the early stages of disease (basilar artery diameter more than 4.3 mm is at risk for stroke, and diameter 10 mm or more is at risk for rupture).

- Clinicians should recognize the potential causes behind vertebrobasilar dolichoectatic artery aneurysm formation, if possible (infection, immunologic, or metabolic diseases).

- Cranial nerve decompression can be done safely in highly specialized centers.

- Sudden changes in flow might lead to catastrophic outcomes.

- Invasive (endovascular or microneurosurgery) treatment should be given at the early stage of the disease by multidisciplinary teams at highly specialized centers.

- Invasive treatment seems to be more effective for younger patients because of vascular plasticity.

DISCLOSURE

Dr B.Rezai Jahromi owns patents and is a shareholder and founder of *Helsinki Surgical Instruments* company which innovates new treatments for vertebrobasilar dolichoectasia and other neurovascular disorders. Drs M. Niemelä and B.Rezai Jahromi have patents pending regarding aneurysm imaging.

REFERENCES

1. Smoker WR, Corbett JJ, Gentry LR, et al. High-resolution computed tomography of the basilar artery: 2. Vertebrobasilar dolichoectasia: clinical-pathologic correlation and review. Am J Neuroradiol 1986; 7(1):61–72.

2. Pico F, Labreuche J, Amarenco P. Pathophysiology, presentation, prognosis, and management of intracranial arterial dolichoectasia. Lancet Neurol 2015; 14(8):833–45.

3. Pico F, Labreuche J, Hauw JJ, et al. Coronary and basilar artery ectasia are associated: results from an autopsy case–control study. Stroke 2016;47(1):224–7.

4. Gutierrez J, Sacco RL, Wright CB. Dolichoectasia—an evolving arterial disease. Nat Rev Neurol 2011; 7(1):41–50.

5. Yu YL, Moseley IF, Pullicino P, et al. The clinical picture of ectasia of the intracerebral arteries. J Neurol Neurosurg Psychiatry 1982;45(1):29–36.

6. Ubogu EE, Zaidat OO. Vertebrobasilar dolichoectasia diagnosed by magnetic resonance angiography and risk of stroke and death: a cohort study. J Neurol Neurosurg Psychiatry 2004;75(1): 22–6.

7. Kurtelius A, Väntti N, Rezai Jahromi B, et al. Association of intracranial aneurysms with aortic aneurysms in 125 patients with fusiform and 4253 patients with saccular intracranial aneurysms and their family members and population controls. J Am Heart Assoc 2019;8(18):e013277.

8. Dandy WE. Intracranial arterial aneurysms. Comstock publishing company. Incorporated, Cornell University; 1947.

9. Nasr DM, Flemming KD, Lanzino G, et al. Natural history of vertebrobasilar dolichoectatic and fusiform aneurysms: a systematic review and meta-analysis. Cerebrovasc Dis 2018;45(1–2):68–77.

10. Nasr DM, Brinjikji W, Rouchaud A, et al. Imaging characteristics of growing and ruptured vertebrobasilar non-saccular and dolichoectatic aneurysms. Stroke 2016;47(1):106–12.

11. Em H, JL P. A systematic analysis of intracranial aneurysms from the autopsy file of the Presbyterian Hospital, 1914 to 1956. J Neuropathol Exp Neurol 1958;17(3):409–23.

12. Ikeda K, Nakamura Y, Hirayama T, et al. Cardiovascular risk and neuroradiological profiles in asymptomatic vertebrobasilar dolichoectasia. Cerebrovasc Dis 2010;30(1):23–8.

13. Yin K, Liang S, Tang X, et al. The relationship between intracranial arterial dolichoectasia and intracranial atherosclerosis. Clin Neurol Neurosurg 2021;200:106408.

14. Flemming KD, Wiebers DO, Brown RD, et al. Prospective risk of hemorrhage in patients with vertebrobasilar nonsaccular intracranial aneurysm. J Neurosurg 2004;101(1):82–7.

15. Flemming KD, Wiebers DO, Brown RD Jr, et al. The natural history of radiographically defined vertebrobasilar nonsaccular intracranial aneurysms. Cerebrovasc Dis 2005;20(4):270–9.

16. Nakatomi H, Segawa H, Kurata A, et al. Clinicopathological study of intracranial fusiform and dolichoectatic aneurysms: insight on the mechanism of growth. Stroke 2000;31(4):896–900.

17. Narsinh KH, Narsinh K, McCoy DB, et al. Endovascular Biopsy of Vertebrobasilar Aneurysm in Patient With Polyarteritis Nodosa. Front Neurol 2021;12: 697105.

18. Rezai Jahromi B, Valori M, Tulamo, et al. (2021). Cancer-Type Somatic Mutations in Saccular Cerebral Aneurysms.

19. Karasozen Y, Osbun JW, Parada CA, et al. Somatic PDGFRB activating variants in fusiform cerebral aneurysms. Am J Hum Genet 2019;104(5): 968–76.

20. de Kok-Mercado F, Habib M, Phelps T, et al. Adaptations of the owl's cervical & cephalic arteries in relation to extreme neck rotation. Science 2013; 339(6119):514.

21. Muskat JC, Rayz VL, Goergen CJ, et al. Hemodynamic modeling of the circle of Willis reveals unanticipated functions during cardiovascular stress. J Appl Physiol 2021;131(3):1020–34.

22. Tanaka M, Sakaguchi M, Miwa K, et al. Basilar artery diameter is an independent predictor of incident cardiovascular events. Arterioscler Thromb Vasc Biol 2013;33(9):2240–4.

23. Mizutani T. A fatal, chronically growing basilar artery: a new type of dissecting aneurysm. J Neurosurg 1996;84(6):962–71.

24. Siddiqui AH, Abla AA, Kan P, et al. Panacea or problem: flow diverters in the treatment of symptomatic large or giant fusiform vertebrobasilar aneurysms. J Neurosurg 2012;116(6):1258–66.

25. Natarajan SK, Lin N, Sonig A, et al. The safety of Pipeline flow diversion in fusiform vertebrobasilar aneurysms: a consecutive case series with longer-term follow-up from a single US center. J Neurosurg 2016;125(1):111–9.

26. Bhogal P, Pérez MA, Ganslandt O, et al. Treatment of posterior circulation non-saccular aneurysms with flow diverters: a single-center experience and review of 56 patients. J NeuroInterv Surg 2017;9(5): 471–81.

27. Wang J, Jia L, Yang X, et al. Outcomes in symptomatic patients with vertebrobasilar dolichoectasia following endovascular treatment. Front Neurol 2019;10:610.

28. Dobrocky T, Piechowiak El, Goldberg J, et al. Absence of pontine perforators in vertebrobasilar dolichoectasia on ultra-high resolution cone-beam computed tomography. J Neurointerv Surg 2021; 13(6):580–4.

29. Saalfeld S, Stahl J, Korte J., et al Can Endovascular Treatment of Fusiform Intracranial Aneurysms Restore the Healthy Hemodynamic Environment?-A Virtual Pilot Study. Front Neurol, 12.

30. Jahromi BR, Hirvela V, Sarpaneva S, et al. Device for applying external pressure on a surface of an anatomical object. U.S. Patent 11,266,419.

31. Drake CG. Bleeding aneurysms of the basilar artery: direct surgical management in four cases. J Neurosurg 1961;18(2):230–8.

32. Drake CG, Peerless SJ. Giant fusiform intracranial aneurysms: review of 120 patients treated surgically from 1965 to 1992. J Neurosurg 1997;87(2):141–62.

33. Kalani MYS, Ramey W, Albuquerque FC, et al. Revascularization and aneurysm surgery: techniques, indications, and outcomes in the endovascular era. Neurosurgery 2014;74(5):482–98.

34. Anson JA, Lawton MT, Spetzler RF. Characteristics and surgical treatment of dolichoectatic and fusiform aneurysms. J Neurosurg 1996;84(2):185–93.

35. Tjahjadi M, Kivelev J, Serrone JC, et al. Factors determining surgical approaches to basilar bifurcation aneurysms and its surgical outcomes. Neurosurgery 2016;78(2):181–91.

36. Lawton MT, Abla AA, Rutledge WC, et al. Bypass surgery for the treatment of dolichoectatic basilar trunk aneurysms: a work in progress. Neurosurgery 2016;79(1):83–99.

37. Nakatomi H, Kiyofuji S, Ono H, et al. Giant fusiform and dolichoectatic aneurysms of the basilar trunk and vertebrobasilar junction—clinicopathological and surgical outcome. Neurosurgery 2021;88(1): 82–95.

38. Jahromi BR, Frösen J, Hernesniemi J. Commentary: bypass surgery for the treatment of dolichoectatic basilar trunk aneurysms: a work in progress. Neurosurgery 2016;79(3):E514–6.

39. Choudhri O, Connolly ID, Lawton MT. Macrovascular decompression of the brainstem and cranial nerves: evolution of an anteromedial vertebrobasilar artery transposition technique. Neurosurgery 2017;81(2): 367–76.

40. Srinivasan VM, Labib MA, Furey CG, Catapano JS, Lawton MT. The "Binder Ring" Bypass: transection, rerouting, and reanastomosis as an alternative to macrovascular decompression of a dolichoectatic vertebral artery. Oper Neurosurg 2022;22(4): 224–30.

41. Zisimopoulou V, Ntouniadaki A, Aggelidakis P, et al. Vertebrobasilar dolichoectasia induced hydrocephalus: the water-hammer effect. Clin Pract 2015; 5(2):47–9.

42. Çelik O, Berkman ZM, Orakdöğen M, et al. Obstructive hydrocephalus due to vertebrobasilar dolichoectasia: diagnostic and therapeutic considerations. J Neurol Surg A Cent Eur Neurosurg 2013;74(S 01):e4–8.

43. Liu Y, Zhu J, Deng X, et al. Serum level of lipoprotein-associated phospholipase A2 is a potential biomarker of vertebrobasilar dolichoectasia and its progression to cerebral infarction. Neurol Sci 2021;42(2):599–605.

Biology and Hemodynamics of Aneurysm Rupture

Casey A. Chitwood, PhD[a,1], Elizabeth D. Shih, BS[a,1], Omid Amili, PhD[b],
Anthony S. Larson, MD[c], Brenda M. Ogle, PhD[a,d], Patrick W. Alford, PhD[a],
Andrew W. Grande, MD[c,d,*]

KEYWORDS

• Intracranial aneurysms • Hemodynamics • Biology • Mechanics • Rupture • Predictive modeling

KEY POINTS

• This is a review of the current state of research in predicting an intracranial aneurysm rupture. Research is summarized into hemodynamics, biology, and tissue/cell mechanics, which contribute to aneurysm stability and rupture. Investigators identify the most pressing needs in each field toward developing a predictive model of rupture with clinical translatability.

• Recent studies on aneurysms would suggest that aneurysm size aand shape alone are not sufficient for predicting growth and rupture.

• Hemodynamics influence aneurysm wall cellular changes which can lead to aneurysm growth.

• Cellular changes in the wall of cerebral aneurysms can either lead to growth and rupture or stabilization. Understanding these is important for aneurysm treatment.

• Future predictive models of aneurysm should incorporate aneurysm hemodynamics, cellular processes and tissue mechanics.

INTRODUCTION

What leads to aneurysm rupture versus stabilization is a question that has perplexed researchers for decades, the answer would unquestionably influence how aneurysms are selected for intervention versus observation. Factually, the risk of intracranial aneurysm (IA) rupture was based primarily on aneurysm size and patient-specific factors such as hypertension, gender, or family history.[1,2] Although these factors continue to be used when determining rupture risk, statistics suggest that their presence is weakly correlated with the actual rupture.[3] Consequently, some IAs undergo intervention when the actual risk of rupture is low, while others are observed when they are at high risk. Although risk assessment does include factors addressed in risk score calculations (ie, PHASES criteria), they are not universally accepted in the clinic.[1] An aneurysm size is still the key factor assessed for determining rupture risk, where aneurysms ≥ 7 mm in the maximal dimension are treated with surgical or endovascular techniques.[4] More sophisticated, "aneurysm-specific" risk factor assessments may appropriately guide intervention decisions.

Recently, there has been emphasis in identifying advanced methods of determining an aneurysm-specific risk for rupture based on evolving research

[a] Department of Biomedical Engineering, University of Minnesota Twin Cities, 312 Church St. SE, 7-105 Nils Hasselmo Hall, Minneapolis, MN 55455, USA; [b] Mechanical, Industrial, and Manufacturing Engineering, The University of Toledo, 2801 Bancroft St, Toledo, OH 43606, USA; [c] Department of Neurosurgery, University of Minnesota Twin Cities, MMC 96, Room D-429 Mayo Memorial Building, 420 Delaware St. SE, Minneapolis, MN 55455, USA; [d] Stem Cell Institute, McGuire Translational Research Facility, 2001 6th Street SE, Mail Code 2873, Minneapolis, MN 55455, USA

[1] Equal contribution.

* Corresponding author. Department of Neurosurgery, 420 Delaware street SE, MMC96, D429 Mayo Memorial Building, Minneapolis, MN 55455.

E-mail address: grande@umn.edu

Neurosurg Clin N Am 33 (2022) 431–441
https://doi.org/10.1016/j.nec.2022.06.002
1042-3680/22/© 2022 Elsevier Inc. All rights reserved.

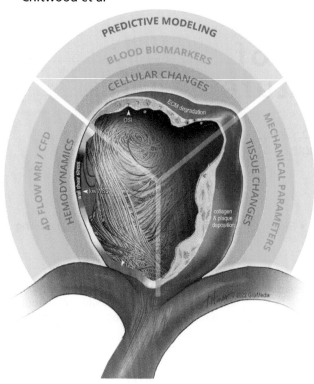

Fig. 1. Overview of the three evolving research domains (*orange*) to understand IA rupture: hemodynamics that influences IA lumen, cellular changes resulting in inflammation and tissue degradation, and the tissue mechanical stability from ECM remodeling. Future therapies (*green*) built on these research areas inform patient-specific risk of rupture: 4D MR imaging, blood biomarkers, and mechanical parameters influence a clinically accurate predictive modeling tool (*blue*) for neurosurgeons to guide that IAs to treat. (Published with permission from Glia Media.)

in aberrant biology, hemodynamics, and tissue mechanics. IA pathobiology is separated into three distinct phases: initiation, growth, and rupture. However, a comprehensive picture of the interplay in hemodynamics, biochemical pathways, and tissue remodeling between these phases is yet to be drawn.

To identify new metrics for improved predictions of rupture, we require a thorough understanding of the molecular and cellular biology of vascular remodeling, the interplay with hemodynamics within the IA sac, and the changes in mechanical properties of the IA wall leading to rupture (**Fig. 1**). Thus, we review advances being made in the fields of biological assessment, complex fluid mechanics, and tissue mechanics in relation to metrics for predicting rupture. We discuss how single metrics do not consider the true complexity of IAs and discuss multiple pathways to identify a clinical tool that considers the true complexity of aneurysm progression to predict rupture. We also propose how novel predictive modeling using hemodynamics and biomarkers could transform future IA treatment and pinpoint current gaps standing between present research and clinical implementation.

FLUID DYNAMICS IN INTRACRANIAL ANEURYSMS

Hemodynamics has been considered a crucial factor in aneurysm progression for decades, but rigorous analyses of these properties are rarely clinically employed. One of the first proposed causes of aneurysm was the weakening of the wall of an artery caused by laceration, inflammation, or increased strain on the artery.[5] It was suggested that rupture was caused by an inability to maintain structural integrity against blood pressure; thus, rupture was linked to aspects of blood flow and hemodynamic stresses. Early hemodynamics studies addressed factors such as turbulence and dilation of the vessel wall, followed by wall shear stress (WSS) as a potential important factor in lesion development.[6–8] Approximately 500 publications on aneurysm hemodynamics are released every year. With decades of study and thousands of publications on the hemodynamics of aneurysm, it is surprising that these findings have not become clinical diagnostic tool. In other vascular diseases such as coronary artery disease, applications such as CT-flow are Food and Drug Administration-approved platforms that incorporate hemodynamic simulations in clinical practice.[9] However, IAs are inherently multi-factored and much more complex, highlighting the need for inclusive metrics. There is also controversy over what exact hemodynamic factors contribute to IA rupture, suggesting that a single metric approach that ignores biological complexity is insufficient.

COMPUTATIONAL FLUID DYNAMICS FOR STUDYING INTRACRANIAL ANEURYSMS

The common method for characterizing vascular hemodynamics is computational fluid dynamics (CFD). Laboratories use either commercially available software (eg, Fluent, COMSOL, ABAQUS), open-source platform (eg, SimVascular, FeniCS, OpenFOAM), or in-house developed program to solve flow governing equations to investigate the blood velocity field and associated derivative quantities such as WSS. To perform robust simulations, a well-defined vascular geometry, and an appropriate boundary conditions are required. This includes determination of several variables such as blood viscosity, density, flow rate, and pressure distribution at different branches. The results of numerical simulations are sensitive to the imposed inputs or the implemented numerical methods (**Fig. 2**). In addition, three-dimensional geometries are limited by the resolution of current imaging modalities such as magnetic resonance angiography and computed tomography angiography. As such, there are inconsistencies or contradicting data leading to different conclusions in the literature.[10–13] For example, studies suggest that high WSS is correlated to areas of rupture whereas many suggest the opposite.[14,15] As both may be true in different circumstances, more inclusive metrics are required to characterize and correlate what those variables so as to use hemodynamic patterns as predictive measures in the clinic.

CFD provides useful insights despite disagreements in the literature. Researchers preliminarily identified parameters that may assist in the creation of a diagnostic tool, such as instantaneous WSS, time-averaged WSS, oscillatory shear index (OSI), number of vortices, relative residence time, and flow impinging zones.[16] Recently, there is an increased agreement that oscillations in WSS, calculated as an OSI, are correlated with growth and rupture, as opposed to solely high or low WSS.[16–18] With advancements in machine learning techniques and physics-informed neural networks, there is growing potential of artificial intelligence (AI) in detecting IAs and assessing rupture risk using preclinical images and CFD measurements.[16,19,20]

CELL-SPECIFIC CONTRIBUTIONS IN INTRACRANIAL ANEURYSM GROWTH AND RUPTURE

Aberrant flow is linked to IA formation and other vascular maladies; thus, the effects of flow on cells in the vascular wall has been vastly explored

(**Fig. 3**). Endothelial cell (EC) activation caused by hemodynamic forces, including but not limited to low, high, and oscillatory WSS, have been characterized by morphologic changes and expression of transcriptional regulators, surface markers, and cytokines. In many studies, upregulation of Vascular cell adhesion protein-1 (VCAM-1), Intercelllular cell adhesion molecule-1 (ICAM-1), E-selectin, P-selectin, and Monocyte chemoattractant protein-1 (MCP-1) that provide anchors for immune infiltration, are observed. Immune cells, including mast cells, macrophages, and neutrophils are significant contributors to IA progression.[21–23] Signaling molecules produced by mast cells including Tumor necrosis factor (TNF)-α, Interlueken (IL)-1β, and IL-6 further bolster immune-associated signaling pathways.[21] In addition, mast cells also produce TGF-β, IL-3, IL-4, IL-8, and IL-13 in granules, and degranulation of the mast cells has been linked to IA formation and rupture.[21,24] Rupture has also been linked to both M1 macrophages outnumbering M2 macrophages,[22] and neutrophil accumulation.[23]

Hemodynamic forces, activated ECs, and immune cells induce smooth muscle cells (SMCs) in the IA wall to switch from a less contractile to more proliferative phenotype. This phenotypic switch in SMCs increases expression of MCP-1, VCAM-1, IL-1, and matrix metalloproteinases (MMPs), reinforcing the responses from ECs and immune cells.[25,26] SMCs undergo different responses depending on the level of activation. Certain levels induce SMC apoptosis or extreme proliferation, resulting in myointimal hyperplasia.[4] Different activation levels result in different regions of the IA having thin or thick walls. Thin-walled regions are likely more susceptible to rupture whereas thick-walled regions act like stiff plaques.[27] Thus, it is important to elucidate the different inflammatory pathways and corresponding key proteins that potentially arise from hemodynamic stimuli, as these mechanisms are integral to IA stabilization or rupture. Although the list of infiltrating cells and signaling molecules is not actually complete, this shows the biological complexity of the phenomena within the IA wall in response to hemodynamic changes, and the subsequent potential in blood biomarkers to better evaluate rupture risk.

IDENTIFYING BIOMARKERS FOR INTRACRANIAL ANEURYSM RUPTURE

Cell products associated with IA progression can be measured but are not currently clinically used. There is considerable potential in the use of biomarkers from blood draws for risk evaluation with

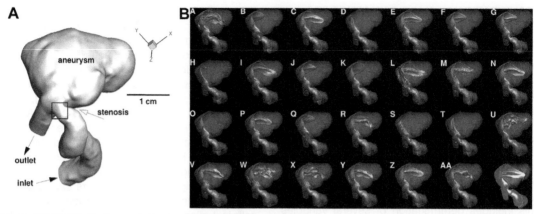

Fig. 2. ASME CFD Challenge. Left: Aneurysm model geometry distributed to challenge participants. Right: Phase I, pulsatile-2 peak systolic (PK2) velocities. Shown are isosurfaces of velocity magnitude at 50 cm/s. Results of the challenge clearly and considerably vary between groups. (*From* Steinman DA, Hoi Y, Fahy P, et al. Variability of computational fluid dynamics solutions for pressure and flow in a giant aneurysm: the ASME 2012 Summer Bioengineering Conference CFD Challenge. J Biomech Eng. 2013;135(2):021016.)

further research. Earlier animal studies to identify biomarkers have investigated proteins of interest in IA rupture such as MMP-2, MMP-9, thrombospondin type 1 domain-containing protein-1, and prostaglandin E2.[28–31] These studies may also test drugs and inhibitors that influence a protein's likeliness to cause rupture. A recent study showed that delivery of increasing dose of Blood pressure

(BP)-1-102, a Signal transducer and activator of transcription3 (STAT3) inhibitor, decreased the incidence of IA rupture in a dose-dependent manner.[32] Challenges with these studies include the evaluation of limited molecules within a system that encompasses multiple signaling pathways including the Janus Kinase (JAK)/STAT3/Nuclear factor Kappa B (NF-κB), HIPPO, and Rho-

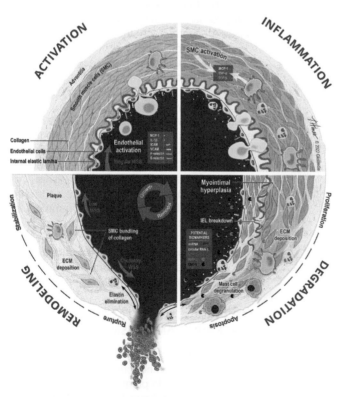

Fig. 3. Aneurysm initiation and growth and remodeling cycles begin with cell activation, most likely due to changes in hemodynamic forces, followed by immune infiltration, tissue degradation, and remodeling. Four phases of intracranial arterial wall are illustrated. Top left: Endothelial activation leads to the upregulation of surface markers responsible for immune attachment and infiltration. Top right: Endothelial and immune cell signaling results in SMC activation where SMCs switch to a less contractile phenotype, whereas upregulated cytokines continue to recruit immune cells. Immune cells and SMCs start producing MMPs and other various cytokines. Bottom right: MMPs degrade both collagen and elastin while cytokine signaling may result in either SMC hyperplasia or apoptosis. This results in some areas of the artery wall thickening or thinning, respectively. Bottom left: Remaining SMCs attempt to stabilize local microenvironment through collagen remodeling. Failure of stabilization at the tissue-scale will result in rupture. (Published with permission from Glia Media.)

associated protein kinase (RhoA)/Rho-associated kinase (ROCK) pathways.[4,28,32–34] Furthermore, specific translatable proteins have not yet been identified as potential clinical biomarkers for IA rupture.

Recently, genomic, transcriptomic, and proteomic studies have begun to garner interest. Transcriptomic studies have reiterated the importance of IL-1(α and β), TNF, and IL-6 to differentiate unruptured and ruptured IAs.[24] Hierarchical clustering of RNA sequencing from unruptured and ruptured IAs has led to the identification of "rupture-like" unruptured IAs. When comparing this group to control unruptured IAs, expression of BCAT1, DSC2, and GALNT6 were upregulated whereas MTRNR2L1 was downregulated in the "rupture-like" group.[24] As the former markers are associated with cell turnover, cell death, and tissue remodeling, they are excellent candidates for identifying IAs with a greater risk of rupture. Their presence suggests that the IA was maladapting toward rupture at the time of collection. Pathway analysis further revealed enrichment of lysosome pathways, cytokine–receptor interactions and toll-like receptor signaling in ruptured versus unruptured IAs.[35,36] In addition, several small micro RNAs (miRNAs) may also serve as potential biomarkers. A promising miRNA metric is downregulation of miRNA-21, which is indicative of loss of vascular protection.[37] Downregulation of miR-513b-5p has been linked to rupture as this results in increased production of COL1A1 and COL1A2.[38] Circular RNAs, including hsa_circ_0005505 and circ_0001947, were found to be more highly expressed whereas circ_0008433 and circ_0001946 showed decreased expression in ruptured IAs.[39,40] Proteomic studies have also focused on identifying biomarkers such as MMP9 and ORM1 for IAs.[41] MMP9 and ORM1 have been linked to the presence of IAs, although these studies have been less successful in identifying those linked directly to the rupture.[41] The plethora of such studies demonstrates the abundance of detectable proteins that might indicate rupture risk with the refinement of corresponding clinical assays. When appropriate biomarkers have been identified, microarray systems can be developed to help determine a patient-specific risk of rupture.

EXTRACELLULAR MATRIX REMODELING ON INTRACRANIAL ANEURYSM MECHANICS

The upstream pathways described above influence IA mechanics, which are primarily governed by fibrous proteins in the extracellular matrix (ECM) and contractile SMCs. Cells actively remodel their ECM by degrading and depositing fibers to suit external loads to combat fatigue and failure in healthy states. This is also observed in maladaptive remodeling that contributes to IA development and rupture. Healthy arteries are structurally organized to maintain mechanical integrity. ECM proteins, primarily collagen and elastin, exist in conjunction to provide structural robustness to tensile loads while providing necessary elasticity. Although SMC-secreted MMPs play a crucial role in ECM remodeling, not all contribute to IA formation and long-term studies on rupture have yet to be performed.[29,42] Aside from degradation, disorientation of newly synthesized ECM proteins, such as changes in fiber alignment, crimping, or bundling play a role in mechanical instability and rupture. The activated SMCs and fibroblasts contribute to the majority of collagen deposition within the IA sac when exposed to TNF-α or TGF-β.[4] Etminan and colleagues have shown that there are large levels of newly deposited collagen in IAs.[43] Other investigations implicate hemodynamic properties in ECM remodeling, suggesting that high collagen turnover is associated with areas of high WSS and low turnover with areas of low WSS.[44]

Deposition and degradation of different fiber constituents evolve over time at different rates, resulting in either the IA maintaining its volume (homeostasis), exhibiting a net growth, or a net atrophy. These outcomes affect IA morphology and mechanics, ultimately leading to stabilization or rupture. Deposition and degradation occur in response to mechanical stimuli through a process known as growth and remodeling (G&R).[45,46] G&R of an IA influences regional geometries, hemodynamics, and tensile wall stress.[47] These in turn result in further biological mechanisms and IA G&R, creating a feedback loop of complex multiscale phenomena governing stabilization or rupture. On the microscale, the phenotypic changes of SMCs[48] and immune infiltration[4] continue to influence ECM reorganization and degradation, and the changing morphology and hemodynamics lead to spatially variant microstructure and G&R throughout the aneurysm.

EXPERIMENTAL CHARACTERIZATION OF THE MECHANICAL PROPERTIES OF INTRACRANIAL ANEURYSMS

Collagen, elastin, and SMCs contribute to tissue stiffness, elasticity, and contractility. Fatigue, damage, and failure are reflected in changes in tissue mechanics due to structural and compositional alterations[49]; thus, the rupture of IAs can be modeled

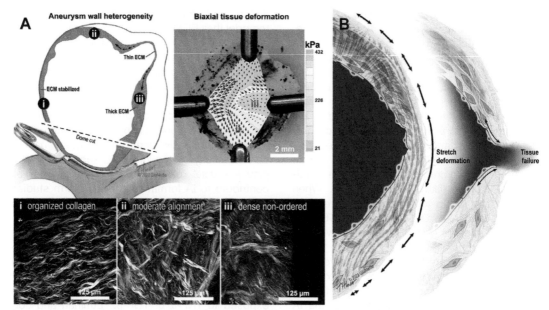

Fig. 4. Mechanics of aneurysm wall remodeling. (*A*) SMCs deposit/degrade fibers to return to a target homeostatic stress. In a cell-sparse aneurysm, in which ECM can only be regulated around the remaining cells, the tissue is likely to be mechanically heterogeneous. To examine aneurysm mechanics, the tissue is removed during clipping surgery and placed into a biaxial stretcher for mechanical characterization. Heterogeneous stiffnesses have been found in sample aneurysms. To examine structural changes in the ECM, the tissue is imaged via multiphoton imaging to examine how collagen structure varies across different regions (i–iii). This is a result from cell G&R and contributes to heterogeneous mechanical properties. (*B*) Cell-mediated G&R and heterogeneous material properties result in aneurysm stabilization or rupture. (Published with permission from Glia Media.)

as a mechanical problem. The G&R of the SMCs and the surrounding ECM in an IA results in a spatially mechanically heterogeneous aneurysm,[50] which is hypothesized to be a considerable factor influencing the failure strength of the tissue. As such, it is necessary to fully characterize stable and ruptured IA wall mechanics for accurate multiphysics simulations for risk diagnoses (**Fig. 4**).

Studies have shown that aneurysm mechanics and microstructure are different from healthy arteries, vary significantly from one aneurysm to another, and are heterogeneous within a single specimen. Constitutive models describe the mechanical properties of a material by relating an applied force to the material deformation. These models have been developed to describe phenomenological and structural properties of aneurysms in detail and implemented into CFD and fluid-structure interaction (FSI) simulations.[51,52]

Owing to their small size and rarity of samples, much of the work conducted on IAs lies in single-axis stretching tests, which provide unique data on the tissue mechanics but cannot fully capture physiologic multi-axis complex behavior.[53,54] From these tests, it is possible to determine preliminary mechanical parameters; however, more complex multi-axis tests are required for improved constitutive modeling. There have been experiments involving cyclic inflation of IAs, which more closely reflect in vivo deformation.[55] Another study records a small number of planar biaxial tests on IAs, but the test size was not sufficient to fully inform subsequent simulations.[54] The current state of experimental reports on IAs suggests that a more detailed study is necessary to pinpoint what mechanical properties (fiber and SMC density, elasticity, etc.) differentiate stable IAs from IAs that rupture. In recent years, there have been considerable efforts that not only capture the multi-axial behavior of human IAs,[56] but also to detect spatial heterogeneity of the regional stiffnesses and fiber organization not otherwise seen in healthy arteries.[50] This marks the identification of a potential new metric—degree of heterogeneity—to be incorporated into simulations to evaluate its effect on mechanical behavior and rupture risk.

MODELING INTRACRANIAL ANEURYSM RUPTURE RISK

The evolving hemodynamics influence extracellular activation of the IA lumen that initiates immune infiltration and SMC activation that remodels the ECM and weakens the IA toward

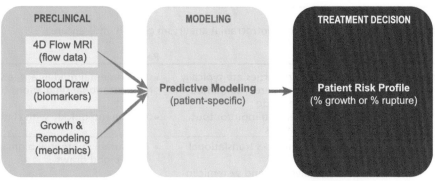

Fig. 5. Summary of the ultimate modeling tool that surgeons can use to evaluate risk.

rupture. Theoretic growth laws estimate how microscale constituents regulate tissue-scale growth to return to a homeostatic stress.[45,57] Mixture theory is a frequent approach to growth models; here, an IA is described as a mixture of collagen, elastin, and smooth muscle. This continuum approach allows the IA simulations to be computationally inexpensive. Deposition and degradation of different fiber constituents evolve over time and influence IA geometry and stresses. Results from these models are compared against clinical and experimental data, so a biologically informed and empirically justified mathematical model holds translational potential in tying experimental findings to predictive laws.[58,59] Many computational models have been proposed to predict future growth of IAs, but current models are not yet accurate enough for clinical use.

Although a clinically relevant, robust, and accurate model that can predict patient-specific rupture has yet to be developed, key factors in IA growth have preliminarily been identified.[60] Sensitivity analyses pinpoint the most important parameters in mathematical models of aneurysm to focus on in future efforts.[61] However, determining such values in specific patients remains a challenge until links to measurable biomarkers are found. The evolution of imaging modalities is integral to other metrics such as IA geometry, thickness, and flow pattern. These concerns reiterate the necessity of further multiphysical aneurysm rupture research.

In the past, computational models have made assumptions on various parameters, especially IA material properties, due to the rarity of experimental data, though these values are critical for accurate simulations of IA mechanics.[62] With continued research, predictive models to evaluate rupture risk and determine treatment are well-positioned to transform clinical care. G&R is now implemented into computational models of patient-specific IAs to evaluate longitudinal growth.[63–65] The recent literature incorporates

the influence of cellular and molecular processes on tissue scale behavior. This is now an overarching hypothesis that mechanical forces and mechanical equilibrium drive IA adaptation through biological pathways.

AI has been proposed as a potential approach to bridge the multiple phenomena that intersect in governing aneurysm rupture risk.[16,19,20] With the increasing acquisition and availability of patient data and the expanding repertoire of experimental and computational research, AI becomes a more worthwhile pursuit for predictive modeling. The complexity and multidisciplinary nature of an aneurysm formation suggests that multiple variables influence rupture, and there is a considerable challenge in bridging the diverse parameters. Further developments in research and clinical reports can aid in the establishment of a data bank to inform AI models. Combined with experimentally validated fluid dynamics, FSI, tissue mechanics, and cell mechanoadaptation, computational models are now an edge closer to improved and realistic predictive capability.

CLINICS CARE POINTS

Original hypotheses and approaches to evaluate risk factors were established on the idea that a single metric could evaluate intracranial aneurysm (IA) stability and transform patient care; however, given the complex and multifaceted nature of IA growth and rupture, we believe that an integrated multimodal approach is more likely to yield predictive results. The advancements in the characterization of IAs are improving the predictability of computational models, though validation is required before clinical translation. Ideally, measurements taken from the clinic would inform key parameters in simulations, thus providing de novo patient-specific data. Preclinical evaluation would include the consistent implementation of four-dimensional-Flow MRI to obtain geometries, vessel wall, and flow data in

Table 1
Pearls and pitfalls of current research in intracranial aneurysm growth and rupture

	Pitfall	Pearls
Hemodynamics	• Wall material properties are typically neglected; if considered, simplified assumptions are made • Highly dependent on input/output boundary conditions	• Experimental models agree with computational simulations to a good extent • Can be run quickly with clinical scans
Biology	• Benchtop system lacks translational parameters • Lack of cell diversity and systemic interactions in studies	• Measurable potential biomarkers from blood draws
Mechanics	• Relating biochemical pathways and biomarkers to mechanics • Further verification and validation before clinical impact	• Advancements in experimental characterization • Mathematical models capture mechanisms from initiation to rupture

conjunction with a blood draw to obtain key biomarkers. A corresponding computational model would take the measured properties and determine the heterogeneous G&R mechanics of the IA wall that leads to rupture or stabilization. This timely workflow results in a comprehensive risk profile provided to neurosurgeons that gives a probability of IA growth or rupture. The combination of multidisciplinary studies informing a computational model could act as the new standard of diagnoses that guide treatment options (**Fig. 5**). However, the most pressing setback in between implementation of this diagnostic pipeline is the lack of connection between hemodynamics, inflammatory biomarkers, and mechanical remodeling. Therefore, the ultimate need in IA research is to bridge the gap between the three phenomena in collaboration with clinicians.

The overarching goal of aneurysm research is to improve risk diagnoses and maximize optimal treatments of aneurysms. With increasing developments in imaging modalities, endovascular and surgical methods, the availability of intervention and treatment also expands. The latter drives open vascular treatments to redefine the necessary risk threshold. All the above emphasize the question of how one should determine a patient-specific risk of rupture, which continues to remain elusive after decades of research. To answer this question, the current state of the literature in IA research is summarized in **Table 1**.

SUMMARY

We describe a complex multiscale process that starts with hemodynamic forces initiating biochemical pathways that ultimately result in tissue remodeling contributing to IA formation,

growth, and rupture. These processes are investigated by four-dimensional-flow MRI, CFD, molecular biology, animal models, mechanical characterization, and mathematical modeling, all of which strive to improve physician decision-making methods in evaluating the necessity of surgical intervention in IAs. Clinical outcomes suggest that a multimodal approach is required in the determination of aneurysm stability or rupture rather than geometric measurements, location, and patient history. However, more research is required to elucidate what factors in the feedback loop described above, or unknown and evasive factors not described, are most crucial in driving an IA toward growth, stability, or failure. We believe that a predictive model that can evaluate hemodynamic, biological, and mechanical phenomena to provide a comprehensive risk profile could transform IA diagnoses and treatment, but the current state of the research is not yet complete to make concrete correlations.

More work is required to fully understand the multi-faceted and multi-scale phenomenon of IA rupture. As explained here, CFD simulations are being improved with novel techniques and imaging modalities. The key biological pathways and measurable biomarkers in blood drawn toward rupture will soon be identified. Experimental characterization of human IAs is a recent stride toward elucidating IA mechanical behavior. The model systems to investigate the complex processes within IAs are limited yet considerably improved in recent years. Future investigations will soon comprehensively elucidate the multimodal feedback loop that drives IA progression and rupture. Ultimately, IA research optimistically points toward the implementation of data-driven and research-supported predictive models to transform future patient care.

DISCLOSURE

The authors have no conflicts of interest to declare.

REFERENCES

1. Greving JP, Wermer MJH, Brown RD, et al. Development of the PHASES score for prediction of risk of rupture of intracranial aneurysms: a pooled analysis of six prospective cohort studies. Lancet Neurol 2014;13(1):59–66.

2. Etminan N, Brown RD Jr, Beseoglu K, et al. The unruptured intracranial aneurysm treatment score: A multidisciplinary consensus. Neurology 2015;85:881–9.

3. Backes D, Vergouwen MD, Velthuis BK, et al. Difference in aneurysm characteristics between ruptured and unruptured aneurysms in patients with multiple intracranial aneurysms. Stroke 2014;45(5): 1299–303.

4. Chalouhi N, Hoh BL, Hasan D. Review of cerebral aneurysm formation, growth, and rupture. Stroke 2013;44(12):3613–22.

5. Holmes T. Pathology of Aneurysm. Br Med J 1886; 2(1354):1146–50.

6. Killian H. [New hemodynamic process in arteriovenous aneurysms and dilatation diseases of the arteries]. Langenbecks Arch Klin Chir Ver Dtsch Z Chir 1951;270:368–72.

7. German WJ, Black SP. Intra-aneurysmal hemodynamics: turbulence. Trans Am Neurol Assoc 1954; 13(79th Meeting):163–5.

8. Nakatani H, Hashimoto N, Kang Y, et al. Cerebral blood flow patterns at major vessel bifurcations and aneurysms in rats. J Neurosurg 1991;74(2): 258–62.

9. Bovenschulte H, Krug B, Schneider T, et al. CT coronary angiography: coronary CT-flow quantification supplements morphological stenosis analysis. Eur J Radiol 2013;82(4):608–16.

10. Steinman DA, Hoi Y, Fahy P, et al. Variability of computational fluid dynamics solutions for pressure and flow in a giant aneurysm: the ASME 2012 Summer Bioengineering Conference CFD Challenge. J Biomech Eng 2013;135(2):021016.

11. Berg P, Roloff C, Beuing O, et al. The Computational Fluid Dynamics Rupture Challenge 2013–Phase II: Variability of Hemodynamic Simulations in Two Intracranial Aneurysms. J Biomech Eng 2015;137(12): 121008.

12. Janiga G, Berg P, Sugiyama S, et al. The Computational Fluid Dynamics Rupture Challenge 2013-Phase I: prediction of rupture status in intracranial aneurysms. AJNR Am J Neuroradiol 2015;36(3): 530–6.

13. Valen-Sendstad K, Bergersen AW, Shimogonya Y, et al. Real-World Variability in the Prediction of Intracranial Aneurysm Wall Shear Stress: The 2015 International Aneurysm CFD Challenge. Cardiovasc Eng Technol 2018;9(4):544–64.

14. Zhang Y, Jing L, Zhang Y, et al. Low wall shear stress is associated with the rupture of intracranial aneurysm with known rupture point: case report and literature review. BMC Neurol 2016;16(1):231.

15. Zhou G, Zhu Y, Yin Y, et al. Association of wall shear stress with intracranial aneurysm rupture: systematic review and meta-analysis. Sci Rep 2017;7(1): 5331.

16. Shi Z, Chen GZ, Mao L, et al. Machine Learning-Based Prediction of Small Intracranial Aneurysm Rupture Status Using CTA-Derived Hemodynamics: A Multicenter Study. AJNR Am J Neuroradiol 2021; 42(4):648–54.

17. Xiang J, Natarajan SK, Tremmel M, et al. Hemodynamic-morphologic discriminants for intracranial aneurysm rupture. Stroke 2011;42(1):144–52.

18. Dabagh M, Nair P, Gounley J, et al. Hemodynamic and morphological characteristics of a growing cerebral aneurysm. Neurosurg Focus 2019;47(1):E13.

19. Aranda A, Valencia A. Study on Cerebral Aneurysms: Rupture Risk Prediction Using Geometrical Parameters and Wall Shear Stress with Cfd and Machine Learning Tools. Machine Learn Appl Int J 2018;5(4):01–13.

20. Arzani A, Dawson STM. Data-driven cardiovascular flow modelling: examples and opportunities. J R Soc Interf 2021;18(175):20200802.

21. Ishibashi R, Aoki T, Nishimura M, et al. Contribution of mast cells to cerebral aneurysm formation. Curr Neurovasc Res 2010;7(2):113–24.

22. Hasan D, Chalouhi N, Jabbour P, et al. Macrophage imbalance (M1 vs. M2) and upregulation of mast cells in wall of ruptured human cerebral aneurysms: preliminary results. J Neuroinflammation 2012;9:222.

23. Kushamae M, Miyata H, Shirai M, et al. Involvement of neutrophils in machineries underlying the rupture of intracranial aneurysms in rats. Sci Rep 2020; 10(1):20004.

24. Tutino VM, Zebraski HR, Rajabzadeh-Oghaz H, et al. RNA Sequencing Data from Human Intracranial Aneurysm Tissue Reveals a Complex Inflammatory Environment Associated with Rupture. Mol Diagn Ther 2021;25(6):775–90.

25. Rizas KD, Ippagunta N, Tilson MD 3rd. Immune cells and molecular mediators in the pathogenesis of the abdominal aortic aneurysm. Cardiol Rev 2009;17(5): 201–10.

26. Sawyer DM, Pace LA, Pascale CL, et al. Lymphocytes influence intracranial aneurysm formation and rupture: role of extracellular matrix remodeling

and phenotypic modulation of vascular smooth muscle cells. J Neuroinflammation 2016;13(1):185.

27. Hosaka K, Downes DP, Nowicki KW, et al. Modified murine intracranial aneurysm model: aneurysm formation and rupture by elastase and hypertension. J Neurointerv Surg 2014;6(6):474–9.

28. Aoki T, Nishimura M, Matsuoka T, et al. PGE(2)-EP(2) signalling in endothelium is activated by haemodynamic stress and induces cerebral aneurysm through an amplifying loop via NF-kappaB. Br J Pharmacol 2011;163(6):1237–49.

29. Nuki Y, Tsou TL, Kurihara C, et al. Elastase-induced intracranial aneurysms in hypertensive mice. Hypertension 2009;54(6):1337–44.

30. Santiago-Sim T, Fang X, Hennessy ML, et al. THSD1 (Thrombospondin Type 1 Domain Containing Protein 1) Mutation in the Pathogenesis of Intracranial Aneurysm and Subarachnoid Hemorrhage. Stroke 2016; 47(12):3005–13.

31. Aoki T, Frosen J, Fukuda M, et al. Prostaglandin E2-EP2-NF-kappaB signaling in macrophages as a potential therapeutic target for intracranial aneurysms. Sci Signal 2017;10(465):eaah6037.

32. Jiang Z, Huang J, You L, et al. Pharmacological inhibition of STAT3 by BP-1-102 inhibits intracranial aneurysm formation and rupture in mice through modulating inflammatory response. Pharmacol Res Perspect 2021;9(1):e00704.

33. Wang KC, Yeh YT, Nguyen P, et al. Flow-dependent YAP/TAZ activities regulate endothelial phenotypes and atherosclerosis. Proc Natl Acad Sci U S A 2016;113(41):11525–30.

34. Nakajima H, Yamamoto K, Agarwala S, et al. Flow-Dependent Endothelial YAP Regulation Contributes to Vessel Maintenance. Dev Cell 2017;40(6): 523–36.e6.

35. Kurki MI, Hakkinen SK, Frosen J, et al. Upregulated signaling pathways in ruptured human saccular intracranial aneurysm wall: an emerging regulative role of Toll-like receptor signaling and nuclear factor-kappaB, hypoxia-inducible factor-1A, and ETS transcription factors. Neurosurgery 2011;68(6): 1667–75 [discussion: 1675–6].

36. Kleinloog R, Verweij BH, van der Vlies P, et al. RNA Sequencing Analysis of Intracranial Aneurysm Walls Reveals Involvement of Lysosomes and Immunoglobulins in Rupture. Stroke 2016;47(5):1286–93.

37. Jin H, Jiang Y, Liu X, et al. Cell-free microRNA-21: biomarker for intracranial aneurysm rupture. Chin Neurosurg J 2020;6:15.

38. Zheng Z, Chen Y, Wang Y, et al. MicroRNA-513b-5p targets COL1A1 and COL1A2 associated with the formation and rupture of intracranial aneurysm. Sci Rep 2021;11(1):14897.

39. Huang Q, Sun Y, Huang Q, et al. Association Between Circular RNAs and Intracranial Aneurysm Rupture Under the Synergistic Effect of Individual Environmental Factors. Front Neurol 2021;12: 594835.

40. Chen X, Yang S, Yang J, et al. The Potential Role of hsa_circ_0005505 in the Rupture of Human Intracranial Aneurysm. Front Mol Biosci 2021;8: 670691.

41. Sharma T, Datta KK, Kumar M, et al. Intracranial Aneurysm Biomarker Candidates Identified by a Proteome-Wide Study. OMICS 2020;24(8):483–92.

42. Kanematsu Y, Kanematsu M, Kurihara C, et al. Critical roles of macrophages in the formation of intracranial aneurysm. Stroke 2011;42(1):173–8.

43. Etminan N, Dreier R, Buchholz BA, et al. Age of collagen in intracranial saccular aneurysms. Stroke 2014;45(6):1757–63.

44. Hackenberg KAM, Rajabzadeh-Oghaz H, Dreier R, et al. Collagen Turnover in Relation to Risk Factors and Hemodynamics in Human Intracranial Aneurysms. Stroke 2020;51(5):1624–8.

45. Valentin A, Holzapfel GA. Constrained Mixture Models as Tools for Testing Competing Hypotheses in Arterial Biomechanics: A Brief Survey. Mech Res Commun 2012;42:126–33.

46. Humphrey JD, Rajagopal KR. A constrained mixture model for growth and remodeling of soft tissues. Math Models Methods Appl Sci 2002;12(03):407–30.

47. Cebral JR, Duan X, Chung BJ, et al. Wall Mechanical Properties and Hemodynamics of Unruptured Intracranial Aneurysms. AJNR Am J Neuroradiol 2015; 36(9):1695–703.

48. Ali MS, Starke RM, Jabbour PM, et al. TNF-alpha induces phenotypic modulation in cerebral vascular smooth muscle cells: implications for cerebral aneurysm pathology. J Cereb Blood Flow Metab 2013; 33(10):1564–73.

49. Humphrey JD, Schwartz MA, Tellides G, et al. Role of mechanotransduction in vascular biology: focus on thoracic aortic aneurysms and dissections. Circ Res 2015;116(8):1448–61.

50. Shih ED, Provenzano PP, Witzenburg CM, et al. Characterizing Tissue Remodeling and Mechanical Heterogeneity in Cerebral Aneurysms. J Vasc Res 2021;1–9.

51. Christian Gasser T. An irreversible constitutive model for fibrous soft biological tissue: a 3-D microfiber approach with demonstrative application to abdominal aortic aneurysms. Acta Biomater 2011; 7(6):2457–66.

52. Holzapfel GA, Gasser TC, Ogden RW. A new constitutive framework for arterial wall mechanics and a comparative study of material models. J Elasticity 2000;61(1/3):1–48.

53. Tóth BK, Raffai G. Analysis of the mechanical parameters of human brain aneurysm. J Vasc Res 2022:59:34-42.

54. Valencia A, Contente A, Ignat M, et al. Mechanical Test of Human Cerebral Aneurysm Specimens

Obtained from Surgical Clipping. J Mech Med Biol 2015;15(05).

55. Seshaiyer P, Hsu FPK, Shah AD, et al. Multiaxial Mechanical Behavior of Human Saccular Aneurysms. Comput Methods Biomech Biomed Engin 2001; 4(3):281–9.

56. Laurence DW, Homburg H, Yan F, et al. A pilot study on biaxial mechanical, collagen microstructural, and morphological characterizations of a resected human intracranial aneurysm tissue. Sci Rep 2021; 11(1):3525.

57. Baek S, Rajagopal KR, Humphrey JD. A theoretical model of enlarging intracranial fusiform aneurysms. J Biomech Eng 2006;128(1):142–9.

58. Kroon M, Holzapfel GA. A model for saccular cerebral aneurysm growth by collagen fibre remodelling. J Theor Biol 2007;247(4):775–87.

59. Braeu FA, Seitz A, Aydin RC, et al. Homogenized constrained mixture models for anisotropic volumetric growth and remodeling. Biomech Model Mechanobiol 2017;16(3):889–906.

60. Cyron CJ, Wilson JS, Humphrey JD. Mechanobiological stability: a new paradigm to understand the enlargement of aneurysms? J R Soc Interf 2014; 11(100):20140680.

61. Brandstaeter S, Fuchs SL, Biehler J, et al. Global Sensitivity Analysis of a Homogenized Constrained Mixture Model of Arterial Growth and Remodeling. J Elasticity 2021;145(1–2):191–221.

62. Davis FM, Luo Y, Avril S, et al. Pointwise characterization of the elastic properties of planar soft tissues: application to ascending thoracic aneurysms. Biomech Model Mechanobiol 2015;14(5):967–78.

63. Kroon M. Simulation of Cerebral Aneurysm Growth and Prediction of Evolving Rupture Risk. Model Simulation Eng 2011;2011:1–10.

64. Teixeira FS, Neufeld E, Kuster N, et al. Modeling intracranial aneurysm stability and growth: an integrative mechanobiological framework for clinical cases. Biomech Model Mechanobiol 2020;19(6): 2413–31.

65. Ghavamian A, Mousavi SJ, Avril S. Computational Study of Growth and Remodeling in Ascending Thoracic Aortic Aneurysms Considering Variations of Smooth Muscle Cell Basal Tone. Front Bioeng Biotechnol 2020;8:587376.

Brain Arteriovenous Malformations
Status of Open Surgery after A Randomized Trial of Unruptured Brain Arteriovenous Malformations

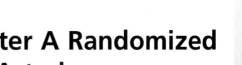

Evan Luther, MD[a],*, Vaidya Govindarajan, BS[a], David J. McCarthy, MD, MS[b],
Joshua Burks, MD[a], Victor Lu, MD, PhD[a], Ian Ramsay, BS[a], Michael Silva, MD[a],
Robert M. Starke, MD, MS[a]

KEYWORDS

- Arteriovenous malformation • ARUBA • Unruptured AVM • Ruptured AVM
- Cerebrovascular surgery • Intracranial hemorrhage • Ischemic stroke

KEY POINTS

- ARUBA was the first prospective, randomized trial evaluating treatment outcomes for unruptured brain arteriovenous malformations (AVMs) and was halted at a mean follow-up period of less than 3 years after an interim analysis demonstrated a significantly higher risk of death and symptomatic stroke in the interventional arm.
- The results of ARUBA led to various criticisms citing selection bias, lack of treatment arm standardization, low enrollment rate, short follow-up, and lack of subgroup analyses as the factors driving the lack of treatment effectiveness in the trial.
- Several subsequent retrospective studies evaluating microsurgical resection of unruptured AVMs in ARUBA-eligible patients demonstrated better outcomes than those in the treatment arm of ARUBA.
- Despite these findings, studies evaluating national trends in AVM treatment suggest that clinicians are less inclined to treat unruptured AVMs with any modality, including microsurgery, following ARUBA.
- Future prospective trials evaluating the role of open surgery for AVMs are needed to confirm the findings of the post-ARUBA studies.

BACKGROUND

In 2014, the results of "A Randomized Trial of Unruptured Brain Arteriovenous Malformations" (ARUBA) were published, suggesting that observation resulted in less morbidity and mortality than intervention for these lesions.[1,2] Although ARUBA was the first prospective, randomized trial evaluating treatment outcomes for unruptured brain arteriovenous malformations (AVMs), these findings were questioned by a large proportion of the cerebrovascular community. Citing flaws in the ARUBA study design, various resultant investigations demonstrated better interventional outcomes than those in the treatment arm of ARUBA with many suggesting that the increased use of microsurgical resection accounted for this improvement in outcomes.[3–10] As such, no standardized AVM treatment guidelines exist.[11–15] However, it is the purpose of this article to provide

a Department of Neurosurgery, University of Miami Miller School of Medicine, Lois Pope Life Center, 2nd Floor, 1095 Northwest 14th Terrace, Miami, FL 33136, USA; b Department of Neurological Surgery, University of Pittsburgh Medical Center, UPMC Presbyterian, Suite B-400, 200 Lothrop Street, Pittsburgh, PA 15213, USA
* Corresponding author.
E-mail address: evan.luther@jhsmiami.org

Neurosurg Clin N Am 33 (2022) 443–448
https://doi.org/10.1016/j.nec.2022.05.006
1042-3680/22/© 2022 Elsevier Inc. All rights reserved.

a detailed overview of ARUBA and the effect that this study has had on open microsurgical resection of AVMs.

DISCUSSION
A Randomized Trial of Unruptured Brain Arteriovenous Malformations Overview

ARUBA was a multi-institutional, prospectively enrolled trial evaluating best medical management (ie, observation alone or observation with medical management of AVM sequelae such as epilepsy) versus treatment of unruptured AVMs. The trial was designed with a follow-up period of up to 12 years and the 2 primary endpoints were death and symptomatic stroke. If randomized to the treatment arm, the trial allowed the enrolling physician to determine an optimal treatment strategy based on their personal expertise.[1]

Although 1740 patients were screened for enrollment, only 13% were randomized into either arm of the trial. At less than 3 years of mean follow-up, randomization was stopped after an interim analysis demonstrated a significantly higher risk of death and symptomatic stroke in the interventional arm.[1,8] In 2020, the final ARUBA analysis continued to demonstrate better outcomes with medical management alone at an average follow-up of slightly over 4 years.[16]

Criticisms of a Randomized Trial of Unruptured Brain Arteriovenous Malformations Overview

The results of ARUBA were at odds with the clinical experience of many cerebrovascular specialists, resulting in a widespread critical review that revealed some noteworthy shortcomings in the trial. Selection bias, lack of treatment arm standardization, low enrollment rate, short follow-up, and lack of subgroup analyses were the most frequently cited criticisms.[17] Many felt that the primary endpoint of symptomatic stroke was inappropriately defined and created an overestimation of treatment morbidity as even headache alone was considered "symptomatic."[1,18–20] With several participating centers enrolling minimal patients, concerns for potential recruitment bias were raised especially given the low rate of low grade AVMs treated with microsurgical resection (**Fig. 1**).[8,17,18] Moreover, partial embolization was included as an acceptable treatment in the intervention arm despite previous studies, suggesting that it increases the risk of AVM rupture (**Fig. 2**).[21–23] The early cessation of ARUBA, and the resultant brevity of the mean follow-up period, left many questioning whether the data could truly compare the upfront risk of intervention to the

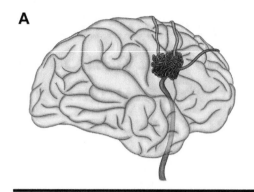

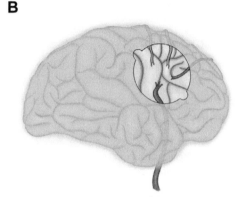

Fig. 1. (*A*) Illustration of a right frontal low-grade AVM before and (*B*) after craniotomy for the resection of the lesion.

overall risk of rupture for an AVM.[1,2,24,25] This doubt was further compounded by the fact that the mean follow-up period was similar to the radiosurgery latency period and thus could not even accurately represent the full risk reduction of such a procedure.[5]

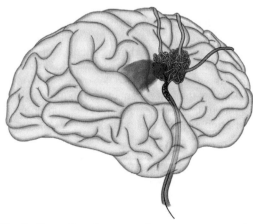

Fig. 2. Illustration demonstrating AVM rupture after partial embolization.

Post-a Randomized Trial of Unruptured Brain Arteriovenous Malformations Overview Studies

These pitfalls were the motivation for several subsequent studies evaluating interventional outcomes for unruptured AVMs in ARUBA-eligible patients. In 2014, *Rutledge and colleagues* retrospectively analyzed 74 ARUBA-eligible patients in which 13 were observed and 61 underwent intervention. With identical ARUBA endpoints, no significant difference in symptomatic stroke or death was observed between the 2 groups. Of note, 70.5% of the interventional group received microsurgical resection as treatment.[8] In the following year, *Nerva and colleagues*[26] retrospectively stratified 61 ARUBA-eligible patients by Spetzler-Martin grade and found that their functional outcomes were similar to the medical arm of ARUBA, especially in lower grade AVMs treated with surgical resection. In 2017, *Wong and colleagues*[10] evaluated 155 ARUBA-eligible patients that underwent surgical excision and presented favorable rates of neurologic disability at last follow-up compared with ARUBA (16.1% vs 46.2%). In the same year, *Schramm and colleagues*[9] attempted to reconcile the differences between ARUBA and those of other unruptured AVM series by subdividing their own series of patients with AVM by Spetzler-Martin grade. Their analysis echoed that of *Nerva and colleagues,*[26] again demonstrating that the microsurgical resection of unruptured AVMs was associated with high obliteration rates and did not result in increased complications, particularly with respect to lower Spetzler-Martin grade AVMs. One year later, *Lang and colleagues*[27] published a retrospective analysis of 105 ARUBA-eligible patients demonstrating that the obliteration rate among patients who underwent microsurgery was 95.5% with postoperative mortality and stroke rates noticeably lower than those reported by the ARUBA trial, once again highlighting the efficacy and safety of microsurgical interventions for AVM. In 2019, *Pulli and colleagues*[28] retrospectively analyzed 142 ARUBA-eligible patients with AVM treated via a multimodal approach and again found significantly lower rates of postoperative stroke relative to the interventional arm of the ARUBA trial.

Although the generalizability of these studies remains limited due to their retrospective nature and the fact that they are single-center series, their findings do consistently demonstrate better outcomes than the those of the ARUBA treatment arm, even in those patients receiving SRS alone.[3–6,9] Many attributed these differences in outcome to both careful patient selection and the increased utilization of microsurgical resection as a treatment modality. While the mounting evidence opposing ARUBA seemingly substantiates the widespread critiques, a comprehensive investigation of the effect of ARUBA on cerebrovascular practice patterns remains limited.

Trends in Overall Arteriovenous Malformation Treatments Post-a Randomized Trial of Unruptured Brain Arteriovenous Malformations Overview

Available studies
Following ARUBA, multiple groups have investigated the effect the trial has had on overall AVM treatment trends. In 2020, *Komatsu and colleagues*[29] evaluated their institutional trends in AVM management before and after ARUBA and identified a significant decline in microsurgery with a concurrent increase in radiosurgery between the 2 epochs. In contrast, 2 other studies used the same publicly available inpatient database, the Nationwide Inpatient Sample (NIS), and produced relatively incongruent findings when assessing elective AVM admissions. The first evaluated elective treatments of AVMs from 2011 to 2015 and found that rates of microsurgical intervention for AVMs increased in the setting of declining overall AVM interventions.[14] The second was more comprehensive looking at elective AVM treatments from 2006 to 2018 and found a significant decline in microsurgical resection post-ARUBA while endovascular treatments and radiosurgery did not change.[30] Given the significant discrepancy in sample size between the 2 studies (2029 vs 40,285, respectively), it is likely that the first study did not appropriately account for database sampling and population changes during the time period in question. As such, the results of the latter study, which seem to mimic those of *Komatsu and colleagues*, seem the most plausible and suggest that the results of ARUBA have made clinicians less likely to commit to an invasive intervention for unruptured AVMs.

Our results
Given these findings, we performed an analysis of the NIS for both ruptured and unruptured AVM admissions from 2003 to 2017 to determine the effect ARUBA had on AVM treatment trends. All patients with a brain AVM were identified using *International Classification of Diseases, Ninth and Tenth Revisions* (ICD-9/10) codes similar to previously published works.[31–33] For unruptured AVMs, a significant decline in overall treatment was seen following ARUBA (−3.71% per year, *P* = .025) (**Fig. 3**). Interestingly, we found no difference in

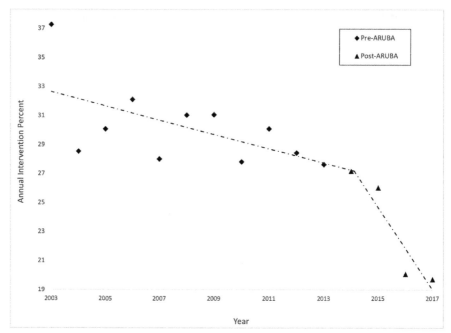

Fig. 3. Unruptured AVM intervention rates pre- and post-ARUBA.

overall treatment numbers in the pre- and post-ARUBA periods for ruptured AVMs. However, when stratified by treatment type, we found a significant increase in endovascular treatments accompanied by a significant decrease in microsurgical resection (*P* = .0039) (**Fig. 4**). For unruptured AVMs, both microsurgery and endovascular treatments declined with a concurrent increase in patients receiving no treatment (*P* < .0001) (see **Fig. 4**).

FUTURE DIRECTIONS

Based on the results above, 2 conclusions can be drawn: (1) microsurgery still seems to be an effective treatment of unruptured AVMs as various single-center series of ARUBA-eligible patients treated with surgical resection seem to have less perioperative morbidity than the treatment arm of ARUBA, and (2) despite the results of these

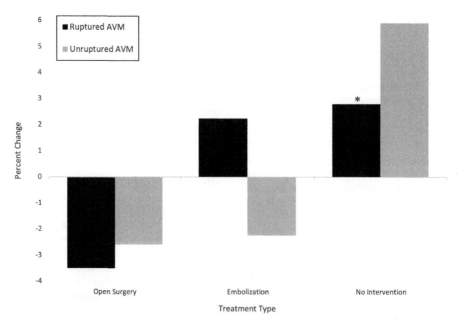

Fig. 4. Percent change in AVM intervention type pre- and post-ARUBA. *denotes nonsignificance.

publications it seems that clinicians are less inclined to treat unruptured AVMs with any modality following ARUBA. These statements seem to be in direct opposition with one another and, as such, should serve as the impetus for future prospective studies evaluating the role of open surgery for these lesions.[34] Moreover, other investigations have also demonstrated promising results with adjuvant medical therapies for otherwise inoperable AVMs; however, further research must be conducted to confirm their effectiveness.[35,36]

SUMMARY

ARUBA was the first, prospective trial evaluating treatment outcomes for unruptured AVMs and found that observation alone resulted in less morbidity and mortality than intervention for these lesions. These findings were inconsistent with the clinical experience of many cerebrovascular specialists and led to the publication of several retrospective studies that demonstrated better outcomes than the treatment arm of ARUBA when using open surgery as a treatment of unruptured AVMs. Despite the results of these post-ARUBA studies, it seems that the ARUBA trial has led to a significant nationwide decrease in interventions, including open surgery, for unruptured AVMs.

CLINICS CARE POINTS

- The results of ARUBA suggested that the treatment of unruptured AVMs was worse than the natural history of these lesions
- Selection bias, lack of treatment arm standardization, low enrollment rate, short follow-up, and lack of subgroup analyses were the most frequently cited ARUBA criticisms
- Subsequent studies evaluating open surgery for ARUBA-eligible patients found much better outcomes than those of the ARUBA treatment arm
- Despite these studies challenging the findings of ARUBA, AVM treatments (including open surgery) seem to have significantly declined in the post-ARUBA period
- Future prospective studies evaluating the role of open surgery for unruptured AVMs are necessary to confirm the value of microsurgical resection for these lesions

ACKNOWLEDGMENTS

Roberto Suazo for creating the illustrations displayed in this article.

DISCLOSURE

The authors have nothing to disclose.

REFERENCES

1. Mohr JP, Parides MK, Stapf C, et al. Medical management with or without interventional therapy for unruptured brain arteriovenous malformations (ARUBA): a multicentre, non-blinded, randomised trial. Lancet 2014;383(9917):614–21.
2. Mohr JP, Moskowitz AJ, Stapf C, et al. The ARUBA trial: current status, future hopes. Stroke 2010; 41(8):e537–40.
3. Link TW, Winston G, Schwarz JT, et al. Treatment of unruptured brain arteriovenous malformations: a single-center experience of 86 patients and a critique of the a randomized trial of unruptured brain arteriovenous malformations (ARUBA) trial. World Neurosurg 2018;120:e1156–62.
4. Karlsson B, Jokura H, Yang HC, et al. The NASSAU (New ASSessment of cerebral Arteriovenous Malformations yet Unruptured) analysis: are the results from the ARUBA trial also applicable to unruptured arteriovenous malformations deemed suitable for gamma knife surgery? Neurosurgery 2019;85(1): E118–24.
5. Tonetti DA, Gross BA, Atcheson KM, et al. The benefit of radiosurgery for ARUBA-eligible arteriovenous malformations: a practical analysis over an appropriate follow-up period. J Neurosurg 2018; 128(6):1850–4.
6. Ding D, Starke RM, Kano H, et al. Stereotactic radiosurgery for ARUBA (A Randomized Trial of Unruptured Brain Arteriovenous Malformations)-eligible spetzler-martin grade I and II arteriovenous malformations: a multicenter study. World Neurosurg 2017;102:507–17.
7. Hong CS, Peterson EC, Ding D, et al. Intervention for a randomized trial of unruptured brain arteriovenous malformations (ARUBA) - Eligible patients: an evidence-based review. Clin Neurol Neurosurg 2016;150:133–8.
8. Rutledge WC, Abla AA, Nelson J, et al. Treatment and outcomes of ARUBA-eligible patients with unruptured brain arteriovenous malformations at a single institution. Neurosurg Focus 2014;37(3):E8.
9. Schramm J, Schaller K, Esche J, et al. Microsurgery for cerebral arteriovenous malformations: subgroup outcomes in a consecutive series of 288 cases. J Neurosurg 2017;126(4):1056–63.
10. Wong J, Slomovic A, Ibrahim G, et al. Microsurgery for ARUBA trial (A Randomized Trial of Unruptured

Brain Arteriovenous Malformation)-eligible unruptured brain arteriovenous malformations. Stroke 2017;48(1):136–44.

11. Cenzato M, Boccardi E, Beghi E, et al. European consensus conference on unruptured brain AVMs treatment (Supported by EANS, ESMINT, EGKS, and SINCH). Acta Neurochir (Wien) 2017;159(6):1059–64.

12. Kato Y, Dong VH, Chaddad F, et al. Expert consensus on the management of brain arteriovenous malformations. Asian J Neurosurg 2019;14(4):1074–81.

13. Zuurbier SM, Al-Shahi Salman R. Interventions for treating brain arteriovenous malformations in adults. Cochrane Database Syst Rev 2019;9:CD003436.

14. Birnbaum LA, Straight M, Hegde S, et al. Microsurgery for Unruptured Cerebral Arteriovenous Malformations in the National Inpatient Sample is More Common Post-ARUBA. World Neurosurg 2020;137:e343–6.

15. Reynolds AS, Chen ML, Merkler AE, et al. Effect of a randomized trial of unruptured brain arteriovenous malformation on interventional treatment rates for unruptured arteriovenous malformations. Cerebrovasc Dis 2019;47(5–6):299–302.

16. Mohr JP, Overbey JR, Hartmann A, et al. Medical management with interventional therapy versus medical management alone for unruptured brain arteriovenous malformations (ARUBA): final follow-up of a multicentre, non-blinded, randomised controlled trial. Lancet Neurol 2020;19(7):573–81.

17. Magro E, Gentric JC, Darsaut TE, et al. Responses to ARUBA: a systematic review and critical analysis for the design of future arteriovenous malformation trials. J Neurosurg 2017;126(2):486–94.

18. Lawton MT, Abla AA. Management of brain arteriovenous malformations. Lancet 2014;383(9929):1634–5.

19. Pierot L, Fiehler J, Cognard C, et al. Will a randomized trial of unruptured brain arteriovenous malformations change our clinical practice? AJNR Am J Neuroradiol 2014;35(3):416–7.

20. Solomon RA, Connolly ES Jr. Management of brain arteriovenous malformations. Lancet 2014;383(9929):1634.

21. Heidenreich JO, Hartlieb S, Stendel R, et al. Bleeding complications after endovascular therapy of cerebral arteriovenous malformations. AJNR Am J Neuroradiol 2006;27(2):313–6.

22. Burks JD, Luther EM, Govindarajan V, et al. Treatment-Associated Stroke in Patients Undergoing Endovascular Therapy in the ARUBA Trial. Stroke 2021;52(11):e710–4.

23. Luther EM, Chagani F, King H, et al. Rupture of a de novo dural AV fistula following adult cerebral AVM resection. BMJ Case Rep 2021;14(12).

24. Amin-Hanjani S. ARUBA results are not applicable to all patients with arteriovenous malformation. Stroke 2014;45(5):1539–40.

25. Gross BA, Scott RM, Smith ER. Management of brain arteriovenous malformations. Lancet 2014;383(9929):1635.

26. Nerva JD, Mantovani A, Barber J, et al. Treatment outcomes of unruptured arteriovenous malformations with a subgroup analysis of ARUBA (A Randomized Trial of Unruptured Brain Arteriovenous Malformations)-eligible patients. Neurosurgery 2015;76(5):563–70 [discussion: 570], [quiz: 570].

27. Lang M, Moore NZ, Rasmussen PA, et al. Treatment outcomes of a randomized trial of unruptured brain arteriovenous malformation-eligible unruptured brain arteriovenous malformation patients. Neurosurgery 2018;83(3):548–55.

28. Pulli B, Chapman PH, Ogilvy CS, et al. Multimodal cerebral arteriovenous malformation treatment: a 12-year experience and comparison of key outcomes to ARUBA. J Neurosurg 2019;133(6):1–10.

29. Komatsu K, Takagi Y, Ishii A, et al. Changes in treatment strategy over time for arteriovenous malformation in a Japanese high-volume center. BMC Neurol 2020;20(1):404.

30. Wahood W, Alexander AY, Doherty RJ, et al. Elective intervention for unruptured cranial arteriovenous malformations in relation to ARUBA trial: a National Inpatient Sample study. Acta Neurochir (Wien) 2021;163(9):2489–95.

31. Davies JM, Yanamadala V, Lawton MT. Comparative effectiveness of treatments for cerebral arteriovenous malformations: trends in nationwide outcomes from 2000 to 2009. Neurosurg Focus 2012;33(1):E11.

32. Luther EM, McCarthy D, Berry KM, et al. Hospital teaching status associated with reduced inpatient mortality and perioperative complications in surgical neuro-oncology. J Neurooncol 2020;146(2):389–96.

33. Luther E, McCarthy DJ, Brunet MC, et al. Treatment and diagnosis of cerebral aneurysms in the post-International Subarachnoid Aneurysm Trial (ISAT) era: trends and outcomes. J Neurointerv Surg 2020;12(7):682–7.

34. Lawton MT. The role of AVM microsurgery in the aftermath of a randomized trial of unruptured brain arteriovenous malformations. AJNR Am J Neuroradiol 2015;36(4):617–9.

35. Gaztanaga W, Luther E, McCarthy D, et al. Giant, symptomatic mixed vascular malformation containing a cavernoma, developmental venous anomaly, and capillary telangiectasia in a 19-month-old infant. Childs Nerv Syst 2021;38:1005–9.

36. Govindarajan V, Burks JD, Luther EM, et al. Medical adjuvants in the treatment of surgically refractory arteriovenous malformations of the head and face: case report and review of literature. Cerebrovasc Dis 2021;50(5):493–9.

Cavernous Malformations
Updates in Surgical Management and Biology

Philipp Dammann, MD*, Alejandro N. Santos, MD, Xue-Yan Wan, MD,
Yuan Zhu, MD, Ulrich Sure, MD

KEYWORDS

• Cavernous malformations • Genetics • Surgical Treatment • Biology • CCM

INTRODUCTION

Cavernous malformations (CMs) are low-flow vascular lesions of the central nervous system prone to symptomatic hemorrhage. CMs are estimated to be present in approximately 0.5% of the population.[1] Usually, they are characterized by a relatively benign clinical course, staying asymptomatic in many patients.[2] However, depending on the anatomic location, CMs can cause significant morbidity due to symptoms such as seizures or focal neurologic deficits (most of the time caused by symptomatic hemorrhage).[3] CMs occur in sporadic or familial form; the latter, characterized by multiple lesions and occurring in approximately 15% to 20% of cases, is inherited in an autosomal dominant manner. Loss-of-function mutations in 3 underlying loci have been identified so far (CCM1−3).[4] The pathogenesis of the sporadic form has not been fully clarified yet, although multiple influencing factors are discussed.[5] A systematic association (up to 30% of cases) of sporadic CMs with the so-called developmental venous anomalies (DVA) has been reported by several investigators.[6,7] The risk of symptomatic hemorrhage during the natural course of the disease has been analyzed in many observational and population-based cohort studies and meta-analyses in both adults and children.[1,2,8,9] Risk factors for hemorrhage have been studied and identified.[1,6,10–15] In 2008, reporting standards were defined by the research community, leading to more homogeneous definitions and terms in CM research.[16] The evidence for treatment of CMs is limited[17–21]; no randomized controlled trials have been completed so far. In 2017, a synopsis of guidelines for the clinical management of cerebral cavernous malformations (CCMs) was published, confirming the overall low levels of clinical evidence (levels B and C according to american heart association (AHA)/american stroke association (ASA) criteria).[21] In 2013, the surgical task force of the International League Against Epilepsy (ILAE) commission on therapeutic strategies published recommendations for the management of cavernoma-related epilepsy (CRE).[22]

This nonsystematic review aims to summarize important recent clinical research focusing on the biology and surgical management of CMs published since 2017.

SURGICAL MANAGEMENT
Scores, Classifications, and Surveys

Brainstem cavernous malformations

Although the surgical treatment of brainstem cavernous malformations (BSCMs) is a balancing between natural history risks and surgical morbidity, its indication is still a matter of debate. Guidelines see evidence for surgical treatment after a second symptomatic hemorrhage (level B), whereas that for treatment following a first disabling symptomatic hemorrhage is considered weaker (level C).[21] To select potential candidates who may benefit most from surgical treatment (vs observation), 2 grading scores have been proposed and recently validated: the Lawton score,[23] based on different clinical parameters, and the Dammann-Sure score[24] proposed by the authors' group, based on MRI data.

Department of Neurosurgery and Spine Surgery, University Hospital Essen, Hufelandstrasse 55, 45147 Essen, Germany
* Corresponding author.
E-mail address: philipp.dammann@uk-essen.de

Neurosurg Clin N Am 33 (2022) 449–460
https://doi.org/10.1016/j.nec.2022.05.001
1042-3680/22/© 2022 Elsevier Inc. All rights reserved.

One study found each score a relatively robust tool to predict the outcome of BSCM surgery; albeit combined, they provided the most reliable results.[25] Another study revealed the Lawton score being suitable to distinguish between low-, intermediate-, and high-grade BSCMs with accuracy comparable to those of other grading scores in widespread use.[26] In a smaller series of 22 patients, the Lawton score was also validated for postoperative quality of life (QOL).[27] To further improve patient selection in BSCM surgery and guide the selection of the specific surgical approach, proposals of different subtypes of midbrain BSCMs based on 151 cases[28] and 72 patients[29] were also recently published.

To address the multiple technical and clinical aspects of a complex surgical procedure such as BSCM resection, an international Delphi consensus on the surgical treatment of BSCMs was performed and published in 2021.[30] A group of 29 experts repetitively rated 99 statements on BSCM surgery, resulting in the definition and interpretation of a vast catalog of various BSCM- and patient-related aspects. Among other aspects, a consensus was reached for surgical timing, handling of associated DVA, handling of postoperative BSCM remnants, assessment of specific anatomic BSCM localizations, and treatment decisions in typical clinical BSCM scenarios.

As an alternative BSCM score, Yang and colleagues[31] published a 12-grade scale for BSCM surgery based on the analysis of various parameters in a unicenter series of 88 cases. **Fig. 1** shows an overview of BSCM-related scores and surveys.

Cerebral cavernous malformations

Fontanella and colleagues[32] proposed a grading system for cerebral and cerebellar CMs based on neuroradiological features, neurologic status, lesion location, and patient age with a score ranging from −1 to 10 to indicate an intrinsic treatment recommendation. The investigators encouraged other sites to externally validate the system.[32]

Another survey on surgical resection of eloquent CMs among 19 specialized centers, including experience with 272 patients with CRE, revealed a strong variety of practice between the participating centers. The survey pointed out relevant controversies regarding overall management, timing of surgery, and optimal extent of hemosiderin resection.[33]

Surgical Outcome

Brainstem cavernous malformations

Although many observational noncomparative studies have assessed outcome after surgery of BSCMs,[34] a randomized controlled trial is still lacking. Modified Rankin scale (mRS) scores less than or equal to 2 are commonly accepted to define a favorable functional outcome. Two recent publications focused on specific subgroups of patients with BSCMs: Yang and colleagues[35] described 6 patients with acute respiratory failure due to BSCM hemorrhage, all of whom were acutely surgically treated and recovered from respiratory failure; Xie and colleagues[36] analyzed a series of surgically treated patients with severe BSCM hemorrhage: whereas the mean mRS on admission was 4.2, a favorable outcome (mRS ≤ 2) was observed in 64% of cases, and treatment in the subacute period after hemorrhage (≥3−8 weeks) was beneficial. Garcia and colleagues[37] analyzed the frequency and significance of recurrent BSCM, finding that 6.6% of 213 patients were reoperated for recurrent/remnant BSCM. The annual hemorrhage risk of remnant BSCM was 5.9%. In comparison, Fontanella and colleagues observed postsurgical remnants in 19% of 126 patients with CCMs with 7 subsequent symptomatic hemorrhage events (29%) within a mean follow-up period of 80.7 months.[38]

Huang and colleagues[39] assessed the postoperative outcome in a unicenter series restricted to midbrain BSCMs. The investigators found no influence of lesion distance from the surface on surgical outcome. Overall functional outcome was reported as improved in 64.9% (absolute functional outcome was not reported); cranial nerve III function was found worse or unchanged in 65.5%. Xie and colleagues,[40] examining the outcome of BSCMs restricted to the medulla oblongata, detected high rates of caudal cranial nerve dysfunction in the acute postoperative phase. Overall long-term outcome was in line with previous reports (80.3% with mRS ≤ 2). Herten and colleagues[41] from our CCM research group meticulously screened patients for the occurrence of neuropathic pain after BSCM surgery. Albeit it was only rarely or not reported in most series, they showed evidence for neuropathic pain in 8% of 74 patients in their cohort, which is in accordance with findings from post-stroke neuropathic pain; the investigators encouraged to raise awareness for this potentially underdiagnosed symptom.[41] The authors also found an impaired QOL related to certain brainstem symptoms in patients with BSCMs following surgery, which was also present in patients with low-level impairment on the mRS scale, reflecting the impact of BSCM hemorrhage and surgery.[42] The authors recommend using absolute outcome measures in BSCM research. Nathal and colleagues[43] analyzed a unicenter series of 50 surgically treated patients with BSCMs focusing on features that may predict unfavorable outcome.

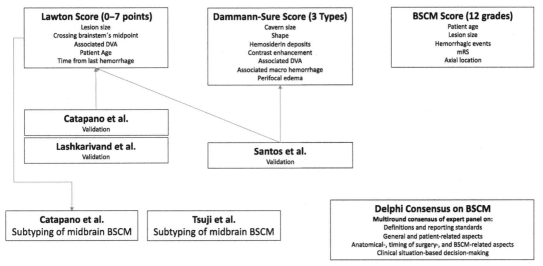

Fig. 1. Available scores (including validation studies) and surveys on BSCM treatment.

BSCM size, compromise of lower cranial nerves, and hemorrhagic recurrence before surgery were identified as risk factors.

Intramedullary spinal cavernous malformations
Evidence for the surgical treatment of intramedullary spinal cavernous malformations (ISCMs) is even more limited compared with CCMs or BSCMs due to the rarity of the disease.[44] Approximately 5% of patients with CM have a spinal CM in larger cohorts,[45] and the lesions account for only around 10% of spinal vascular malformations.[46] Natural history studies suggest that ISCMs have a more aggressive course compared with other locations,[45,46] although surgical removal may also be associated with significant morbidity. Recently, several relatively large observational and partially comparative surgical series have described surgical outcomes. Including 73 surgically and 39 conservatively treated patients, Liu and colleagues[47] identified associated subarachnoid hemorrhage, lesion size and morphology, hemosiderin deposition, and motor dysfunction-independent risk factors that may help to select surgical candidates and predict outcome. Zhang and colleagues[48] described a unicenter series of long-term results of 111 surgically treated patients. The investigators found "good" preoperative neurologic function and improvement immediately after surgery predictors for long-term favorable outcome and argue for surgical removal of symptomatic ISCMs to avoid further deterioration; comparable findings and conclusions were reported by Li and colleagues[49] (83 patients) and Nagoshi and colleagues[50] (66 patients). In addition, Li and colleagues[49] observed better results in patients treated within 3 months after

hemorrhage when compared with those treated thereafter. The so far largest single-center series of Ren and colleagues[51] (219 patients) showed a "favorable" outcome in 86.1% of patients. Deep-seated lesions were associated with worse long-term outcomes, and cervical lesions yielded better results than thoracic lesions. The same group also reported more aggressive clinical courses of ISCMs in children.[52] Overall, most investigators agree (in the context of very limited evidence) that the potentially devastating consequences of a severe intramedullary hemorrhage justify surgical treatment of symptomatic ISCMs in selected cases.

Cavernoma-related epilepsy
Based on excellent surgical treatment results in CRE cases and a strong tendency to develop epilepsy after an initial CCM-related seizure,[53] the ILAE task force has published relatively "prosurgery" recommendations.[22] Surgery seems justified after an initial seizure if antiepileptic drug treatment is refused, the patient is incompliant, or the risk of (re-)hemorrhage is high. Moreover, surgery is also an option in drug-resistant CRE. There remains debate about the extent of surgery, especially in temporal lobe CCMs,[54,55] in addition to information gaps regarding longer-term seizure control. Recently, He and colleagues[56] confirmed high rates of postoperative seizure control (80% Engel class I after 5 years) in a large cohort (181 cases); Lin and colleagues[57] reported comparable long-term results in pediatric patients.

Miscellaneous
Numerous studies address other aspects of surgical outcome in CMs. Padarti and colleagues[58] searched

the US National Readmission Database to assess reasons for readmission following CM surgery: 14.9% of patients were readmitted within 30 days after surgery, mostly due to neurologic (33.9%) and infectious (14.6%) causes. Risk factors for readmission were substance abuse and metabolic disease spectrum. Protective factors were age group 65 to 74 years, private insurance, and treatment in a metropolitan teaching institute. Shoubash and colleagues[59] analyzed long-term QOL and functional outcome after surgical treatment of eloquent and noneloquent CCMs. In eloquent CCMs, functional outcome was worse in 14.6% of patients at long-term follow-up; functional impairment was negligible in noneloquent CCMs. Although QOL was comparable to healthy controls, general health perception and physical and emotional roles were affected in eloquent CCMs. La Rocca and colleagues[60] compared results of a transsulcal versus a transparenchymal approach in 177 patients with CCMs of 2 neurosurgical centers. The investigators discovered higher rates of postoperative seizures and longer lengths of hospital stay in the transsulcal cohort, concluding that a transparenchymal approach is preferable. Clinical features and surgical outcome of the very rare entity of hypothalamic CCMs were reported by Khahera and colleagues.[61] The investigators also provided a systematic review of published cases, leading to an overall number of 28 analyzed datasets, including their own unicenter series of 12 patients from a period of roughly 30 years.

Technical and Anatomic Aspects

Surgical approaches
Several new or particularly challenging approaches to CMs have been described: the transsylvian, transanterior sulcus approach to basal ganglia CMs[62]; the contralateral supracerebellar-transtentorial approach to posterior mediobasal CMs[63]; the supracerebellar infratentorial infratrochlear transquadrangular lobule approach to pontine CM[64]; and the medial tonsillar telovelar approach for resection of a superior medullary velum CM.[65] Woodall and colleagues[66] described approaches for CMs in and around the third ventricle, Campero and colleagues[67] summarized approaches and anatomy of CMs in the mesial temporal region, and Bertanlanffy and colleagues[68] demonstrated optimal access routes for pontine CM resection with preservation of abducens and facial nerve function, concluding that posterolateral approaches may be superior to posteromedial approaches.

Neuromonitoring
Hardian and colleagues[69] described their experience with intraoperative facial motor evoked potential monitoring through the suprafacial triangle approach. In a feasibility study including 11 patients, Le and colleagues[70] reported their technique of direct stimulation of the primary somatosensory pathways helpful in mapping distorted brainstem anatomy. Rauschenbach and colleagues[71] shared their experience with the predictive value of the "standard" neuromonitoring techniques in BSCMs. The investigators found that pneumatocephalus due to semisitting procedures may interfere with the reliability of neuromonitoring.

Imaging
In a prospective randomized clinical trial including 47 patients with BSCMs, Li and colleagues[72] demonstrated that diffusion tensor imaging and diffusion tensor tractography allowed for visualization of anatomic relationships, improving of surgical approach and entry point decision making, and reducing of surgical morbidity in BSCMs. Ille and colleagues[73] investigated the feasibility of noninvasive functional mapping (navigated transcranial magnetic stimulation) in decision making in eloquent CCMs (n = 40); in 90% of cases, the mapping results influenced the indication/strategy for CCM resection, leading to excellent functional outcome results. In a prospective study assessing the reliability of early postoperative MRI to predict CCMs/hemosiderin remnants, the author's group found that imaging, often hampered by artifacts, led to false-positive results in a significant number of patients.[74] In contrast, the reliability of a negative result on early postoperative T2-weighted MRI was relatively high, regarding both hemosiderin and CCM remnants.

Miscellaneous
Malcolm and colleagues[75] performed a feasibility study of MRI-guided laser interstitial thermal therapy on 4 patients with CCMs (poor surgical candidates or refusal of surgery). The investigators found the treatment feasible but associated with high risk of procedure-related complications; several research groups commented on the study.[76–78] Lin and colleagues[79] published their experience with endoscopic resection of deep-seated CCMs adjacent to the pyramidal tract in 6 patients in a technical note. Singh and colleagues[80] described their resection technique of BSCMs in a unicenter series of 46 consecutive patients.

Systematic Reviews and Meta-analyses

Harris and colleagues[20] performed a systematic review and meta-analysis of surgery for CCMs including 70 cohorts with a total of 5098 patients. The primary outcome was a composite of death attributed to CCMs or surgery, nonfatal symptomatic intracerebral hemorrhage, or new/worsened persistent nonhemorrhagic focal neurologic deficit. The investigators found the overall risk of the primary outcome to be 4%, with BSCMs having a higher risk than supratentorial CMs (6% vs 2.4%). Kearns and colleagues[34] performed a systematic review on outcomes of BSCM surgery including 86 studies with 2493 patients. The investigators found that complete resection was achieved in 92.3%, rehemorrhage of residual postoperative BSCMs occurred in 58.6%, and postoperative morbidity occurred in 34.8% of cases; 16.2% of patients had a worsened functional status after surgery, whereas the mortality rate was 1.6%. Mortality in patients with BSCMs was also analyzed by Velz and colleagues,[81] who observed a rate of 2.3% (n = 1251) in conservatively treated patients and 1.3% (n = 3275) in those undergoing surgery. In a decision model, Rinkel and colleagues[82] aimed to evaluate the preferred treatment strategy (radiosurgery, microsurgery, conservative) for patients with symptomatic CCMs by estimating the expected number of quality-adjusted life years and the intracerebral hemorrhage recurrence risk over 5 years. In their model, for CCMs presenting with intracerebral hemorrhage or focal neurologic deficit, conservative management was the first option, whereas for CCMs presenting with epilepsy, CCM intervention should be considered. Another meta-analysis[83] examined the conservative treatment of symptomatic spinal cavernomas and evaluated the efficacy and safety of surgical management of spinal cord CMs in 396 cases (264 surgical vs 132 conservative). The meta-analysis concluded that patients who have experienced a hemorrhagic episode should consider surgical intervention, thereby decreasing the risk of recurrent hemorrhage and further neurologic deterioration. In nonhemorrhagic ISCMs, conservative treatment may be optimal to avoid surgery-related morbidity risks. Shang-Guan and colleagues[84] performed a meta-analysis on the question whether extended compared with standard lesionectomy including hemosiderin rim is required for patients with CRE. No significant differences were identified in the analyzed cohorts, suggesting that extended lesionectomy does not contribute to better seizure control.

CEREBRAL CAVERNOUS MALFORMATION GENES IN THE BIOLOGY OF CEREBRAL CAVERNOUS MALFORMATIONS

CCMs can be classified as sporadic and familial. The familial form is an autosomal dominant disorder, attributable to loss-of-function mutations in any of the 3 CCM genes, *CCM1/KRIT1* (*KREV interaction trapped-1*), *CCM2* (*malcavernin*), and *CCM3/PDCD10* (*programmed cell death 10*). Although *CCM1*, *CCM2*, and *CCM3* are normally expressed in a variety of cell types including neurons, astrocytes, and vascular endothelium,[85,86] loss of individual CCM proteins was found in the affected endothelial cells of all forms of familial CCM.[87] Furthermore, somatic mutations in *CCM1* were also detected in the endothelium of CCM lesions.[88] Increasing evidence identifies the vascular endothelium as the primarily targeted compartment in human CCMs.

The 3 CCM proteins could either function in protein complexes or act individually in a distinct manner.[89] CCM1 interacts with the small Ras-like guanosine triphosphatase RAP1A[90] and integrin cytoplasmic domain-associated protein-1α (ICAP1α)[91] to maintain the integrity of endothelial junctions and regulate integrin ß1-dependent angiogenesis. CCM2 may directly interact with CCM1, whereas CCM2 binds CCM3, assembling a CCM protein complex that is important for protein stability and normal vascularization. Studies carried out in transgenic animal models reported that neuroepithelial expression of *CCM2* is dispensable for vascular development, whereas endothelial-specific ablation of *CCM2* leads to midgestation embryonic death due to failed angiogenesis, and these vascular defects are endothelial autonomous.[92–94] CCM2 regulates p38 and Erk5 mitogen-activated protein kinase (MAPK) via binding the N terminus of MEKK3 and MEKK3-MEK5-Erk5 signaling, which is involved in cell proliferation, cardiovascular development, and CCM pathology.[95,96] *CCM3* was discovered in 2005,[97] the latest among the 3 CCM genes. The functions of the CCM3 protein rely on its N-terminal dimerization domain and its C-terminal focal adhesion targeting homology domain; whereas the former is required for its interaction with the germinal-center kinase (GCK) III protein, the latter is responsible for the direct interactions with CCM2 and other protein partners, such as striatin-interacting phosphatase and kinase (STRIPAK) complexes, phosphatidylinositides, and paxillin. The signaling pathway affected by individual CCM proteins and their complex has been intensively studied.[89,98] CCM genes commonly trigger RhoA-ROCK signaling that is important for controlling cell migration and junction integrity. Activation of RhoA-ROCK is induced on mutation of any one of the CCM genes, indicating the involvement of this signaling in the pathology of CCMs. In addition, the CCM protein complex inhibits MEKK3-MEK5-Erk5 signaling. MAPK signaling activates KLF2/4, which causes CCM lesion formation and endothelial-to-mesenchymal transition (EndMT) in multiple animal models of CCMs.

Angiogenesis is the primary mode of vascularization in the brain, requiring the precise coordination of multiple steps.[99] Aberrant angiogenesis is a typical histologic feature of CCMs. The role of *CCM* genes in the maintenance of vascular integrity and angiogenesis has been intensively studied in the past decades.[93,94,100,101] Immunohistochemistry studies have shown a complete inactivation of CCM1, CCM2, and CCM3 proteins in affected endothelial cells,[87] and somatic mutations in CCM tissue are exclusively present in the affected endothelial cells in all forms of inherited CCMs.[88] A recent study reported that inactivation of *CCM* genes results in accumulation of von Willebrand factor and redistribution of Weibel-Palade bodies in endothelial cells.[102] Silencing individual *CCM* genes in endothelial cells results in a proangiogenesis effect and also reveals distinct endothelial functions of individual *CCM* genes.[103–106] Loss of *CCM3* leads to the most significant stimulation of endothelial angiogenesis among the *CCM* genes; this is consistent with the observation that patients with *CCM3* mutations present earlier onset[107] and a more aggressive form of CCM than those harboring *KRIT1/CCM1* or *CCM2* mutations,[108] suggesting a distinct pathomechanism underlying *CCM3* deficiency. Thus, in spite of the lower mutation rate of *CCM3* (approximately 10%) in patients with familial CCMs,[4] increasing

attention has been paid to CCM3 recently.[109] CCM3 deletion leads to a cell-autonomous deregulated activation of the β-catenin pathway resulting in disorganized cell-cell junctions.[110] He and colleagues[111] demonstrated that vascular endothelial cell-specific deletion of *CCM3* caused defects in embryonic angiogenesis and disrupted the vascular integrity via blocking VEGFR2-dependent signaling and angiogenesis in mice. Knockdown of *CCM3* induced RhoA overexpression and persistent RhoA activation, resulting in inhibition of endothelial cell vessellike tube formation and invasion.[112] Increasing evidence highlights the involvement of endothelial CCM3 in EndMT,[113] apoptosis,[103] and autophagy[114] via various signaling pathways.[115,116] CCM3 and the CCM complex have been shown to regulate the MEKK3-KLF2/4 pathway,[117] of which Rho/ROCK, TGF-β/BMP, and PI3K/Akt/mTOR have been identified as the downstream effectors; this association explains why *CCM3* deficiency affects endothelial junctions, cell proliferation, and autophagy, in addition to inducing EndMT.[118] Inhibition of this pathway has been shown to prevent the formation and progression of CCMs.[119] Loss of CCM3 impairs DLL4-Notch signaling, thereby activating angiogenesis. A further study identified EphB4 forward signaling to be downstream of DLL4-Notch in CCM3-deficient endothelial cells.[105] Inhibition of EphB4 by a specific EphB4 kinase inhibitor rescues the angiogenesis

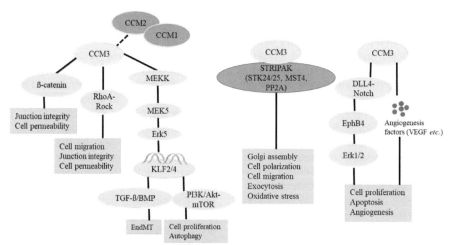

Fig. 2. The key endothelial functions and signaling pathways of CCM3 in CCM. CCM3 alone or in complex with CCM1 and CCM2 (*dashed line*) regulates multiple cellular functions, including cell-cell junction, cell permeability, polarization, migration, and proliferation, apoptosis, autophagy, angiogenesis, and endothelial-to-mesenchymal transition (EndMT) via various signaling pathways. The most well-defined signaling pathways driven by CCM3 or CCM-protein complexes include β-catenin, RhoA-ROCK signaling, MEKK3-MEK5-ERK5-KLF2/4-TGF-β/BMP signaling, and DLL4/Notch-EphB4-Erk1/2 signaling. In addition, CCM3 is a component of the SRIPAK complex that contains multiple proteins such as STK24/25, MST4, and PP2A. Through SRIPAK signaling, CCM3 regulates Golgi assembly, cell migration, neutrophil exocytosis, apoptosis, and oxidative stress.

phenotype in vitro and reduces vascular density in vivo.[104] These studies established a signaling axis of DLL4-Notch/EphB4/Erk1/2 underlying the activated angiogenesis upon *CCM3* deficiency, which provides the potential targets for future therapeutic intervention of CCM. Moreover, an angiogenesis array demonstrated an increase in the release of multiple angiogenesis proteins by *CCM3*-silenced endothelial cells,[102] which may relay upstream signaling pathways as regulators; alternatively, at least in part, it may be the consequence of alterations in pathways mediated by *CCM3* silencing. In addition to forming CCM1-CCM2-CCM3 protein complexes, CCM3 is also a component of the STRIPAK, a multiprotein complex including PP2A, STK24/25, and MST4.[26] Through binding with other proteins in this complex, CCM3 regulates Golgi assembly, cell migration, neutrophil exocytosis, apoptosis, and oxidative stress. The key roles and the underlying signaling pathways affected by CCM3 in CCM are outlined in **Fig. 2**.

Besides the mutation of individual CCM genes, it is most likely that the additional genetic, epigenetic, or local microenvironmental factors determine whether *CCM* gene mutations predispose individuals to CCMs.[88,120] The finding that frequent epigenetic alterations within the PTEN promoter lead to deficiency of its expression in the endothelial cells of familial CCM may support this notion.[106,121] Endothelial cells from the operative specimens of sporadic human CCM exhibit unique angiogenesis properties, suggesting an intrinsic alteration in this CCM type.[99,103] In line with the observation that mice with heterozygous knockout of neither *CCM1*[101,122] nor *CCM2*[92,123] develop vascular lesions in the brain, Gault and colleagues[124] proposed a "two-hit" mechanism in the vascular endothelia of patients with familial CCMs. In addition, nongenetic factors such as oxidative stress, hypoxia, blood flow dynamics, and innate immunity may act as the third hit to activate quiescent *CCM*-deficient endothelial cells. This mechanism may explain the growth of lesions in patients with CCMs and long-term asymptomatic status of many patients with CCMs before bleeding occurs.[98]

At present, surgical treatment of CCMs is the first choice as therapy for symptomatic CCMs. Nevertheless, researchers have attempted pharmacologic intervention of CCMs based on identified mechanisms and signaling pathways. A recent paper has reviewed past and recent developments and concepts in blocking signal pathways to treat CCMs.[14] Among the drugs, the ROCK inhibitor fasudil, β-catenin inhibitor sulindac sulfonate, EphB4 inhibitor NVP-BHG712, and antioxidant tempol have been effective in attenuating different phenotypes including vascular remodeling, cell permeability, angiogenesis, and oxidative stress in cultured endothelial cells; additionally, these molecules also reduced CCM-like lesions in in vivo models of CCMs. Albeit using clinical medications such as statins (atorvastatin and simvastatin) and the nonselective β-adrenergic blocker propanol has been an alternative approach to suppress CCM progression, they have yielded conflicting results. Further screening of small molecules and exploration of approved drugs based on identified altered signaling may be effective for intervention of CCMs in the future.

CLINICS CARE POINTS

- Systematically using and validating available clinical scores for BSCM treatment deepens understanding of and awareness for surgical risk factors in the longterm.

- CRE is a strong argument for surgical treatment of supratentorial CCM.

- DTI seems a helpful tool in planning of BSCM resection.

DISCLOSURE

The authors have nothing to disclose and received no specific funding for this work.

REFERENCES

1. Horne MA, Flemming KD, Su IC, et al. Clinical course of untreated cerebral cavernous malformations: a meta-analysis of individual patient data. Lancet Neurol 2016;15(2):166–73.

2. Taslimi S, Modabbernia A, Amin-Hanjani S, et al. Natural history of cavernous malformation: Systematic review and meta-analysis of 25 studies. Neurology 2016;86(21):1984–91.

3. Dammann P, Jabbarli R, Wittek P, et al. Solitary Sporadic Cerebral Cavernous Malformations: Risk Factors of First or Recurrent Symptomatic Hemorrhage and Associated Functional Impairment. World Neurosurg 2016;91:73–80.

4. Denier C, Labauge P, Bergametti F, et al. Genotype-phenotype correlations in cerebral cavernous malformations patients. Ann Neurol 2006;60(5): 550–6.

5. Dammann P, Saban DV, Herten A, et al. Cerebral cavernous malformations: Prevalence of

cardiovascular comorbidities and allergic diseases compared to the normal population. Eur J Neurol 2021;28(6):2000–5.

6. Chen B, Herten A, Saban D, et al. Hemorrhage from cerebral cavernous malformations: The role of associated developmental venous anomalies. Neurology 2020;95(1):e89–96.

7. Dammann P, Wrede K, Zhu Y, et al. Correlation of the venous angioarchitecture of multiple cerebral cavernous malformations with familial or sporadic disease: a susceptibility-weighted imaging study with 7-Tesla MRI. J Neurosurg 2017;126(2):570–7.

8. Santos AN, Rauschenbach L, Saban D, et al. Natural course of cerebral cavernous malformations in children: a five-year follow-up study. Stroke 2022;53(3):817–24.

9. Al-Shahi Salman R, Hall JM, Horne MA, et al. Untreated clinical course of cerebral cavernous malformations: a prospective, population-based cohort study. Lancet Neurol 2012;11(3):217–24.

10. Zuurbier SM, Hickman CR, Tolias CS, et al. Long-term antithrombotic therapy and risk of intracranial haemorrhage from cerebral cavernous malformations: a population-based cohort study, systematic review, and meta-analysis. Lancet Neurol 2019; 18(10):935–41.

11. Joseph NK, Kumar S, Lanzino G, et al. The Influence of Physical Activity on Cavernous Malformation Hemorrhage. J Stroke Cerebrovasc Dis 2020; 29(4):104629.

12. Joseph NK, Kumar S, Brown RD Jr, et al. Influence of Pregnancy on Hemorrhage Risk in Women With Cerebral and Spinal Cavernous Malformations. Stroke 2021;52(2):434–41.

13. Flemming KD, Kumar S, Brown RD Jr, et al. Predictors of Initial Presentation with Hemorrhage in Patients with Cavernous Malformations. World Neurosurg 2020;133:e767–73.

14. Flemming KD, Brown RD, Link MJ. Seasonal variation in hemorrhage and focal neurologic deficit due to intracerebral cavernous malformations. J Clin Neurosci 2015;22(6):969–71.

15. Chen B, Saban D, Rauscher S, et al. Modifiable Cardiovascular Risk Factors in Patients With Sporadic Cerebral Cavernous Malformations: Obesity Matters. Stroke 2021;52(4):1259–64.

16. Al-Shahi Salman R, Berg MJ, Morrison L, et al. Hemorrhage from cavernous malformations of the brain: definition and reporting standards. Angioma Alliance Scientific Advisory Board. Stroke. 2008; 39(12):3222–30.

17. Moultrie F, Horne MA, Josephson CB, et al. Outcome after surgical or conservative management of cerebral cavernous malformations. Neurology 2014;83(7):582–9.

18. Poorthuis MH, Klijn CJ, Algra A, et al. Treatment of cerebral cavernous malformations: a systematic review and meta-regression analysis. J Neurol Neurosurg Psychiatry 2014;85(12):1319–23.

19. Poorthuis M, Samarasekera N, Kontoh K, et al. Comparative studies of the diagnosis and treatment of cerebral cavernous malformations in adults: systematic review. Acta Neurochir (Wien) 2013;155(4):643–9.

20. Harris L, Poorthuis MHF, Grover P, et al. Surgery for cerebral cavernous malformations: a systematic review and meta-analysis. Neurosurg Rev 2022; 45(1):231–41.

21. Akers A, Al-Shahi Salman R, I AA, et al. Synopsis of Guidelines for the Clinical Management of Cerebral Cavernous Malformations: Consensus Recommendations Based on Systematic Literature Review by the Angioma Alliance Scientific Advisory Board Clinical Experts Panel. Neurosurgery 2017;80(5): 665–80.

22. Rosenow F, Alonso-Vanegas MA, Baumgartner C, et al. Cavernoma-related epilepsy: review and recommendations for management–report of the Surgical Task Force of the ILAE Commission on Therapeutic Strategies. Epilepsia 2013;54(12): 2025–35.

23. Garcia RM, Ivan ME, Lawton MT. Brainstem cavernous malformations: surgical results in 104 patients and a proposed grading system to predict neurological outcomes. Neurosurgery 2015;76(3): 265–77 [discussion: 277–8].

24. Dammann P, Wrede K, Jabbarli R, et al. Of Bubbles and Layers: Which Cerebral Cavernous Malformations are Most Difficult to Dissect From Surrounding Eloquent Brain Tissue? Neurosurgery 2017;81(3): 498–503.

25. Santos AN, Rauschenbach L, Darkwah Oppong M, et al. Assessment and validation of proposed classification tools for brainstem cavernous malformations. J Neurosurg 2020;1–7. https://doi.org/10.3171/2020.6.JNS201585.

26. Catapano JS, Rutledge C, Rumalla K, et al. External validation of the Lawton brainstem cavernous malformation grading system in a cohort of 277 microsurgical patients. J Neurosurg 2021;1–9. https://doi.org/10.3171/2021.3.JNS204291.

27. Lashkarivand A, Ringstad G, Eide PK. Surgery for Brainstem Cavernous Malformations: Association between Preoperative Grade and Postoperative Quality of Life. Oper Neurosurg (Hagerstown) 2020;18(6):590–8.

28. Catapano JS, Rumalla K, Srinivasan VM, et al. A taxonomy for brainstem cavernous malformations: subtypes of midbrain lesions. J Neurosurg 2021;1–20. https://doi.org/10.3171/2021.8.JNS211694.

29. Tsuji Y, Kar S, Bertalanffy H. Microsurgical management of midbrain cavernous malformations: predictors of outcome and lesion classification in 72

patients. Oper Neurosurg (Hagerstown) 2019; 17(6):562–72.

30. Dammann P, Abla AA, Al-Shahi Salman R, et al. Surgical treatment of brainstem cavernous malformations: an international Delphi consensus. J Neurosurg 2021;1–11.

31. Yang Y, Velz J, Neidert MC, et al. The BSCM score: a guideline for surgical decision-making for brainstem cavernous malformations. Neurosurg Rev 2021;45(2):1579–87.

32. Fontanella MM, Bacigaluppi S, Doglietto F, et al. An international call for a new grading system for cerebral and cerebellar cavernomas. J Neurosurg Sci 2021;65(3):239–46.

33. Zanello M, Meyer B, Still M, et al. Surgical resection of cavernous angioma located within eloquent brain areas: International survey of the practical management among 19 specialized centers. Seizure 2019;69:31–40.

34. Kearns KN, Chen CJ, Tvrdik P, et al. Outcomes of Surgery for Brainstem Cavernous Malformations: A Systematic Review. Stroke 2019;50(10):2964–6.

35. Yang Z, Yu G, Zhu W, et al. The benefit and outcome prediction of acute surgery for hemorrhagic brainstem cavernous malformation with impending respiratory failure. J Clin Neurosci 2021; 93:213–20.

36. Xie S, Xiao XR, Xiao SW, et al. Surgical managements and patient outcomes after severe hemorrhagic events from brainstem cavernous malformations. Neurosurg Rev 2021;44(1):423–34.

37. Garcia RM, Oh T, Cole TS, et al. Recurrent brainstem cavernous malformations following primary resection: blind spots, fine lines, and the right-angle method. J Neurosurg 2020;135(3):671–82.

38. Fontanella MM, Agosti E, Zanin L, et al. Cerebral cavernous malformation remnants after surgery: a single-center series with long-term bleeding risk analysis. Neurosurg Rev 2021;44(5):2639–45.

39. Huang C, Bertalanffy H, Kar S, et al. Microsurgical management of midbrain cavernous malformations: does lesion depth influence the outcome? Acta Neurochir (Wien) 2021;163(10):2739–54.

40. Xie MG, Xiao XR, Guo FZ, et al. Surgical Management and Functional Outcomes of Cavernous Malformations Involving the Medulla Oblongata. World Neurosurg 2018;119:e643–52.

41. Herten A, Saban D, Santos AN, et al. The occurrence of neuropathic pain following surgery of brainstem cavernous malformations. Eur J Neurol 2021;29(3):865–72.

42. Dammann P, Herten A, Santos AN, et al. Multimodal outcome assessment after surgery for brainstem cavernous malformations. J Neurosurg 2020; 1–9. https://doi.org/10.3171/2020.6.JNS201823.

43. Nathal E, Patino-Rodriguez HM, Arauz A, et al. Risk Factors for Unfavorable Outcomes in Surgically Treated Brainstem Cavernous Malformations. World Neurosurg 2018;111:e478–84.

44. Al-Shahi Salman R, Kitchen N, Thomson J, et al. Top ten research priorities for brain and spine cavernous malformations. Lancet Neurol 2016; 15(4):354–5.

45. Santos AN, Rauschenbach L, Darkwah Oppong M, et al. Natural course of untreated spinal cord cavernous malformations: a follow-up study within the initial 5 years after diagnosis. J Neurosurg Spine 2021;1–5. https://doi.org/10.3171/2021.9. SPINE211052.

46. Goyal A, Rinaldo L, Alkhataybeh R, et al. Clinical presentation, natural history and outcomes of intramedullary spinal cord cavernous malformations. J Neurol Neurosurg Psychiatry 2019;90(6): 695–703.

47. Liu T, Li K, Wang Y, et al. Treatment strategies and prognostic factors for spinal cavernous malformation: a single-center retrospective cohort study. J Neurosurg Spine 2021;35(6):824–33.

48. Zhang L, Yu X, Qiao G, et al. Long-term surgical outcomes and prognostic factors of adult symptomatic spinal cord cavernous malformations. J Clin Neurosci 2021;90:171–7.

49. Li J, Chen G, Gu S, et al. Surgical Outcomes of Spinal Cord Intramedullary Cavernous Malformation: A Retrospective Study of 83 Patients in a Single Center over a 12-Year Period. World Neurosurg 2018; 118:e105–14.

50. Nagoshi N, Tsuji O, Nakashima D, et al. Clinical outcomes and prognostic factors for cavernous hemangiomas of the spinal cord: a retrospective cohort study. J Neurosurg Spine 2019;31(2):271–8.

51. Ren J, Hong T, He C, et al. Surgical approaches and long-term outcomes of intramedullary spinal cord cavernous malformations: a single-center consecutive series of 219 patients. J Neurosurg Spine 2019;31(1):123–32.

52. Ren J, Hong T, Zeng G, et al. Characteristics and Long-Term Outcome of 20 Children With Intramedullary Spinal Cord Cavernous Malformations. Neurosurgery 2020;86(6):817–24.

53. Josephson CB, Leach JP, Duncan R, et al. Seizure risk from cavernous or arteriovenous malformations: prospective population-based study. Neurology 2011;76(18):1548–54.

54. Yang PF, Pei JS, Jia YZ, et al. Surgical Management and Long-Term Seizure Outcome After Surgery for Temporal Lobe Epilepsy Associated with Cerebral Cavernous Malformations. World Neurosurg 2018;110:e659–70.

55. Schuss P, Marx J, Borger V, et al. Cavernoma-related epilepsy in cavernous malformations located within the temporal lobe: surgical management and seizure outcome. Neurosurg Focus 2020; 48(4):E6.

56. He K, Jiang S, Song J, et al. Long-Term Outcomes of Surgical Treatment in 181 Patients with Supratentorial Cerebral Cavernous Malformation-Associated Epilepsy. World Neurosurg 2017;108: 869–75.

57. Lin Q, Yang PF, Jia YZ, et al. Surgical Treatment and Long-Term Outcome of Cerebral Cavernous Malformations-Related Epilepsy in Pediatric Patients. Neuropediatrics 2018;49(3):173–9.

58. Padarti A, Amritphale A, Eliyas JK, et al. Readmissions in patients with Cerebral Cavernous Malformations (CCMs): a National Readmission Database (NRD) study. J Neurosurg Sci 2021. https://doi.org/10.23736/S0390-5616.21.05605-8.

59. Shoubash L, Baldauf J, Matthes M, et al. Long-term outcome and quality of life after CNS cavernoma resection: eloquent vs. non-eloquent areas. Neurosurg Rev 2022;45(1):649–60.

60. La Rocca G, Ius T, Mazzucchi E, et al. Trans-sulcal versus trans-parenchymal approach in supratentorial cavernomas. A multicentric experience. Clin Neurol Neurosurg 2020;197:106180.

61. Khahera AS, Li Y, Steinberg GK. Cavernous malformations of the hypothalamus: a single-institution series of 12 cases and review of the literature. J Neurosurg 2021;1–10.

62. Kalani MYS, Yagmurlu K, Martirosyan NL, et al. Transsylvian, Transanterior Sulcus Approach to Basal Ganglia Cavernous Malformations. Oper Neurosurg (Hagerstown) 2017;13(6):756.

63. Frisoli FA, Baranoski JF, Catapano JS, et al. Contralateral Supracerebellar-Transtentorial Approach for Posterior Mediobasal Temporal Cavernous Malformation Resection. World Neurosurg 2021;158:166.

64. Rutledge C, Raper DMS, Rodriguez Rubio R, et al. Supracerebellar Infratentorial Infratrochlear Trans-Quadrangular Lobule Approach to Pontine Cavernous Malformations. Oper Neurosurg (Hagerstown) 2021;20(3):268–75.

65. Brogna C, Lavrador JP, Kandeel HS, et al. Medial-tonsillar telovelar approach for resection of a superior medullary velum cerebral cavernous malformation: anatomical and tractography study of the surgical approach and functional implications. Acta Neurochir (Wien) 2021;163(3):625–33.

66. Woodall MN, Catapano JS, Lawton MT, et al. Cavernous Malformations in and Around the Third Ventricle: Indications, Approaches, and Outcomes. Oper Neurosurg (Hagerstown) 2020;18(6):736–46.

67. Campero A, Ajler P, Rica C, et al. Cavernomas and Arteriovenous Malformations in the Mesial Temporal Region: Microsurgical Anatomy and Approaches. Oper Neurosurg (Hagerstown) 2017; 13(1):113–23.

68. Bertalanffy H, Ichimura S, Kar S, et al. Optimal access route for pontine cavernous malformation resection with preservation of abducens and facial nerve function. J Neurosurg 2020;1–10. https://doi.org/10.3171/2020.7.JNS201023.

69. Hardian RF, Goto T, Fujii Y, et al. Intraoperative facial motor evoked potential monitoring for pontine cavernous malformation resection. J Neurosurg 2019;132(1):265–71.

70. Le S, Nguyen V, Lee L, et al. Direct brainstem somatosensory evoked potentials for cavernous malformations. J Neurosurg 2021;1–7. https://doi.org/10.3171/2021.7.JNS21317.

71. Rauschenbach L, Santos AN, Dinger TF, et al. Predictive value of intraoperative neuromonitoring in brainstem cavernous malformation surgery. World Neurosurg 2021;156:e359–73.

72. Li D, Jiao YM, Wang L, et al. Surgical outcome of motor deficits and neurological status in brainstem cavernous malformations based on preoperative diffusion tensor imaging: a prospective randomized clinical trial. J Neurosurg 2018;130(1): 286–301.

73. Ille S, Schroeder A, Hostettler IC, et al. Impacting the Treatment of Highly Eloquent Supratentorial Cerebral Cavernous Malformations by Noninvasive Functional Mapping-An Observational Cohort Study. Oper Neurosurg (Hagerstown) 2021;21(6): 467–77.

74. Chen B, Goricke S, Wrede K, et al. Reliable? The Value of Early Postoperative Magnetic Resonance Imaging after Cerebral Cavernous Malformation Surgery. World Neurosurg 2017;103:138–44.

75. Malcolm JG, Douglas JM, Greven A, et al. Feasibility and morbidity of magnetic resonance imaging-guided stereotactic laser ablation of deep cerebral cavernous malformations: a report of 4 cases. Neurosurgery 2021;89(4):635–44.

76. Traylor JI, Lega B. Commentary: feasibility and morbidity of magnetic resonance imaging-guided stereotactic laser ablation of deep cerebral cavernous malformations: a report of 4 cases. Neurosurgery 2021;89(4):E211–2.

77. Robert SM, Chiang VL. Commentary: feasibility and morbidity of magnetic resonance imaging-guided stereotactic laser ablation of deep cerebral cavernous malformations: a report of 4 cases. Neurosurgery 2021;89(4):E209–10.

78. Awad IA. Commentary: feasibility and morbidity of magnetic resonance imaging-guided stereotactic laser ablation of deep cerebral cavernous malformations: a report of 4 cases. Neurosurgery 2021; 89(4):E207–8.

79. Lin F, Li C, Yan X, et al. Endoscopic Surgery for Supratentorial Deep Cavernous Malformation Adjacent to Cortical Spinal Tract: Preliminary Experience and Technical Note. Front Neurol 2021;12: 678413.

80. Singh H, Elarjani T, da Silva HB, et al. Brain Stem Cavernous Malformations: Operative Nuances of

a Less-Invasive Resection Technique. Oper Neurosurg (Hagerstown) 2018;15(2):153–73.

81. Velz J, Neidert MC, Yang Y, et al. Mortality in Patients with Brainstem Cavernous Malformations. Cerebrovasc Dis 2021;50(5):574–80.

82. Rinkel LA, Al-Shahi Salman R, Rinkel GJ, et al. Radiosurgical, neurosurgical, or no intervention for cerebral cavernous malformations: A decision analysis. Int J Stroke 2019;14(9):939–45.

83. Fotakopoulos G, Kivelev J, Andrade-Barazarte H, et al. Outcome in Patients with Spinal Cavernomas Presenting with Symptoms Due to Mass Effect and/or Hemorrhage: Conservative versus Surgical Management: Meta-analysis of Direct Comparison of Approach-Related Complications. World Neurosurg 2021;152:6–18.

84. Shang-Guan HC, Wu ZY, Yao PS, et al. Is Extended Lesionectomy Needed for Patients with Cerebral Cavernous Malformations Presenting with Epilepsy? A Meta-Analysis. World Neurosurg 2018; 120:e984–90.

85. Petit N, Blecon A, Denier C, et al. Patterns of expression of the three cerebral cavernous malformation (CCM) genes during embryonic and postnatal brain development. Gene Expr Patterns 2006;6(5):495–503.

86. Seker A, Pricola KL, Guclu B, et al. CCM2 expression parallels that of CCM1. Stroke 2006;37(2): 518–23.

87. Pagenstecher A, Stahl S, Sure U, et al. A two-hit mechanism causes cerebral cavernous malformations: complete inactivation of CCM1, CCM2 or CCM3 in affected endothelial cells. Hum Mol Genet 2009;18(5):911–8.

88. Akers AL, Johnson E, Steinberg GK, et al. Biallelic somatic and germline mutations in cerebral cavernous malformations (CCMs): evidence for a two-hit mechanism of CCM pathogenesis. Hum Mol Genet 2009;18(5):919–30.

89. Su VL, Calderwood DA. Signalling through cerebral cavernous malformation protein networks. Open Biol 2020;10(11):200263.

90. Glading A, Han J, Stockton RA, et al. KRIT-1/CCM1 is a Rap1 effector that regulates endothelial cell cell junctions. J Cell Biol 2007;179(2):247–54.

91. Dashti SR, Hoffer A, Hu YC, et al. Molecular genetics of familial cerebral cavernous malformations. Neurosurg Focus 2006;21(1):e2.

92. Kleaveland B, Zheng X, Liu JJ, et al. Regulation of cardiovascular development and integrity by the heart of glass-cerebral cavernous malformation protein pathway. Nat Med 2009;15(2): 169–76.

93. Whitehead KJ, Chan AC, Navankasattusas S, et al. The cerebral cavernous malformation signaling pathway promotes vascular integrity via Rho GTPases. Nat Med 2009;15(2):177–84.

94. Boulday G, Blecon A, Petit N, et al. Tissue-specific conditional CCM2 knockout mice establish the essential role of endothelial CCM2 in angiogenesis: implications for human cerebral cavernous malformations. Dis Model Mech 2009;2(3–4):168–77.

95. Uhlik MT, Abell AN, Johnson NL, et al. Rac-MEKK3-MKK3 scaffolding for p38 MAPK activation during hyperosmotic shock. Nat Cell Biol 2003;5(12): 1104–10.

96. Fisher OS, Deng H, Liu D, et al. Structure and vascular function of MEKK3-cerebral cavernous malformations 2 complex. Nat Commun 2015;6: 7937.

97. Bergametti F, Denier C, Labauge P, et al. Mutations within the programmed cell death 10 gene cause cerebral cavernous malformations. Am J Hum Genet 2005;76(1):42–51.

98. Abdelilah-Seyfried S, Tournier-Lasserve E, Derry WB. Blocking Signalopathic Events to Treat Cerebral Cavernous Malformations. Trends Mol Med 2020;26(9):874–87.

99. Risau W. Mechanisms of angiogenesis. Nature 1997;386(6626):671–4.

100. Voss K, Stahl S, Hogan BM, et al. Functional analyses of human and zebrafish 18-amino acid in-frame deletion pave the way for domain mapping of the cerebral cavernous malformation 3 protein. Hum Mutat 2009;30(6):1003–11.

101. Whitehead KJ, Plummer NW, Adams JA, et al. Ccm1 is required for arterial morphogenesis: implications for the etiology of human cavernous malformations. Development 2004;131(6):1437–48.

102. Much CD, Sendtner BS, Schwefel K, et al. Inactivation of Cerebral Cavernous Malformation Genes Results in Accumulation of von Willebrand Factor and Redistribution of Weibel-Palade Bodies in Endothelial Cells. Front Mol Biosci 2021;8:622547.

103. Zhu Y, Wu Q, Xu JF, et al. Differential angiogenesis function of CCM2 and CCM3 in cerebral cavernous malformations. Neurosurg Focus 2010;29(3):E1.

104. You C, Zhao K, Dammann P, et al. EphB4 forward signalling mediates angiogenesis caused by CCM3/PDCD10-ablation. J Cell Mol Med 2017; 21(9):1848–58.

105. You C, Sandalcioglu IE, Dammann P, et al. Loss of CCM3 impairs DLL4-Notch signalling: implication in endothelial angiogenesis and in inherited cerebral cavernous malformations. J Cell Mol Med 2013;17(3):407–18.

106. Zhu Y, Peters C, Hallier-Neelsen M, et al. Phosphatase and tensin homolog in cerebral cavernous malformation: a potential role in pathological angiogenesis. J Neurosurg 2009;110(3):530–9.

107. Riant F, Bergametti F, Fournier HD, et al. CCM3 Mutations Are Associated with Early-Onset Cerebral Hemorrhage and Multiple Meningiomas. Mol Syndromol 2013;4(4):165–72.

108. Shenkar R, Shi C, Rebeiz T, et al. Exceptional aggressiveness of cerebral cavernous malformation disease associated with PDCD10 mutations. Genet Med 2015;17(3):188–96.

109. Valentino M, Dejana E, Malinverno M. The multifaceted gene. Genes Dis 2021;8(6):798–813.

110. Bravi L, Rudini N, Cuttano R, et al. Sulindac metabolites decrease cerebrovascular malformations in CCM3-knockout mice. Proc Natl Acad Sci U S A 2015;112(27):8421–6.

111. He Y, Zhang H, Yu L, et al. Stabilization of VEGFR2 signaling by cerebral cavernous malformation 3 is critical for vascular development. Sci Signal 2010; 3(116):ra26.

112. Borikova AL, Dibble CF, Sciaky N, et al. Rho kinase inhibition rescues the endothelial cell cerebral cavernous malformation phenotype. J Biol Chem 2010;285(16):11760–4.

113. Maddaluno L, Rudini N, Cuttano R, et al. EndMT contributes to the onset and progression of cerebral cavernous malformations. Nature 2013; 498(7455):492–6.

114. Marchi S, Corricelli M, Trapani E, et al. Defective autophagy is a key feature of cerebral cavernous malformations. EMBO Mol Med 2015;7(11): 1403–17.

115. Jenny Zhou H, Qin L, Zhang H, et al. Endothelial exocytosis of angiopoietin-2 resulting from CCM3 deficiency contributes to cerebral cavernous malformation. Nat Med 2016;22(9):1033–42.

116. Zhou Z, Tang AT, Wong WY, et al. Cerebral cavernous malformations arise from endothelial gain of MEKK3-KLF2/4 signalling. Nature 2016; 532(7597):122–6.

117. Renz M, Otten C, Faurobert E, et al. Regulation of beta1 integrin-Klf2-mediated angiogenesis by CCM proteins. Dev Cell 2015;32(2):181–90.

118. Snellings DA, Hong CC, Ren AA, et al. Cerebral Cavernous Malformation: From Mechanism to Therapy. Circ Res 2021;129(1):195–215.

119. Choi JP, Wang R, Yang X, et al. Ponatinib (AP24534) inhibits MEKK3-KLF signaling and prevents formation and progression of cerebral cavernous malformations. Sci Adv 2018;4(11): eaau0731.

120. Patterson C. Torturing a blood vessel. Nat Med 2009;15(2):137–8.

121. Zhu Y, Wloch A, Wu Q, et al. Involvement of PTEN promoter methylation in cerebral cavernous malformations. Stroke 2009;40(3):820–6.

122. Plummer NW, Gallione CJ, Srinivasan S, et al. Loss of p53 sensitizes mice with a mutation in Ccm1 (KRIT1) to development of cerebral vascular malformations. Am J Pathol 2004;165(5):1509–18.

123. Plummer NW, Squire TL, Srinivasan S, et al. Neuronal expression of the Ccm2 gene in a new mouse model of cerebral cavernous malformations. Mamm Genome 2006;17(2):119–28.

124. Gault J, Awad IA, Recksiek P, et al. Cerebral cavernous malformations: somatic mutations in vascular endothelial cells. Neurosurgery 2009; 65(1):138–44 [discussion: 144–5].

Cavernous Malformations and Artificial Intelligence
Machine Learning Applications

Benjamin K. Hendricks, MD[a], Kavelin Rumalla, MD[a], Dimitri Benner, BS[a], Michael T. Lawton, MD[b],*

KEYWORDS

- Artificial intelligence • Cavernoma • Cavernous malformation • Deep learning • Machine learning
- Model • Statistics • Vascular

KEY POINTS

- Artificial intelligence (AI), comprising machine learning (ML) and deep learning applications, has a demonstrated ability to augment clinical decision-making.
- Enhanced developments in AI are positioned to expand its role in routine clinical and subspecialty care.
- Quantifiable schemes for clinical pathology characterization and decision-making enable the future application of AI, such as the brainstem cavernous malformation (BSCM) approach triangles and anatomic taxonomy.
- Combining applications of augmented reality with ML provides a promising frontier for intraoperative surgical guidance using algorithms or possibly fully automated shared-control or supervisory-controlled surgical robotics.

INTRODUCTION

To effectively discuss the applications of artificial intelligence (AI) to treating cerebral cavernous malformations (CCMs), we must first define the concepts covered within the realm of AI. AI is generically referred to as the methodology by which machines achieve a simulated intelligence to permit decision-making by using explicit algorithms that determine how data are processed.[1] A subset of algorithms designed to be used in AI can be classified as machine learning (ML) applications; these applications represent a developmental outgrowth of AI. To be categorized as ML, the algorithm must provide sufficient complexity to permit it to learn from the experience provided by exposure to data, without explicitly programming the learned behaviors.[1]

Importantly, both AI and ML applications are encountered within multiple aspects of daily life—common examples include online shopping suggestions, self-driving cars, speech recognition, and an email spam filter.[2] The type of this application that is more relevant to the field of science places central importance on the probabilistic framework and allows for sufficiently programmed algorithms to surpass human capabilities of data analysis to uncover predictions and elucidate consequences hidden within large data sets. The critical effectors for applying ML are the data inputs and the type of learning adopted by the algorithm; therefore, each application can be unique, based on differing data inputs and learning models.[2] Learning models can be generically grouped into 4 main types: supervised, semi-supervised, unsupervised, and

Financial Support: None.

[a] Department of Neurosurgery, Barrow Neurological Institute, St. Joseph's Hospital and Medical Center, Phoenix, AZ, USA; [b] Department of Neurosurgery, c/o Neuroscience Publications, Barrow Neurological Institute, St. Joseph's Hospital and Medical Center, 350 West Thomas Road, Phoenix, AZ 85013, USA

* Corresponding author.

E-mail address: Neuropub@barrowneuro.org

reinforcement.[3] The type of learning model determines the method by which input variables are analyzed and translated into predicted outcomes.

ML algorithms have been used in clinical applications recently, with speculation that the use of ML can positively impact all phases of clinical care: diagnosis, treatment, clinical workflow, availability of clinical expertise, and prognosis.[4] The neurosurgery literature is rich with interest in AI and ML applications, in large part because the morbid nature of many neurosurgical pathologies and the data-rich clinical care record bait scientific interest and exploration to advance the management of neurosurgical pathologies. A systematic review in 2018 using the terms "artificial intelligence" and "neurosurgery" revealed 23 evaluated studies that discussed 34 ML models.[2] In each study analyzed, the comparison of results of the ML model with clinicians' results showed a median absolute improvement of prediction accuracy of 13% and area under the curve of 0.14 (range: 0.03–0.27; interquartile range: 0.07–0.21).[2] Some examples of the outputs included were differentiating pituitary adenoma, craniopharyngioma, and Rathke cleft cyst[5]; differentiating between benign and malignant soft-tissue tumors, including neural tumors[6]; and automated seizure detection in patients with epilepsy.[7] These findings highlight the potential ML models have for making more accurate and efficacious clinical predictions than humans.

Given the promise that ML models hold for clinical medicine and neurosurgery, our discussion will focus on the potential applications of ML within vascular neurosurgery. Recent ML applications emerging in vascular neurosurgery include models to detect aneurysm rupture or predictive features of rupture,[8] identify risk factors for cerebral or myocardial infarction after carotid endarterectomy,[9] and conduct the differential diagnosis of moyamoya disease.[10] ML applications, particularly for CCMs, were not represented within the 2018 systematic review[2] or our literature review. In fact, only 1 published study adopted an ML algorithm for CCMs.[11] In that study, an ML algorithm was used to weight and cluster candidate biomarkers to determine a diagnosis of CCM, predict risk for future hemorrhage, and monitor for a response to therapy.[11]

In this article, we discuss the future of ML applications within CCM, expanding beyond what has been published or discussed within the literature. This discussion will hopefully stimulate future developments to enhance the role of AI in patients with CCMs and ultimately translate to enhanced clinical care.

DISCUSSION

ML applications have a large role within the field of vascular neurosurgery and, more specifically, in the care of patients with CCMs. In the era of "big data," patient-centered outcomes research provides the essential building blocks for designing ML algorithms. The management of CCMs can be grouped by the answers to 2 major questions: Should the lesion be observed or resected microsurgically? How should the CCM be approached safely? ML algorithms could potentially address both of these questions and work adjunctively with clinical insight and judgment. Recent studies provide the mathematical ingredients in terms of supervised inputs and outputs.[12–15] These inputs are relevant to the desired output from the model, such that if the model has the goal of predicting the optimal cranial approach and intracranial path to the lesion, the inputs include preoperative baseline characteristics, radiographic anatomic metrics, and postoperative characteristics. These types of data permit the model to make a differential assessment between preoperative and postoperative characteristics to identify the ideal clinical outcome and determine the anatomic corollary features that portend a better clinical outcome.

Brainstem Cavernous Malformation Classifications

Brainstem cavernous malformation grading system

The brainstem cavernous malformation (BSCM) grading system proposed in 2015[14] collapses numerous variables into a manageable list of factors proven to influence neurologic outcomes after surgery. The grading system is scored on a scale of 0 to 7 with points assigned for patient age (0 for ≤40 years; 2 for >40), lesion size (0 for ≤2 cm; 1 for >2 cm), lesion crossing brainstem midpoint (0 for no; 1 for yes), presence of developmental venous anomaly (0 for no; 1 for yes), and time from most recent hemorrhage to surgery (0 for acute [0–3 weeks]; 1 for subacute [3–8 weeks]; and 2 for chronic [>8 weeks]).[14] To date, the BSCM grading system has been both internally and externally validated with an area under the curve of 0.74, which is considered adequate by commonly accepted statistical standards.[16]

The validated quantitative scoring system provides the necessary ingredients for a complete ML algorithm that predicts the likelihood of favorable outcomes after surgery for BSCM. The grading system based on the supervised ML model favors surgery for patients with low-grade BSCMs and observation of patients with high-grade BSCMs, with varying boundaries of operability and nonoperability for intermediate-grade BSCMs. The generalizability of such grading systems has major limitations, particularly considering that outcomes data were derived from surgeons with a combined experience of more than 700 BSCM resections. Future advanced applications may integrate image recognition software to capture the radiologic components automatically (eg, BSCM size, presence of developmental venous anomaly, crossing the axial midpoint) and thus allow the BSCM score to be automatically calculated. A continuous input data stream would ultimately enhance the algorithm's ability to predict outcomes and possibly identify novel associations between patient and lesion characteristics and surgical outcomes.

Brainstem cavernous malformation anatomic taxonomy

The adoption of BSCM and CCM subtyping that encompasses the surgical approach (ie, cranial approach and intracerebral pathway components, such as cranial triangles and safe entry zones) can categorically divide data to permit ML analyses, recommendations, and predictions, which will further enhance the role of ML in surgical CCM management. This subtyping was recently proposed in a novel anatomic taxonomy for BSCMs aiming to improve diagnostic acumen at the bedside, help identify the optimal surgical approach and preferred entry zone, enhance consistency of academic communications, and improve patient outcomes.[15] Variables of the taxonomy may serve as inputs for ML algorithms. The taxonomy consists of the type or brainstem level (midbrain, pons, medulla) and subtype or closest surface presentation (based on the direction on a horizontal plane, named according to regional anatomy). We found that each subtype of BSCM was associated with a recognizable constellation of neurologic symptoms or signs that were explained by the involvement of specific tracts and cranial nerve nuclei within the brainstem. The taxonomy defines 5 midbrain, 6 pontine, and 5 medullary subtypes (**Table 1**).

Midbrain lesions A single surgical approach unique to each subtype was favored for greater than 90% of cases in a series of 151 surgically resected midbrain BSCMs classified into 5 subtypes.[15] Interpeduncular midbrain lesions were located anteriorly in the interpeduncular fossa, and patients were most likely to present with ipsilateral oculomotor nerve palsy and contralateral cerebellar ataxia or dyscoordination. Peduncle midbrain lesions were associated with contralateral hemiparesis and ipsilateral oculomotor nerve

palsy. Tegmental midbrain lesions were most likely to cause a variety of contralateral hemisensory deficits. Patients with quadrigeminal midbrain lesions presented with features of Parinaud syndrome. Periaqueductal lesions were most likely to cause obstructive hydrocephalus. For midbrain lesions, favorable outcomes with a modified Rankin Scale score of 2 or lower were observed in 81% of patients with follow-up data (110 of 136).

Pontine lesions By studying 323 surgically resected pontine lesions, a classification of 6 subtypes was developed.[15] Basilar pontine lesions, although rare, were located in the anteromedial pons and associated with hemiparesis. Peritrigeminal pontine lesions (anterolateral pons) were associated with hemiparesis and hemibody sensory symptoms. Middle peduncular pontine lesions (lateral pons) were associated with a milder form of anterior inferior cerebellar artery syndrome with contralateral hemisensory loss, ipsilateral ataxia, ipsilateral facial numbness, and hemiparesis without cranial neuropathies. Inferior peduncular lesions (inferolateral pons) were associated with acute vestibular syndrome, ataxia, and sensory deficits. Rhomboid lesions presented to the superior portion of the 4th ventricular floor and were associated with diplopia, dysconjugate eye movements, and ipsilateral facial weakness for larger lesions. Supraolivary lesions surface at the ventral pontine underbelly, for which ipsilateral abducens palsy was a strong localizing sign.

Medullary lesions Medullary lesions were classified into 5 subtypes based on 77 surgically resected cases.[15] Pyramidal lesions (anterior medulla) were associated with hemiparesis and hypoglossal nerve palsy. Olivary lesions (anterolateral medulla) were associated with ataxia related to damage to the olivary nuclei. Cuneate lesions (posterolateral medulla) were associated with ipsilateral upper extremity sensory symptoms. Gracile lesions (posterior medulla) were associated with ipsilateral lower extremity sensory deficits. Trigonal lesions presented to the medullary surface of the 4th ventricle floor and were associated with severe nausea and vomiting (area postrema) and occasionally diplopia.

Two-point method

These symptom-subtype correlates can serve as distinct inputs to guide ML lesion location predictions that facilitate surgical approach planning. In addition, established concepts such as the "two-point-method"[17] can be integrated into ML applications. These variables, however, are thus far able to be used only to calculate the most favorable craniotomy and angle to the lesion, which

Table 1
Brainstem cavernous malformation taxonomy

Location	Lesion Types
Midbrain	Interpeduncular, peduncular, tegmental, quadrigeminal, periaqueductal
Pons	Basilar, peritrigeminal, middle peduncular, inferior peduncular, rhomboid, supraolivary
Medulla	Pyramidal, olivary, trigonal, gracile, cuneate

introduces the first and guides the final steps of the surgery, without appropriate consideration of the subarachnoid and cisternal and parenchymal components of a successful BSCM resection.

Cranial Approach Triangles

To safely navigate the long and delicate corridors that need to be traversed to reach the brainstem, a specific set of anatomic triangles for BSCM resection was defined. These triangles add an additional "iron-sight," based on surrounding anatomic structures, that guides the microsurgeon toward the lesion. Importantly, this type of navigation is not affected by the brain shift that frequently renders neuronavigation technology inaccurate, especially in deep approaches. Furthermore, the anatomic triangles provide vision and a trajectory based on borders toward a target that is often clouded by the sequelae of previous hemorrhages and parenchymal distortion.

Five triangles were previously known and most notably used for skull-base approaches to vascular structures in and around the cavernous sinus.[18–22] These 5 are the carotid-oculomotor triangle, oculomotor-tentorial triangle, postero-medial (Kawase) triangle, glossopharyngeal-cochlear triangle, and vagoaccessory triangle (with its 3 encompassing triangles: supra-hypoglossal triangle, hypoglossal-hypoglossal triangle, and infrahypoglossal triangle). Nine triangles were newly defined for BSCM resection: the supracerebellar-supratrochlear, supracerebellar-infratrochlear, infragalenic, supratrigeminal, infratrigeminal, interlobular, vertebrobasilar junction, subtonsillar, and the vallecular triangles. These triangles provide an incredibly accurate layer of data entry for ML systems to characterize the dissection pathway and fill in the blank between craniotomy and lesion, with a set number of variables as 3 (or at times 4) borders, and their specific contents.

The anatomic triangles were further conceptualized in a way to supplement the BSCM taxonomy, such that each subtype is assigned to a set

number of triangles, with specific craniotomies and surgical approaches between these 2 variables. In the example of midbrain lesions, a quadrigeminal subtype is to be resected only through the infragalenic triangle (after torcular craniotomy and supracerebellar-infratentorial [SCIT]-midline approach), whereas tegmental subtypes can be resected through supracerebellar-supratrochlear and supracerebellar-infratrochlear triangles, based on the laterality of the lesion and the prior decision to use a torcular craniotomy and SCIT-paramedian approach, or lateral suboccipital craniotomy and SCIT-lateral approach. Additionally, the resection of peduncular subtypes is guided through either a supracerebellar-infratrochlear or a carotid-oculomotor triangle, whereas the interpeduncular subtype should be approached only through the carotid-oculomotor triangle.

Brainstem triangles provide the last coordinates of subarachnoid trajectory after the craniotomy and surgical approach have been executed. These 3 components can feed the ML system enough information to define an accurate and safe approach to a lesion on a parenchymal surface.

Safe Entry Zones

For ML to guide the resection of deep CMs covered by eloquent tissue, a final component needs to be added to a system that aims to replicate or improve on current microsurgical capabilities. Safe entry zones (SEZs), often defined in anatomic laboratories based on cadaveric dissection, enable the transgression of brainstem tissue with minimal postoperative deficits. The 21 originally defined SEZs, however, have a limited level of evidence due to their cadaveric origin and the scarcity of clinical cases in which they have been used.

A separate, single-surgeon series analyzed 154 BSCM resections whereby SEZs were used in 72 cases (unpublished data). Importantly, no differences in postoperative outcomes were found between patients who underwent brainstem transgression through SEZs and those who had superficial or exophytic lesions (final modified Rankin Scale score >2 in 19.7% and 21.2%, respectively; $P = .83$). In this series, the new middle cerebellar peduncle SEZ was also defined. For the purposes of ML applications, we emphasize that all 22 SEZs were matched to their respective triangles in an effort to streamline the surgical excision model and to add the final component that enables safe parenchymal transgression.

For midbrain lesions, the infragalenic triangle leads to the infracollicular, supracollicular, and intercollicular SEZs. The supracerebellar-infratrochlear and supracerebellar-supratrochlear triangles both lead to the lateral mesencephalic sulcus SEZ, whereas the carotid-oculomotor triangle guides the surgeon toward the interpeduncular zone. Pontine lesions show triangle-SEZ correlates as follows: oculomotor-tentorial triangle and anterior mesencephalic zone, posteromedial and supratrigeminal triangles and supratrigeminal SEZ, interlobular triangle and middle cerebellar peduncle SEZ, infratrigeminal triangle and infratrigeminal SEZ, glossopharyngo-cochlear triangle and pontomedullary sulcus SEZ, and vallecular triangle leading toward the median sulcus SEZ as well as the superior foveal and suprafacial collicular zones. Medullary lesions are also resected through the vallecular triangle, but they are accessed through the posterior median sulcus SEZ or the infrafacial collicular zone. Additional medullary triangle and SEZ connections were the subtonsillar triangle and posterior intermediate sulcus and area acustica SEZs; the vagoaccessory triangles and lateral medullary, olivary, retro-olivary, and pontomedullary sulcus SEZs; and the junctional triangle with the anterolateral sulcus.

Another nominal variable, the SEZ, which complements all previously described inputs can thus be added to the ML algorithm, as can each SEZ's specific associations to the respective anatomic triangles.

Future Development

ML algorithms could be used to inform a neurosurgeon's decision of surgical resection versus conservative observation to enhance this decision. An article by Girard and colleagues[11] presented an ML algorithm for predicting the risk for future symptomatic hemorrhage within CCMs based on a biomarker panel. A more extensive repository of input data could conceivably generalize the predictive capability of this model to allow a neurosurgeon to make hemorrhage risk predictions that are personalized to patients based on demographic and radiographic features and could potentially be serum-biomarker driven. This hemorrhage risk score could be contrasted to the likelihood of a clinical adverse event associated with the resection of a CCM within the region of the patient's specific lesion and predict the optimal treatment strategy (ie, conservative observation vs surgical resection).

Augmented reality (AR) is a critical component of many neurosurgical operating rooms today, given the prolific use of neuronavigation with a multitude of supportive publications since its introduction in 1996.[23] Other investigations within the realm of AR devices for surgical applications include overlaying patient anatomy within a head-mounted display (HMD).[24] Given that ML would be capable of inputting immense data sets, such as those capacitating surgical procedure techniques, it is conceivable that this type of application could provide real-time feedback to the surgeon regarding the surgical approach or technique through an HMD output. This feedback could take the form of an in situ visualization of anatomy with guidance markers along a CCM approach path, such that the guidance markers have been generated based on an ML analysis of cranial approach trajectories provided in learning data sets. This information would permit an ML algorithm to output planned trajectory paths based on simple inputs, such as the lesion location and, optionally, the entry site, and guide the surgeon through AR markers within the HMD. This combined application of AR and ML within the operating room for surgical guidance could be the next step toward automated or semi-automated robotic surgery. If the ML algorithms had enough surgeon-guided test cases, the model would be capable of predicting and outputting the appropriate compensatory response to an operative event, such as a vascular injury.

CCM resection surgeries provide the ideal test case environment for ML algorithms to learn, given that many of the patients with CCM have relatively normal adjacent anatomy and can be approached in a standardized manner (as described in the "Cranial Approach Triangles" section above). This reduced variability within the data set would enhance the predictive capabilities of such an algorithm. Overall, the functional logic for educating the ML model is seemingly identical to that of a surgeon-trainee, who must observe the appropriate response to various operative events to output the correct response to future events. Given the rapid development of more capable ML learning models and capabilities even within the field of neurosurgery, we believe that this lofty goal is within the reach of the field of neurosurgery in the near future.

ML models certainly face an immense challenge within the realm of clinical practice, given changing treatment paradigms and sometimes sparse data to support model generation. The availability of high-quality data poses a significant barrier to model generation. When the model is being generated, it must be trained with data that resemble the real-world it is expected to input. Within the realm of clinical care, this model generation requires a diverse data set originating from a system notorious for poor data quality, such as the quality of traditional electronic health records. If the ML model is expected to input this poor quality data for predictive outcomes, it will be trained with low-quality noisy data, which will translate to noisy outputs.[4] Given the need for access to large data sets for ML algorithm training, the issue of data privacy and regulatory hurdles also pose a barrier to developing these efforts.

SUMMARY

Neurosurgeons use an immense number of inputs to make clinical care decisions each day, whether it is the decision to operate on the patient or the technique with which to remove a CCM from the brainstem. As ML capabilities continue to be enhanced, the inputs being analyzed by the neurosurgeon's brain to inform clinical decisions can be augmented or perhaps replaced in some scenarios by computer-based ML models. ML models represent an opportunity for neurosurgeons to enhance their data-driven decision-making to facilitate enhanced clinical outcomes for patients. Model concepts must combine the realm of surgical approach planning, decision-making surrounding surgical management that balances hemorrhage risk with surgical resection risk, and the role of augmented reality with ML to enhance future clinical care for patients with CCMs.

CLINICS CARE POINTS

- Although no ML-based clinical tools are currently used in standard care for neurosurgical pathologies, ML applications have a promising role across numerous pathologies, including CCM.

- With recent developments in the BSCM grading system, anatomic subtype taxonomy, and triangle and safe entry zone structure, future efforts may strive for multi-institutional cross-validation and design of ML algorithms to assist patient counseling and surgical decision-making.

ACKNOWLEDGMENTS

The authors thank the staff of Neuroscience Publications at Barrow Neurological Institute for assistance with article preparation.

DISCLOSURE

B.K. Hendricks and M.T. Lawton are inventors on a pending patent related to an ML application for technical intraoperative guidance.

REFERENCES

1. Ghahramani Z. Probabilistic machine learning and artificial intelligence. Nature 2015;521(7553):452–9.
2. Senders JT, Arnaout O, Karhade AV, et al. Natural and artificial intelligence in neurosurgery: a systematic review. Neurosurgery 2018;83(2):181–92.
3. Obermeyer Z, Emanuel EJ. Predicting the future - big data, machine learning, and clinical medicine. N Engl J Med 2016;375(13):1216–9.
4. Rajkomar A, Dean J, Kohane I. Machine learning in medicine. N Engl J Med 2019;380(14):1347–58.
5. Kitajima M, Hirai T, Katsuragawa S, et al. Differentiation of common large sellar-suprasellar masses effect of artificial neural network on radiologists' diagnosis performance. Acad Radiol 2009;16(3):313–20.
6. Juntu J, Sijbers J, De Backer S, et al. Machine learning study of several classifiers trained with texture analysis features to differentiate benign from malignant soft-tissue tumors in T1-MRI images. J Magn Reson Imaging 2010;31(3):680–9.
7. Duun-Henriksen J, Kjaer TW, Madsen RE, et al. Channel selection for automatic seizure detection. Clin Neurophysiol 2012;123(1):84–92.
8. Silva MA, Patel J, Kavouridis V, et al. Machine learning models can detect aneurysm rupture and identify clinical features associated with rupture. World Neurosurg 2019;131:e46–51.
9. Bai P, Zhou Y, Liu Y, et al. Risk Factors of cerebral infarction and myocardial infarction after carotid endarterectomy analyzed by machine learning. Comput Math Methods Med 2020;2020:6217392.
10. Akiyama Y, Mikami T, Mikuni N. Deep learning-based approach for the diagnosis of moyamoya disease. J Stroke Cerebrovasc Dis 2020;29(12):105322.
11. Girard R, Li Y, Stadnik A, et al. A roadmap for developing plasma diagnostic and prognostic biomarkers of cerebral cavernous angioma with symptomatic hemorrhage (CASH). Neurosurgery 2021;88(3):686–97.
12. Santos AN, Rauschenbach L, Darkwah Oppong M, et al. Assessment and validation of proposed classification tools for brainstem cavernous malformations. J Neurosurg 2020;16:1–7.

13. Lashkarivand A, Ringstad G, Eide PK. Surgery for brainstem cavernous malformations: association between preoperative grade and postoperative quality of life. Oper Neurosurg (Hagerstown) 2020;18(6): 590–8.

14. Garcia RM, Ivan ME, Lawton MT. Brainstem cavernous malformations: surgical results in 104 patients and a proposed grading system to predict neurological outcomes. Neurosurgery 2015;76(3): 265–77 [discussion: 277-268].

15. Catapano JS, Rumalla K, Srinivasan VM, et al. A taxonomy for brainstem cavernous malformations: subtypes of midbrain lesions. J Neurosurg 2021;17: 1–20.

16. Catapano JS, Rutledge C, Rumalla K, et al. External validation of the Lawton brainstem cavernous malformation grading system in a cohort of 277 microsurgical patients. J Neurosurg 2021;1–9.

17. Brown AP, Thompson BG, Spetzler RF. The two-point method: evaluating brain stem lesions. Barrow Q 1996;12(1).

18. Youssef AS, Abdel Aziz KM, Kim EY, et al. The carotid-oculomotor window in exposure of upper basilar artery aneurysms: a cadaveric morphometric study. Neurosurgery 2004;54(5):1181–7 [discussion: 1187-1189].

19. Tayebi Meybodi A, Gandhi S, Mascitelli J, et al. The oculomotor-tentorial triangle. Part 1: microsurgical anatomy and techniques to enhance exposure. J Neurosurg 2018;1:1–9.

20. Kanzaki J, Kawase T, Sano K, et al. A modified extended middle cranial fossa approach for acoustic tumors. Arch Otorhinolaryngol 1977;217(1): 119–21.

21. Surek CC, Van Ess M, Stephens R. Acousticofacial-glossopharyngeal triangle: an anatomic model for rapid surgical orientation. Skull Base 2010;20(3): 139–42.

22. Rodriguez-Hernandez A, Lawton MT. Anatomical triangles defining surgical routes to posterior inferior cerebellar artery aneurysms. J Neurosurg 2011; 114(4):1088–94.

23. Meola A, Cutolo F, Carbone M, et al. Augmented reality in neurosurgery: a systematic review. Neurosurg Rev 2017;40(4):537–48.

24. Nguyen NQ, Cardinell J, Ramjist JM, et al. An augmented reality system characterization of placement accuracy in neurosurgery. J Clin Neurosci 2020;72:392–6.

Application of Big Data in Vascular Neurosurgery

Moleca M. Ghannam, MD[a], Jason M. Davies, MD, PhD[a,b,c],*

KEYWORDS

- Big data • Machine learning • Artificial intelligence • Vascular neurosurgery • Registry
- Intracranial aneurysm • Carotid stenosis • Moyamoya

KEY POINTS

- Big data is characterized by the 5 Vs—volume, variety, velocity, value, and veracity—all of which are important in the consideration of study design.
- Randomized controlled trials are the gold standard, but due to the demanding nature, pragmatic research designs, including registries and registry-based randomized controlled trial, are growing in popularity.
- More than 50% of big data studies are focused on intracranial aneurysms, although in less frequency, studies also focus on arteriovenous malformation, carotid stenosis, intracranial atherosclerotic disease, and moyamoya.
- Big data studies have a key role in quality improvement studies assessing outcomes data, hospital acquired condition/patient safety indicators, and developing precision medicine.
- There is significant opportunity for big data application in global vascular neurosurgery to better understand barriers in access and providing solutions in the eradication of such disparities.

INTRODUCTION

The practice of medicine has always been a mixture of art and science, in large part because good data to guide practice can be difficult to generate and interpret. Particularly in fields like neurosurgery in which the types of disease processes treated are relatively rare, there is a real need for means to obtain meaningful insights from our data. Instead, case reports, single-institution or surgeon series, and increasingly multiinstitutional series comprise the majority of our literature, and yet the strength of conclusions drawn from these is limited. The field of data science may help to overcome the common issues of noise, heterogeneity, and multiple confounders to help meaningfully guide practice.

Big data, a term popularized by John Mashey in the 1990s, refers both to the accrual of large datasets and the subsequent data analysis.[1] A large

sample size supports a high-powered study and through the process can focus on nuances of more common disease and capture more rare illnesses in greater frequency. Big data techniques allow for multidimensional investigation of large patient datasets, including multiinstitution sets collected over long periods, and across greater territories. Due to the increased power of these methods, the larger scale techniques allow researchers to have increasingly fine focus on disease processes, supporting precision medicine.

Big data is characterized by the 5 Vs—volume, variety, velocity, value, and veracity (**Fig. 1**).[1]

- Volume, perhaps the most straight forward, refers to the large sample size.
- Variety refers to the heterogeneity of the collected data forms.
- Velocity describes the speed at which data are created, which is powered by the switch

a Department of Neurosurgery, Jacobs School of Medicine and Biomedical Sciences, University at Buffalo, 100 High Street, Suite B4, Buffalo, NY 14203, USA; b Department of Biomedical Informatics, Jacobs School of Medicine and Biomedical Sciences, University at Buffalo, Buffalo, NY, USA; c Jacobs Institute, Buffalo, NY, USA
* Corresponding author. University at Buffalo Neurosurgery, 100 High Street, Suite B4, Buffalo, NY 14203.
E-mail address: jdavies@ubns.com

Neurosurg Clin N Am 33 (2022) 469–482
https://doi.org/10.1016/j.nec.2022.06.001

to electronic record-keeping, as well as the increasing numbers of data elements stored in modern Electronic Medical Record (EMR)s.
- Value is the potential benefit big data can provide and applications, which are only made possible by
- Veracity or the quality and accuracy of the data.

No single researcher or even team of researchers will be able to keep up with the goliath of data output provided by current health care systems. The development of AI and ML algorithms is our conduit with its insatiable thirst for information. Data scientists and trained clinicians are necessary in the integration of big data and its applications into the clinical workflow of health care systems. They are needed to apply complex algorithms, manage big data, and harmonize data. Expectedly, there has been an increase in recruitment and support for scientists and clinicians with this academic interest.

In the following review, we will address the larger data series in vascular neurosurgery and highlight growth potential wherein big data may help overcome current limitations to answer important questions.

TRIALS AND REGISTRIES

Between 1958 and 1965, a group from London, UK, set out to perform the first randomized controlled trial (RCT) of vascular neurosurgery. McKissock and his colleagues in Atkinson Morley Hospital, St. George's Hospital asked whether there was a difference in mortality of patients with aneurysms treated with surgery compared with those advised bedrest. This pioneering study was designed in response to contradicting and controversial conclusions of prior observational studies by the same group, one of which concluded that surgical treatment offered a definite lowering of mortality whereas the second found that there was no proof surgical treatment was superior to conservative measures. McKissock and colleagues wrote, "we have been forced to the conclusion that the truth of this controversial matter can only be established by a pre-planned campaign," and so began the preparation for the first ever RCT of vascular neurosurgery.[2-8]

Although RCTs have been accepted as the gold standard in defining best practices, there has been increasing concern regarding the pace at which these studies are conducted. They are expensive, labor intensive, and take years to complete at times falling behind innovations in technique and technology becoming outdated at the time of

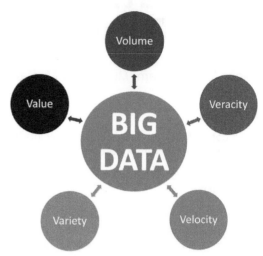

Fig. 1. Big data is characterized by the 5 Vs—volume, variety, velocity, value, and veracity. All parts are necessary for useful and accurate studies.[1]

completion.[9] Further pragmatic trial design sometimes favors numbers over standardization; for example, in the study led by McKissock the surgical technique used varied widely including aneurysm clipping and proximal artery ligation. In addition, RCTs can be unmasked and use strict inclusion and exclusion criteria that are not always representative of the whole population and raise ethical concerns regarding generalizability.[9]

Large administrative datasets are an attractive data source that can powerfully answer certain kinds of questions due to patient cohorts that are much larger than what is available at a single institution. These derive from administrative sampling efforts, such as the Nationwide Inpatient Sample (NIS)—sponsored by the Agency for Healthcare Research and Quality—the largest all-payer inpatient care database of US hospitals. This has been widely used to report inpatient mortality, complications, and outcomes. The NIS does not include hospitals from all states; however, the hospitals included are still diverse with respect to size, region, and academic status, which supports the generalizability of findings. One shortcoming is that the NIS relies on billing data and does not provide detailed patient-level and disease-specific information, such as structure, size, or location of the disease, which is important in vascular neurosurgery research.

With the advent of EMRs and the ready availability of data, alternatives to RCT have arisen with the goal of generating high-quality data and robust conclusions but without the expense and time that are often required for RCT, for instance, registries that have grown in popularity.[10] They collect

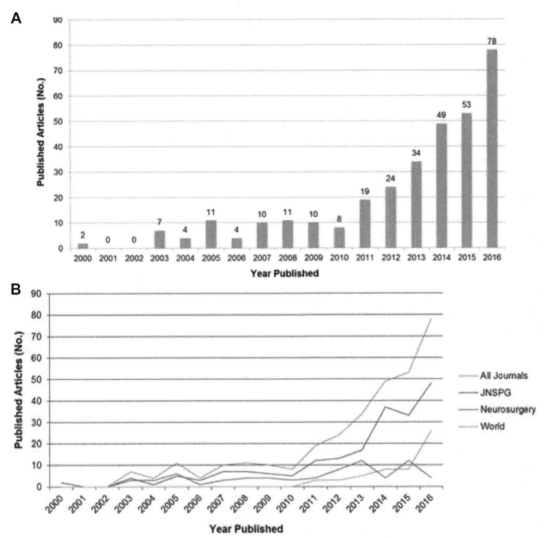

Fig. 2. (*A*) Neurosurgical related big data studies published from 2000 to 2016. (*B*) Neurosurgical related big data studies published from 2000 to 2016 in total compared to those in journal JNSPG, Neurosurgery, and World Neurosurgery. (*From* Oravec CS, Motiwala M, Reed K, Kondziolka D, Barker FG 2nd, Michael LM 2nd, Klimo P Jr. Big Data Research in Neurosurgery: A Critical Look at this Popular New Study Design. Neurosurgery. 2018 May 1;82(5):728-746. https://doi.org/10.1093/neuros/nyx328. PMID: 28973512.)

prospective data using modified observational methods with faster turnover and analysis. Registries are often flexibly designed to capture real-world data and can adapt or grow as necessity dictates with changing practices.

The use of both registry and administrative data is fraught with scrutiny and with due cause. Its greatest challenge is that of veracity. These are large pools of data that require strict validation and monitoring to ensure that the information is complete and accurate.[11] Caution with registries was encouraged by Woodworth and colleagues when they compared the quality of data from the State of Maryland administrative database to the

Johns Hopkins Hospital departmental database on patients diagnosed with intracranial aneurysms (IAs). The authors found that the administrative dataset missed 16% of cases and for those that were caught, 10 of the 12 categories of factors reviewed were deficient in sensitivity, specify, and positive predictive value.[12] We must be critical of the datasets used in the growing number of big data studies conducted despite the alluringly large sample sizes and the complex statistics.[11]

The "preplanned campaigns"—both RCTs and registries—have fallen short of the goal in vascular neurosurgery both in quality and quantity. Dr Fred Barker II concluded in his editorial on the current condition of neurosurgery research published in the *Journal of Neurosurgery*, "In Harvey Cushing's day, learning the subtleties of neurological diagnosis was the challenge for neurosurgeons, so they could choose their own operations and work to improve them. For our generation, learning how to master clinical studies—of every kind—is the equivalent challenge."[13] This similar dissatisfaction with the current structure of clinical research was echoed by Lauer and colleagues in 2013. The group published an editorial in the *New England Journal of Medicine* in which they criticized the present clinical research paradigm. RCTs held as the holy grail, have left all parties wanting with major gaps in conclusions. Similarly, registries are not devoid of bias or standardization that is integral when deciding on instituting new treatments as the standard of care. They advocated for the increasing use of a new "disruptive" technology in clinical research called the registry-based randomized controlled trial (RRCT).[14]

An RRCT is a form of pragmatic trials in which eligible patients are identified and recruited from the registry along with intervention and outcomes. Depending on the question, randomization can be applied at any point following enrollment. This study design is still in its infancy and has seen early success in cardiac research. It will be up to the researchers to define opportunities for its implementation in neurosurgery. RRCTs have attracted increasing attention to address questions of comparative effectiveness in real-world settings.[15–18]

Vascular neurosurgery has seen an exponential increase in big data studies (**Fig.2**) expanding beyond IAs to include arteriovenous malformations (AVMs), intracranial hemorrhage (ICH), and intracranial atherosclerotic disease (ICAD).[9] For the purposes of this review, we will focus on studies related to open vascular neurosurgery. Endovascular neurosurgical treatment of intracranial vascular pathology has welcomed big data quite readily as both fields are relatively new and results from big data research has further bolstered the popularity of endovascular treatment.

DISEASE-BASED MODULES
Intracranial Aneurysms and Subarachnoid Hemorrhage

Over 50% of big data studies in vascular neurosurgery pertain to aneurysms—their treatment, natural history, and associated illnesses.[9] One of the most notable RCTs performed is that of Molyneux and colleagues in the International Subarachnoid Aneurysm Trial (ISAT) which compared neurosurgical clipping versus endovascular coiling in 2143 patients. They found that those treated endovascularly had better outcomes in terms of disability-free survival.[19] A landmark trial, this study altered the trend in aneurysm treatment as proven by Quershi and colleagues who found that following the publication of ISAT there was a swift change in practice with an increase in endovascular treatment and a decrease in-hospital mortality.[20] In a separate study, reviewing over 300,000 cases of ruptured and unruptured IA from the National Hospital Discharge Survey data, Qureishi and colleagues found that between 1986 and 2001 there was a significant reduction in mortality for unruptured intracranial aneurysms (UIAs).[21] Criticisms of ISAT abound, and arguments for consideration of surgical clipping of a number of cohorts including good-grade subarachnoid hemorrhage (SAH), small anterior circulation aneurysms, surgeon expertise, and patient recruitment. On a smaller scale, the Barrow Ruptured Aneurysm Trial attempted to address some of these concerns; however, as the authors shared, the trial was statistically underpowered, which in effect is a call for big data.[22]

UIAs are found in 2% to 3% of the general US population. Registries are playing a critical role in their study.[23] For example, using the American College of Surgeons National Surgical Quality Improvement Program, McCutcheon and colleagues found that of 662 patients who underwent surgical treatment of UIAs, 8.61% developed major neurologic complication in the form of coma or stroke within 30 days post operation.[24] A corrigendum was published shortly to address a coding error for postoperative coma.[25] Although this did not alter the results on repeat analysis, it served as an example of the strict monitoring and review that registries must undergo. Hoh and colleagues, found those who undergo clipping of UIA from NIS data were found to have a significant increased risk of seizures or epilepsy compared to those who underwent coiling.[26]

As demonstrated by the International Study of Unruptured Intracranial Aneurysms, there is priceless information that can be gathered by observational studies.[27] Observational studies can offer insight into the natural history of disease. This particular group assessed 4060 patients with UIAs comparing those who were untreated and treated (open and endovascular). They were able to share 5-year cumulative rupture rates according to size and location of UIAs, information that remains front and center in clinical decision making today.[27] Similarly, Gonda and colleagues used observational study methods to compare rupture rates following UIA treatment. They used the California

Office of Statewide Health Planning and Development database to follow patients with repaired UIAs for an average of 7 years. They found that between the coil and clipping groups, rates of rupture were similar. Those who underwent coiling were more likely to undergo subsequent hospitalizations for additional treatment.[28] Lawson and colleagues sought to understand age groups best served by clipping, coiling, or neither—a step toward precision medicine. They reviewed 14,050 hospitalizations and found a treatment benefit for clipping in patients less than 70 years and for coiling in patients less than 81 years.[29]

Big data has also helped guide patient treatment destinations. Cross and colleagues looked at 16,399 cases of SAH across 18 states concluding that hospitals that treat higher volumes of SAH had lower mortality rates.[30] This was further corroborated by Penday and colleagues who identified 32,336 patients using the NIS concluding high-volume hospitals had more favorable outcomes.[31] Interestingly, Leake and colleagues found the national trend of care paralleled these findings. Patients with ruptured aneurysms are increasingly being treated at high-volume centers and less so at low-volume centers.[32] Bekelis and colleagues went on to ask whether there was a difference in outcomes of UIA treatment between hybrid neurosurgeons compared with proceduralist, to which they found none.[33]

Identifying associations between aneurysmal SAH (aSAH) with other medical conditions has been another major success extracted from registry data. Rumalla and colleagues for example, found that the rate of acute renal failure (ARF) in patients with aSAH has increased overall. This is particularly alarming as there was an association with increased mean length of stay (LOS), hospitalization cost, and risk of disability/in-hospital death in those who suffered from both aSAH and concomitant ARF.[34] Dasenbrock and colleagues used the NIS data to assess for independent predictors of clostridium difficile infection (CDI) in 18,007 patient with aSAH. They concluded Medicaid payer status, ventriculostomy, mechanical ventilation, and other site infections were independent predictors of developing CDI, which is associated with increased LOS and nonroutine hospital discharge.[35] Of hospital acquired infections in aSAH, urinary tract infections and pneumonia were most common, pneumonia and central venous catheters being associated with an increased likelihood of poor outcome.[35] Morbid obesity was associated with increased venous thromboembolic events, renal disease, infection, and nonroutine hospital discharge.[36] Generalized convulsive status epilepticus and cardiac failure

have been linked to higher mortality in this patient population.[37,38]

Sorting through NIS and similar databases poses a daunting task for researchers who are curious enough to approach it. Teams have sought to develop validated methods of data interpretation and stratification. For example, Washington and colleagues developed the SAH Severity Score (NIH-SSS) and SAH Outcome Measure (NIH-SOM), which when applied to the over 150,000 cases of SAH were comparable to the Hunt–Hess grading and modified Rankin Score.[39] Rawal and colleagues further validated this finding on aSAH cases from a Canadian registry.[40]

Variations in coding, data mining, and patient identification may introduce bias. Dasenbrock and colleagues looked at the impact of aspirin and anticoagulant usage on outcomes of patients with aSAH. They identified their patient population by looking at all those diagnosed with SAH that underwent microsurgical or endovascular aneurysm repair. Of the 11,549 hospital admissions, those on aspirin and anticoagulant were mined. These patients were generally older with a greater burden of comorbid conditions. The team concluded that neither long-term aspirin nor anticoagulant use was associated with differences in mortality or complication rates.[41] This study excluded those who did not undergo treatment, which may include patients of higher-grade disease on arrival.

Looking at the less-common presentations of aSAH in increasing frequency has been possible by aggregating such cases from a large dataset. For example, Kim and colleagues used the NIS data to review hundreds of cases of aSAH in pregnancy and delivery concluding that there was no discernible association with risk of aneurysm rupture, thus challenging elective cesarean section deliveries.[42] Bekelis and colleagues compared clipping and coiling of UIA in 8705 elderly patients. There was no difference in mortality or the readmission rate between clipping and coiling, although clipping was associated with a higher rate of discharge to a rehabilitation facility and a longer LOS.[43]

Big data has purchased intellectual shares in IA and SAH research with interest only accruing. It is important researchers move toward standardizing practices in registry use and work toward using them prospectively and pragmatically in conjunction with RCTs.

Arteriovenous Malformations

Big data is an excellent study option as it can collect rare disease, such as AVM, in larger numbers, allowing for more meaningful conclusions and understanding. The Multicenter AVM Research Study (MARS) and the Gross and Du study are the best cited for understanding AVM natural history. The Gross and Du study was a meta-analysis of a number of cohorts.[44] The MARS was formulated from a combination of two large cohort studies (UCSF AVM database and Columbia AVM database) and two population-based studies (Scottish Intracranial Vascular Malformation Study and the Kaiser Permanente of Northern California).[45–47] They projected the cumulative incidence of a patient experiencing a first intraventricular hemorrhage. There was a significant difference in percentage. Smaller cohort studies found values that lie in the middle.[45,47] The differences in these results cannot be attributed to differences in statistical analysis alone. What we can conclude definitively is larger scale studies with longer term follow-up are needed in AVM research.

Endovascular treatment of AVM has grown in popularity, more complex in technique, and more ambitious in treatment goal. Davies and colleagues looked at nearly 34,000 admissions for AVM using the NIS. Patients with unruptured AVMs treated radiosurgically fared the best—no reported mortalities, lowest LOS, and the highest discharge rate. Those treated endovascularly had the highest mortality rate. Patients treated surgically had the longest LOS and lowest discharge rates. Juxtaposed to those with ruptured AVMs, the outcomes differed marginally. The endovascularly treated group had the highest mortality. Surgery plus angiography had the lowest mortality rate.[48] The same group used NIS data to assess for differences in outcome of AVM treatment based on center and surgeon volume. For patients treated at high-volume centers, there was significantly lower morbidity and, for high-volume surgeons, with lower mortality.[49]

The authors advocate for the creation of care paradigms that triage patients to high-volume institutions and surgeons.[48,49] Improvement in outcomes at high-volume centers was similarly seen in IA treatment and ICH which would further support a shift in treatment model.

Spontaneous Intracerebral Hemorrhage

The landmark RCT Surgical Trial in Intracerebral Haemorrhage (STICH) and STICH II, in summary, concluded that in patients with supratentorial spontaneous intracerebral hemorrhage (sICH) there was no significant difference in outcome between those who underwent early hematoma evacuation compared with those who were managed conservatively. These trials involved 1033 and 601 participants respectively. Subgroup analysis in STICH did reveal a favorable outcome following surgery for hematomas less than 1 cm from the cortical surface.[50,51] Concern has been raised regarding the general use of subgroup analyses that are not powered to allow for definitive conclusions. This is yet another call for advancing big data studies.

Andaluz and colleagues used the NIS to evaluate trends in the treatment of sICH following the publication of STICH.[52] There was no significant progress in the treatment or prevention of sICH. Mortality rate from sICH remained unchanged (31.6%), which was similarly found by Russell and colleagues Of those who survived, they were increasingly being discharged to other than home.[53] Arterial hypertension was the most frequently associated comorbidity. Obstructive hydrocephalus was fatal in almost half of the patients who had this associated diagnosis, and it was associated with the lowest incidence of good outcomes in this cohort. Finally, only about 6% of the 905,152 cases received surgical treatment. Craniotomy was associated with decreased mortality but increased morbidity.[53–55]

Treatment and management of nontraumatic ICH is met with pessimism by the neurosurgical community. Less than one-third of patients with sICH make a good functional recovery. Within 30 days of the sICH ictus, 35% to 52% of patients are likely to die, and only 20% are expected to be functionally independent at 6 months.[53–55] In 1999, a special writing committee appointed by the American Heart Association (AHA) issued treatment guidelines for sICH. They published an update in 2007 that was based on 24 relatively small RCTs reviewing medical and surgical interventions. They were unable to issue a single Class IA recommendation. The only Class IB recommendation was offering surgical intervention for evacuation of cerebellar hemorrhages that were either greater than 3 cm, showed evidence of hydrocephalus, or brainstem compression.[54]

Big data has the potential to fill in a sizable void in our understanding of sICH. Presently, treatment of sICH is not standardized and differs according to individual interpretations of present studies and anecdotal evidence. This is an important consideration as the most common cause of death in patients with sICH is the limitation or withdrawal of life-sustaining intervention (68%) followed by brain death (28%).[55] As the literature stands, we cannot advocate for a single line of intervention in all cases, but we can encourage continued thoughtful inquiry in the surgical treatment options for ICH.

Carotid Artery Stenosis

In 1987, the North American Symptomatic Carotid Endarterectomy Trial (NASCET) began recruiting for what was the first large-scale clinical trial to evaluate the efficacy of carotid endarterectomy (CEA) for patients with symptomatic carotid stenosis, a surgery that had been present and in practice for over 50 years. Fast forward 4 years, the team published a clinical alert in Stroke sharing their preliminary results. They reported that of the 659 patients with severe stenosis (70%–99%), CEA was associated with an absolute reduction of 17% in the risk of ipsilateral stroke at 2 years.[56] Three decades later and this study remains relevant. Following its completion, large-scale trials were performed to further refine best practices in the management of carotid stenosis considering intervention style, timing, and symptomatology.

NASCET was followed by a number of studies that put carotid artery stenting (CAS), CEA, and best medical therapy up against one another. These contests have often left the medical community questioning without declaration of a clear or consistent winner. Treatment for high-grade symptomatic carotid artery stenosis (SCS) is undisputed. NASCET was followed by the European Carotid Surgery Trial which concluded that CEA was indicated in patients with SCS of greater than 80%.[57] In this group, the immediate risk of surgery was worth the trade off against the long-term risk of stroke without surgery. Using these combined results, Class 1A recommendation made by the AHA and American Stroke Association is that those with severe stenosis of 70% to 99% should be treated within 6 months.[58,59] Variations in treatment of SCS usually relate to the method and timing of intervention. Carotid Revascularization Endarterectomy Versus Stenting Trial (CREST), published in 2010, showed no significant difference in the rates of stroke, myocardial infarction, or death between CAS and CEA although there was a higher risk of stroke with stenting and a higher risk of MI with CEA.[60]

Big data has been essential in observing and modeling national trends. For example, unlike the observed changes following the discriminating results published in ISAT, expectedly the equivocal results of CREST had no change on rates of CEA versus CAS.[58] This was at odds with a pre-CREST prediction by Dumont and colleagues who anticipated CREST would result in continued increase in CAS based on early trends.[59]

Asymptomatic carotid artery stenosis (ACS) management has eluded the curious probe of big data. The Asymptomatic Carotid Atherosclerosis Study (ACAS) and the Asymptomatic Carotid Surgery Trial (ACST) were performed in an attempt to guide practice.[61,62] ACAS results led to major increases in rates of endarterectomy for ACS in the United States. At least half of the approximate 150,000 endarterectomies performed were done for ACS.[62–65] ACST, which was conducted using a larger sample than ACAS, similarly demonstrated that CEA compared with medical treatment alone reduces the risk of stroke in asymptomatic patients with carotid stenosis. The risk of stroke from asymptomatic stenosis has been estimated at between 0.3% and 1% over 2 years by recent meta-analyses and population-based studies in the United States, United Kingdom, and Canada.[61–63,65] Keeping in mind that the complication rate of CEA or CAS lies between 1% and 5% across multiple trials over many decades, intervention in all patients with asymptomatic stenosis greater than 60% becomes difficult to justify.[61–66] Recent advances in antihypertensive and lipid-lowering medication in conjunction with antiplatelet therapy may nullify the small benefit of CEA, but this is for future big data studies to determine.[62–66]

Defining high risk patients has been greatly served by using big data research methods. This was well demonstrated by Qureshi and colleagues who measured 5-year survival of those greater than 65 years who underwent CEA or CAS for asymptomatic carotid artery stenosis. They found that those with concurrent atrial fibrillation and chronic renal failure had higher mortality rates and encouraged providers to consider this when offering intervention.[67]

Intracranial Atherosclerotic Disease

In 1985, the ECIC (Extracranial–Intracranial) Bypass study group asked whether bypass surgery would offer benefit to patients with symptomatic atherosclerotic disease. 1377 patients were studied with symptomatic ICAD. Nearly half were randomized to best medical therapy and the other to superficial temporal artery and middle cerebral artery bypass. Nonfatal and fatal stroke occurred both more frequently and earlier in the bypass group.[68] The Carotid Occlusion Surgery Study (COSS) was performed to test the hypothesis that ECIC bypass would be of benefit in patients with symptomatic atherosclerotic carotid artery occlusion, excluding those with acute occlusion. COSS failed to show a benefit of surgery in these patients.[69] One of the major criticisms is that the studies were underpowered to identify benefit in subgroup analysis.[70–72]

Despite maximal medical therapy, there remains a high rate of recurrent stroke rate in this group.

Vascular and endovascular neurosurgeons are still in pursuit of a better treatment option. The Stenting Versus Aggressive Medical Therapy for Intracranial Arterial Stenosis study terminated enrollment early as there was a 30-day rate of stroke or death of 14.7% in the group that underwent Wingspan stent placement compared with 5.8% in the medical-management group.[73] This study has resulted in a shift in endovascular treatment of ICAD although critics claim that the technology used in the study is now outdated and newer studies are needed to evaluate more novel methods, a shortcoming of RCTs.[70–72]

Intervention cannot be justified in treatment of all patients with ICAD. Big data research will aid in identifying target populations that may benefit from intervention and if so, guide intervention choice. The AANS–CNS Joint Cerebrovascular Section recently reviewed the results of the ECIC bypass versus medical therapy trials and concluded that specific patient populations with hemispheric ischemia might benefit from surgery. The committee advocated for a registry module to study the effectiveness of ECIC bypass by center volume, careful patient selections, and type of approach on an ongoing basis.[70]

Moyamoya

Moyamoya is a rare disease making it difficult to capture. Big data studies if and when performed can provide key insight into epidemiology, natural history, and treatment.

It is predicted that there are nearly 11,000 admissions annually in the United States. Over time, Starke and colleagues found an increase in diagnosis, associated ischemic stroke, and treatment with ECIC bypass. Moyamoya diagnosis in the United States is more common in women and white patients. Both adults and children were more likely to be diagnosed with ischemic versus hemorrhagic stroke.[74]

Owing to the small population this disease affects, evaluating a subset is challenging. Kainth and colleagues used the NIS data and found increased prevalence of concurrent down syndrome in patients with Moyamoya disease. Similar to general population trends, they were more commonly white and to present with an ischemic event. This association was never previously so strongly reported.[75]

QUALITY IMPROVEMENT

Reviewing large volumes of real time patient data can help hospital administrators better understand care trends and performance. This knowledge will allow for targeted opportunities for improvement in patient care. A leading example of quality improvement powered by big data is the NeuroPoint Alliance (NPA). It was founded to provide data platforms for national registry participation by all neurosurgeons in the United States. The National Neurosurgery Quality and Outcomes Database (N^2QOD) was one of the first efforts focused solely on spinal neurosurgery.[76] They are intended to serve as the principal practice science infrastructure for each neurosurgical subspecialty. This will require significant coordination and cooperation.[76]

Vascular neurosurgery is associated with higher morbidity and mortality and reducing these rates is an ever-present goal. Hospital acquired conditions (HACs) and patient safety indicators (PSIs) are important in quality control. In neurosurgical patients, falls/trauma and catheter-associated urinary tract infections are the most common HACs. Age and greater than 2 comorbidities were strongly linked to HAC.[77–80] This is important because patients with at least 1 HAC were 10 times more likely to have prolonged LOS, and 8 times more likely to have high inpatient costs. In a large observational study of patients with SAH, those treated by either clipping or coiling and had at least one PSI during their hospitalization had significantly longer LOS, higher hospital costs, and higher in-hospital mortality rates. Admission during weekdays was also linked with better outcomes.[77–80]

In patients with cerebrovascular disease, significant predictors of complications include preoperative ventilator dependence, emergency surgery, bleeding disorders, diabetes mellitus, and alcohol abuse.[80] Predictors of mortality included postoperative coma greater than 24 hours, preoperative or postoperative ventilator dependence, black or Asian race, and stroke. The most common complications were ventilator dependence, bleeding requiring transfusion, reoperation within 30 days, pneumonia, and stroke.[80] Specifically in patients who underwent CEA had a 6.0% unplanned readmission rate. The most common comorbidities in the readmitted patients included hypertension, diabetes, and bleeding disorder.[81] These findings allow for more customized care and improved preoperative planning.

Resident training is important but may raise concerns of quality of operative care. Large data studies do not support such claims. In the review of over 8000 operative cases, resident involvement was associated with longer operative duration but was not significantly linked to complication of any type including mortality, reoperation, or unplanned readmission.[82] Further, in review of approximately 35,000 hospitalizations for UIA and ruptured IA, teaching status of a hospital was determined to be an independent factor for favorable outcome in the treatment of ruptured aneurysms.[83]

Big data studies have allowed for short- and long-term cost comparison studies. Looking at 1 year follow-up, endovascular treatment is lower cost up front as surgical clipping is associated with higher complication rates and intervention cost. However, at 2- and 5-year expenses balanced out due to the significantly higher number of follow-up angiograms and outpatient costs in coiling groups.[84,85]

Finally, big data has allowed for more personalized care and precision medicine. One group ventured to develop a predictive model of complications in patients undergoing cerebral aneurysm clipping for ruptured and unruptured aneurysms using NIS data.[86] A validated model for outcome prediction based on individual patient characteristics was developed. The model can provide individualized estimates of the risks of postoperative complications based on preoperative conditions.[86] Big data challenges the definition of "normal," making it relative.[87–89] It is important in development of such models that population differences are accounted for. Obermeyer and colleagues demonstrated that prediction tools are not objective and can exhibit racial or gender biases.[90] Biases such as these must be addressed and accounted for.

Quality improvement, precision medicine, and cost-effective care are all opportunities for continued big data efforts in vascular neurosurgery allowing for the creation of tools which can be used as adjuncts in care.

INNOVATION

Big data in its current and most efficient form is the collection of large volumes of data analyzed by machine learning algorithms to extract meaningful and complex associations which when applied, can be transformative. Advanced computer processing power combined with the vast amounts of digitized data collected and stored by the EMR will augment machine learning and deep learning algorithms and their application—artificial intelligence (AI).[91–96]

Clinically applied AI is expected to grow. AI can enhance and accelerate clinical practice by pushing the limits of diagnostics, clinical decision making, and prognostication. Moreover, it can be combined with surgical robotics and other surgical adjuncts such as image guidance. Automation may potentially reduce medical errors, lower costs, expand access to healthcare, and increase patient autonomy.[91–96] For example, a deep learning algorithm detected cerebral aneurysms in radiologic reports with high sensitivity.[97] One of the most successful examples has been Viz.AI, which was listed as one of *Forbes'* Next Billion-Dollar Startups. The group has been successful in using AI in early stroke and ICH detection with plans to expand to pulmonary embolism and aortic dissection.[98] Furthermore, because of the realtime accesss to data across a large number of institutions, these apps are able to address urgent questions, such as was demonstrated with stroke incidence in the face of the COVID crisis.

Despite the hype surrounding the impending medical AI revolution, considerable caution must be exercised upfront. Garbage in, garbage out—faulty, inadequately trained, or poorly understood algorithms may produce erroneous models.[11] In the longer term, automation risks de-skilling of neurosurgeons due to over-reliance, poor understanding, overconfidence, and lack of necessary vigilance. AI and robotics cannot replace the versatility of human analytical ability and capacity for dynamic troubleshooting.[91–96]

Several steps can be taken to streamline the translation of favorable AI applications into medical practice. Interinstitutional cooperation, critical appraisal of data, and generalizability will be necessary along with increased collaboration between neurosurgeons and scientists.[91–96]

GLOBAL VASCULAR NEUROSURGERY

Although some global neurosurgical outreach programs have intelligently implemented big data, there is still significant opportunity for growth. Big data can play a role in assessing the overall burden of disease, designing cost-effective methods of access, and collecting data on conditions which are rare in developed countries. This will surely be met with skepticism from participating countries and must be a partnership guided by ethical global neurosurgical practice.[1,99–101]

The Duke East Africa neurosurgery program is one successful example. The team has assessed the epidemiology of road traffic injuries and access to pediatric neurosurgical care by geographic distances in low-income countries in East Africa.[1]

Global is local. Big data allows for better understanding and access to cultural silos within the United States. Attenello and colleagues found that of a total of 78,070 aSAH admissions treated with coiling or clipping, Hispanic race and Medicaid payer status were associated with increased time to treatment.[102] Wen and colleagues used NIS data and found minorities and Medicaid payers had increased frequency of HACs, LOS, and inpatient costs in cerebrovascular neurosurgical patients.[103]

Awareness is the first step to providing better access. Big data has a strong role in improving care and extending the reach of global vascular neurosurgery.

FUTURE DIRECTIONS

Since the start of 2020, there have been over 100 submissions to the FDA for AI enabled medical devices and software, cerebrovascular disease a clear focus. The last decade has seen an intellectual race to create the next and most accurate ML model across all fields in neurosurgery. This race is fueled by our inherent impatience to provide prompt care and the large volume of data output produced by the EMR.[104–110] Innovators have quickly carved out niches in the marriage of technology and medicine—radiomics, proteomics, genomics and leaving doors wide open for interdisciplinary communication. Big data both augments and supplies these efforts.

We have seen tremendous and exponential development in vascular neurosurgery since the days of McKissock.[9] Big data will continue to propel the field forward in understanding of individual disease processes, research design, quality care, innovation, and global outreach.

CLINICS CARE POINTS

- There is an exponential rise in available databases and the neurosurgical literature that is published using them.
- Care must be taken using large databases to ensure validity of results, this requires careful ongoing screening of data that is input.
- To better keep up with the large volumes of data that are being created with electronic medical record, registry based randomized control trials are a pragmatic option for big data study designs that could potentially lead to higher level evidence results.
- AI and ML are finding more roles in neurosurgical practice and will prove to be very useful tools moving forward in mining through large data.

REFERENCES

1. West JL, Fargen KM, Hsu W, et al. A review of Big Data analytics and potential for implementation in the delivery of global neurosurgery. Neurosurg Focus FOC 2018;45(4):E16.

2. McKissock KW, Paine K, Walsh L, et al. Further observations on subarachnoid haemorrhage. J Neurol Neurosurg Psychiatry 1958;21:239–48.

3. McKissock W. Subarachnoid haemorrhage. Ann R Coll Surg Engl 1956;19:361–70.

4. McKissock W, Walsh L. Subarachnoid haemorrhage due to intracranial aneurysms; results of treatment of 249 verified cases. Br Med J 1956;2:559–65.

5. McKissock W, Richardson A, Walsh L, et al. Anterior communicating aneurysms: a trial of conservative and surgical treatment. Lancet 1965;1:874–6.

6. McKissock WRA, Walsh L. Middle-cerebral aneurysms further results in the controlled trial of conservative and surgical treatment of ruptured intracranial aneurysms. Lancet 1962;280:417–21.

7. McKissock WRA, Walsh L. Posterior communicating aneurysms. Lancet 1960;275:1203–56.

8. Darsaut TE, Raymond J. RCTs in determining treatment indications for intracranial aneurysms: What can we learn from history? Neurochirurgie 2012;58(2–3):76–86 [English, French].

9. Oravec CS, Motiwala M, Reed K, et al. Big Data Research in Neurosurgery: A Critical Look at this Popular New Study Design. Neurosurgery 2018;82(5):728–46.

10. Sutzko DC, Mani K, Behrendt C-A, et al. AW (University of Alabama at Birmingham, Birmingham, AB, USA; Uppsala University, Uppsala, Sweden; and University Medical Center Hamburg-Eppendorf, Hamburg, Germany). Big data in vascular surgery: registries, international collaboration and future directions (Review Symposium). J Intern Med 2020;288:51–61.

11. Grimes DA. Epidemiologic research using administrative databases: garbage in, garbage out. Obstet Gynecol 2010;116(5):1018–9.

12. Woodworth GF, Baird CJ, Garces-Ambrossi G, et al. Inaccuracy of the administrative database: comparative analysis of two databases for the diagnosis and treatment of intracranial aneurysms. Neurosurgery 2009;65(2):251–6 [discussion: 256-7].

13. Barker FG II. Editorial: Randomized clinical trials and neurosurgery. J Neurosurg 2016;124(2):552–7.

14. Lauer MS, D'Agostino RB Sr. The randomized registry trial–the next disruptive technology in clinical research? N Engl J Med 2013;369(17):1579–81.

15. Frobert O, Lagerqvist B, Olivecrona GK, et al. Thrombus aspiration during ST-segment elevation myocardial infarction. N Engl J Med 2013;369(17):1587–97.

16. Rao SV, Hess CN, Barham B, et al. A registry-based randomized trial comparing radial and femoral approaches in women undergoing percutaneous coronary intervention: the SAFE-PCI for Women (Study of Access Site for Enhancement of

PCI for Women) trial. JACC Cardiovasc Interv 2014;7(8):857–67.

17. Li G, Sajobi TT, Menon BK, et al. 2016 Symposium on Registry-Based Randomized Controlled Trials in Calgary. Registry-based randomized controlled trials- what are the advantages, challenges, and areas for future research? J Clin Epidemiol 2016; 80:16–24.

18. Mansouri A, Cooper B, Shin SM, et al. Randomized controlled trials and neurosurgery: the ideal fit or should alternative methodologies be considered? J Neurosurg 2016;124(2):558–68.

19. Molyneux AJ, Kerr RS, Yu LM, et al. International Subarachnoid Aneurysm Trial (ISAT) Collaborative Group. International subarachnoid aneurysm trial (ISAT) of neurosurgical clipping versus endovascular coiling in 2143 patients with ruptured intracranial aneurysms: a randomised comparison of effects on survival, dependency, seizures, rebleeding, subgroups, and aneurysm occlusion. Lancet 2005;366(9488):809–17.

20. Qureshi AI, Vazquez G, Tariq N, et al. Impact of International Subarachnoid Aneurysm Trial results on treatment of ruptured intracranial aneurysms in the United States. J Neurosurg 2011;114(3):834–41.

21. Qureshi AI, Suri MFK, Nasar A, et al. Trends in hospitalization and mortality for subarachnoid hemorrhage and unruptured aneurysms in the United States. Neurosurgery 2005;57(1):1–8.

22. Spetzler RF, McDougall CG, Zabramski JM, et al. The Barrow Ruptured Aneurysm Trial: 6-year results. J Neurosurg 2015;123(3):609–17.

23. Vlak MH, Algra A, Brandenburg R, et al. Prevalence of unruptured intracranial aneurysms, with emphasis on sex, age, comorbidity, country, and time period: a systematic review and meta-analysis. Lancet Neurol 2011;10(7):626–36.

24. McCutcheon BA, Kerezoudis P, Porter AL, et al. Coma and Stroke Following Surgical Treatment of Unruptured Intracranial Aneurysm: An American College of Surgeons National Surgical Quality Improvement Program Study. World Neurosurg 2016;91:272–8 [Erratum in: World Neurosurg. 2017 Dec 26;: PMID: 27108027].

25. McCutcheon BA, Kerezoudis P, Porter AL, et al. Corrigendum to "Coma and Stroke Following Surgical Treatment of Unruptured Intracranial Aneurysm: An American College of Surgeons National Surgical Quality Improvement Program Study" [World Neurosurgery (2016) 91:272-278]. World Neurosurg 2018;110:614–5 [Erratum for: World Neurosurg. 2016;91:272-8].

26. Hoh BL, Nathoo S, Chi YY, et al. Incidence of seizures or epilepsy after clipping or coiling of ruptured and unruptured cerebral aneurysms in the nationwide inpatient sample database: 2002-

2007. Neurosurgery 2011;69(3):644–50 [discussion: 650].

27. Wiebers DO, Whisnant JP, Huston J 3rd, et al. International Study of Unruptured Intracranial Aneurysms Investigators. Unruptured intracranial aneurysms: natural history, clinical outcome, and risks of surgical and endovascular treatment. Lancet 2003;362(9378):103–10.

28. Gonda DD, Khalessi AA, McCutcheon BA, et al. Long-term follow-up of unruptured intracranial aneurysms repaired in California. J Neurosurg 2014; 120(6):1349–57.

29. Lawson MF, Neal DW, Mocco J, et al. Rationale for treating unruptured intracranial aneurysms: actuarial analysis of natural history risk versus treatment risk for coiling or clipping based on 14,050 patients in the Nationwide Inpatient Sample database. World Neurosurg 2013;79(3–4):472–8.

30. Cross DT 3rd, Tirschwell DL, Clark MA, et al. Mortality rates after subarachnoid hemorrhage: variations according to hospital case volume in 18 states. J Neurosurg 2003;99(5):810–7.

31. Pandey AS, Gemmete JJ, Wilson TJ, et al. High Subarachnoid Hemorrhage Patient Volume Associated With Lower Mortality and Better Outcomes. Neurosurgery 2015;77(3):462–70.

32. Leake CB, Brinjikji W, Kallmes DF, et al. Increasing treatment of ruptured cerebral aneurysms at high-volume centers in the United States. J Neurosurg 2011;115(6):1179–83.

33. Bekelis K, Gottlieb D, Labropoulos N, et al. The impact of hybrid neurosurgeons on the outcomes of endovascular coiling for unruptured cerebral aneurysms. J Neurosurg 2017;126(1):29–35.

34. Rumalla K, Mittal MK. Acute Renal Failure in Aneurysmal Subarachnoid Hemorrhage: Nationwide Analysis of Hospitalizations in the United States. World Neurosurg 2016;91:542–7.e6.

35. Dasenbrock HH, Rudy RF, Smith TR, et al. Hospital-Acquired Infections after Aneurysmal Subarachnoid Hemorrhage: A Nationwide Analysis. World Neurosurg 2016;88:459–74.

36. Dasenbrock HH, Nguyen MO, Frerichs KU, et al. The impact of body habitus on outcomes after aneurysmal subarachnoid hemorrhage: a Nationwide Inpatient Sample analysis. J Neurosurg 2017;127(1):36–46.

37. Claassen J, Bateman BT, Willey JZ, et al. Generalized convulsive status epilepticus after nontraumatic subarachnoid hemorrhage: the nationwide inpatient sample. Neurosurgery 2007;61(1):60–4 [discussion: 64–5].

38. Kim YW, Neal D, Hoh BL. Risk factors, incidence, and effect of cardiac failure and myocardial infarction in aneurysmal subarachnoid hemorrhage patients. Neurosurgery 2013;73(3):450–7 [quiz: 457].

39. Washington CW, Derdeyn CP, Dacey RG Jr, et al. Analysis of subarachnoid hemorrhage using the Nationwide Inpatient Sample: the NIS-SAH Severity Score and Outcome Measure. J Neurosurg 2014; 121(2):482–9.

40. Rawal S, Rinkel GJE, Fang J, et al. External Validation and Modification of Nationwide Inpatient Sample Subarachnoid Hemorrhage Severity Score. Neurosurgery 2021;89(4):591–6.

41. Dasenbrock HH, Yan SC, Gross BA, et al. The impact of aspirin and anticoagulant usage on outcomes after aneurysmal subarachnoid hemorrhage: a Nationwide Inpatient Sample analysis. J Neurosurg 2017;126(2):537–47.

42. Kim YW, Neal D, Hoh BL. Cerebral aneurysms in pregnancy and delivery: pregnancy and delivery do not increase the risk of aneurysm rupture. Neurosurgery 2013;72(2):143–9 [discussion: 150].

43. Bekelis K, Gottlieb DJ, Su Y, et al. Comparison of clipping and coiling in elderly patients with unruptured cerebral aneurysms. J Neurosurg 2017; 126(3):811–8.

44. Gross BA, Du R. Natural history of cerebral arteriovenous malformations: a meta-analysis. J Neurosurg 2013;118(2):437–43.

45. Kim H, Al-Shahi Salman R, McCulloch CE, et al. Untreated brain arteriovenous malformation: patient-level meta-analysis of hemorrhage predictors. Neurology 2014;83(7):590–7.

46. Hernesniemi JA, Dashti R, Juvela S, et al. Natural history of brain arteriovenous malformations: a long-term follow-up study of risk of hemorrhage in 238 patients. Neurosurgery 2008;63(5):823–9 [discussion: 829–31].

47. Al-Shahi Salman R, White PM, Counsell CE, et al. Scottish Audit of Intracranial Vascular Malformations Collaborators. Outcome after conservative management or intervention for unruptured brain arteriovenous malformations. JAMA 2014;311(16): 1661–9.

48. Davies JM, Yanamadala V, Lawton MT. Comparative effectiveness of treatments for cerebral arteriovenous malformations: trends in nationwide outcomes from 2000 to 2009. Neurosurg Focus 2012;33(1):E11.

49. Davies JM, Lawton MT. Improved outcomes for patients with cerebrovascular malformations at high-volume centers: the impact of surgeon and hospital volume in the United States, 2000–2009. J Neurosurg 2017;127(1):69–80.

50. Mendelow AD, Gregson BA, Fernandes HM, et al. Early surgery versus initial conservative treatment in patients with spontaneous supratentorial intracerebral haematomas in the International Surgical Trial in Intracerebral Haemorrhage (STICH): a randomised trial. Lancet 2005;365(9457): 387–97.

51. Mendelow AD, Gregson BA, Rowan EN, et al. Early surgery versus initial conservative treatment in patients with spontaneous supratentorial lobar intracerebral haematomas (STICH II): a randomised trial. Lancet 2013;382(9890):397–408 [Erratum in: Lancet. 2013;382(9890):396. Erratum in: Lancet. 2021 Sep 18;398(10305):1042. PMID: 23726393; PMCID: PMC3906609].

52. Andaluz N, Zuccarello M. Recent trends in the treatment of spontaneous intracerebral hemorrhage: analysis of a nationwide inpatient database. J Neurosurg 2009;110(3):403–10.

53. Russell MW, Joshi AV, Neumann PJ, et al. Predictors of hospital length of stay and cost in patients with intracerebral hemorrhage. Neurology 2006; 67(7):1279–81 [Erratum in: Neurology. 2007; 69(19):1889-1281. PMID: 17030767].

54. Broderick J, Connolly S, Feldmann E, et al. Guidelines for the Management of Spontaneous Intracerebral Hemorrhage in Adults: 2007 Update: A Guideline From the American Heart Association/ American Stroke Association Stroke Council, High Blood Pressure Research Council, and the Quality of Care and Outcomes in Research Interdisciplinary Working Group. Stroke 2007;38: 2001–23.

55. Zurasky JA, Aiyagari V, Zazulia AR, et al. Early mortality following spontaneous intracerebral hemorrhage. Neurology 2005;64(4):725–7.

56. North American Symptomatic Carotid Endarterectomy Trial Collaborators. Beneficial effect of carotid endarterectomy in symptomatic patients with high-grade carotid stenosis. N Engl J Med 1991;325(7): 445–53.

57. Farrell B, Fraser A, Sandercock P, et al. Randomised trial of endarterectomy for recently symptomatic carotid stenosis: final results of the MRC European Carotid Surgery Trial (ECST). Lancet 1998;351(9113):1379–87.

58. Siddiq F, Adil MM, Malik AA, et al. Effect of Carotid Revascularization Endarterectomy Versus Stenting Trial Results on the Performance of Carotid Artery Stent Placement and Carotid Endarterectomy in the United States. Neurosurgery 2015;77(5): 726–32 [discussion: 732].

59. Dumont TM, Rughani AI. National trends in carotid artery revascularization surgery. J Neurosurg 2012; 116(6):1251–7.

60. Mantese VA, Timaran CH, Chiu D, et al, CREST Investigators. The Carotid Revascularization Endarterectomy versus Stenting Trial (CREST): stenting versus carotid endarterectomy for carotid disease. Stroke 2010;41(10 Suppl):S31–4.

61. Halliday A, Harrison M, Hayter E, et al. Asymptomatic Carotid Surgery Trial (ACST) Collaborative Group. 10-year stroke prevention after successful carotid endarterectomy for asymptomatic stenosis

(ACST-1): a multicentre randomised trial. Lancet 2010;376(9746):1074–84.

62. Endarterectomy for asymptomatic carotid artery stenosis. Executive Committee for the Asymptomatic Carotid Atherosclerosis Study. JAMA 1995; 273(18):1421–8.

63. Hobson RW, Weiss DG, Fields Goldstone J, et al. Wright CB, and the Veterans Affairs Cooperative study group. Efficacy of carotid endarterectomy for asymptomatic carotid stenosis. N Engl J Med 1993;328:221–7.

64. Tu JV, Hannan EL, Anderson GM, et al. The fall and rise of carotid endarterectomy in the United States and Canada. N Engl J Med 1998;339:1441–7.

65. Chambers BR, Donnan GA. Carotid endarterectomy for asymptomatic carotid stenosis. Cochrane Database Syst Rev 2005;2005(4):CD001923.

66. Bulbulia R, Halliday A. The Asymptomatic Carotid Surgery Trial-2 (ACST-2): an ongoing randomised controlled trial comparing carotid endarterectomy with carotid artery stenting to prevent stroke. Health Technol Assess 2017;21(57):1–40.

67. Qureshi AI, Chaudhry SA, Qureshi MH, et al. Rates and predictors of 5-year survival in a national cohort of asymptomatic elderly patients undergoing carotid revascularization. Neurosurgery 2015; 76(1):34–40 [discussion: 40–1].

68. EC/IC Bypass Study Group. Failure of extracranial-intracranial arterial bypass to reduce the risk of ischemic stroke. Results of an international randomized trial. N Engl J Med 1985;313(19): 1191–200.

69. Powers WJ, Clarke WR, Grubb RL Jr, et al, COSS Investigators. Extracranial-intracranial bypass surgery for stroke prevention in hemodynamic cerebral ischemia: the Carotid Occlusion Surgery Study randomized trial. JAMA 2011;306(18): 1983–92 [Erratum in: JAMA. 2011;306(24):2672. Obviagele, Bruce [corrected to Ovbiagele, Bruce]. PMID: 22068990; PMCID: PMC3601825].

70. Amin-Hanjani S, Barker FG 2nd, Charbel FT, et al. Cerebrovascular Section of the American Association of Neurological Surgeons; Congress of Neurological Surgeons. Extracranial-intracranial bypass for stroke-is this the end of the line or a bump in the road? Neurosurgery 2012;71(3):557–61.

71. Amin-Hanjani S, Butler WE, Ogilvy CS, et al. Extracranial—intracranial bypass in the treatment of occlusive cerebrovascular disease and intracranial aneurysms in the United States between 1992 and 2001: a population-based study. J Neurosurg 2005;103(5):794–804.

72. William J, Powers, William R, et al. Commentary: Extracranial-Intracranial Bypass for Stroke in 2012: Response to the Critique of the Carotid Occlusion Surgery Study "It was déjà vu all over again". Neurosurgery 2012;71(Issue 3):E772–6.

73. Chimowitz MI, Lynn MJ, Derdeyn CP, et al, SAMMPRIS Trial Investigators. Stenting versus aggressive medical therapy for intracranial arterial stenosis. N Engl J Med 2011;365(11):993–1003 [Erratum in: N Engl J Med. 2012;367(1):93. PMID: 21899409; PMCID: PMC3552515].

74. Starke RM, Crowley RW, Maltenfort M, et al. Moyamoya disorder in the United States. Neurosurgery 2012;71(1):93–9.

75. Kainth DS, Chaudhry SA, Kainth HS, et al. Prevalence and characteristics of concurrent down syndrome in patients with moyamoya disease. Neurosurgery 2013;72(2):210–5 [discussion: 215].

76. Karhade AV, Larsen AMG, Cote DJ, et al. National Databases for Neurosurgical Outcomes Research: Options, Strengths, and Limitations. Neurosurgery 2018;83(3):333–44.

77. Wen T, He S, Attenello F, et al. The impact of patient age and comorbidities on the occurrence of "never events" in cerebrovascular surgery: an analysis of the Nationwide Inpatient Sample. J Neurosurg 2014;121(3):580–6.

78. Fargen KM, Neal D, Rahman M, et al. The prevalence of patient safety indicators and hospital-acquired conditions in patients with ruptured cerebral aneurysms: establishing standard performance measures using the Nationwide Inpatient Sample database. J Neurosurg 2013;119(6): 1633–40.

79. Fargen KM, Rahman M, Neal D, et al. Prevalence of patient safety indicators and hospital-acquired conditions in those treated for unruptured cerebral aneurysms: establishing standard performance measures using the Nationwide Inpatient Sample database. J Neurosurg 2013;119(4): 966–73.

80. Michalak SM, Rolston JD, Lawton MT. Incidence and Predictors of Complications and Mortality in Cerebrovascular Surgery: National Trends From 2007 to 2012. Neurosurgery 2016;79(2):182–93.

81. Rambachan A, Smith TR, Saha S, et al. Reasons for readmission after carotid endarterectomy. World Neurosurg 2014;82(6):e771–6.

82. Lim S, Parsa AT, Kim BD, et al. Impact of resident involvement in neurosurgery: an analysis of 8748 patients from the 2011 American College of Surgeons National Surgical Quality Improvement Program database. J Neurosurg 2015;122(4): 962–70.

83. Lai PM, Lin N, Du R. Effect of teaching hospital status on outcome of aneurysm treatment. World Neurosurg 2014;82(3–4):380–5.e6.

84. Maud A, Lakshminarayan K, Suri MFK, et al. Cost-effectiveness analysis of endovascular versus neurosurgical treatment for ruptured intracranial aneurysms in the United States. J Neurosurg 2009;110(5):880–6.

85. Lad SP, Babu R, Rhee MS, et al. Long-term economic impact of coiling vs clipping for unruptured intracranial aneurysms. Neurosurgery 2013;72(6):1000–11 [discussion: 1011–3].

86. Bekelis K, Missios S, MacKenzie TA, et al. Predicting inpatient complications from cerebral aneurysm clipping: the Nationwide Inpatient Sample 2005–2009. J Neurosurg 2014;120(3):591–8.

87. Moscatelli M, Manconi A, Pessina M, et al. An infrastructure for precision medicine through analysis of big data. BMC Bioinformatics 2018;19:351.

88. Asher AL, Parker SL, Rolston JD, et al. Using clinical registries to improve the quality of neurosurgical care. Neurosurg Clin N Am 2015;26(2):253–63. ix-x.

89. Manrai AK, Patel CJ, Ioannidis JPA. In the Era of Precision Medicine and Big Data, Who Is Normal? JAMA 2018;319(19):1981–2.

90. Obermeyer Z, Topol EJ. Artificial intelligence, bias, and patients' perspectives. Lancet 2021;397(10289):2038.

91. Panesar SS, Kliot M, Parrish R, et al. Promises and Perils of Artificial Intelligence in Neurosurgery. Neurosurgery 2020;87(1):33–44.

92. Senders JT, Arnaout O, Karhade AV, et al. Natural and Artificial Intelligence in Neurosurgery: A Systematic Review. Neurosurgery 2018;83(2):181–92.

93. Tewarie IA, Hulsbergen AFC, Gormley WB, et al. Artificial Intelligence in Clinical Neurosurgery: More than Machinery. World Neurosurg 2021;149:302–3.

94. Dagi TF, Barker FG, Glass J. Machine Learning and Artificial Intelligence in Neurosurgery: Status, Prospects, and Challenges. Neurosurgery 2021;89(2):133–42.

95. Lim MJR. Letter: Machine Learning and Artificial Intelligence in Neurosurgery: Status, Prospects, and Challenges. Neurosurgery 2021;89(6):E333–4.

96. Dagi TF, Barker Ii FG, Glass J. In Reply: Machine Learning and Artificial Intelligence in Neurosurgery: Status, Prospects, and Challenges. Neurosurgery 2021;89(6):E335.

97. Ueda D, Yamamoto A, Nishimori M, et al. Deep Learning for MR Angiography: Automated Detection of Cerebral Aneurysms. Radiology 2019;290(1):187–94.

98. Hassan AE, Ringheanu VM, Rabah RR, et al. Early experience utilizing artificial intelligence shows significant reduction in transfer times and length of stay in a hub and spoke model. Interv Neuroradiol 2020;26(5):615–22.

99. Kondziolka D, Cooper BT, Lunsford LD, et al. Development, Implementation, and Use of a Local and Global Clinical Registry for Neurosurgery. Big Data 2015;3(2):80–9.

100. Meara JG, Leather AJ, Hagander L, et al. Global Surgery 2030: evidence and solutions for achieving health, welfare, and economic development. Lancet 2015;386(9993):569–624.

101. Garcia RM, Yoon S, Potts MB, et al. Investigating the Role of Ethnicity and Race in Patients Undergoing Treatment for Intracerebral Aneurysms Between 2008 and 2013 from a National Database. World Neurosurg 2016;96:230–6.

102. Attenello FJ, Wang K, Wen T, et al. Health disparities in time to aneurysm clipping/coiling among aneurysmal subarachnoid hemorrhage patients: a national study. World Neurosurg 2014;82(6):1071–6.

103. Wen T, Attenello FJ, He S, et al. Racial and socioeconomic disparities in incidence of hospital-acquired complications following cerebrovascular procedures. Neurosurgery 2014;75(1):43–50.

104. Walicke P, Abosch A, Asher A, et al. Workshop Participants. Launching Effectiveness Research to Guide Practice in Neurosurgery: A National Institute Neurological Disorders and Stroke Workshop Report. Neurosurgery 2017;80(4):505–14.

105. Siddiq F, Chaudhry SA, Tummala RP, et al. Factors and outcomes associated with early and delayed aneurysm treatment in subarachnoid hemorrhage patients in the United States. Neurosurgery 2012;71(3):670–7 [discussion: 677–8].

106. Bekelis K, Gottlieb DJ, Su Y, et al. Medicare expenditures for elderly patients undergoing surgical clipping or endovascular intervention for subarachnoid hemorrhage. J Neurosurg 2017;126(3):805–10.

107. Holland CM, Foley KT, Asher AL. Editorial. Can big data bridge the chasm? Issues, opportunities, and strategies for the evolving value-based health care environment. Neurosurg Focus FOC 2015;39(6):E2.

108. Das P, Abuhusain HJ, Reka A, et al. Letter: Harnessing Big Data: The Need for Datathon Research in Neurosurgery. Neurosurgery 2020;86(4):E402.

109. Shakir HJ, Shakir MA, Sharan AD, et al. The Future Currency of Neurosurgery is Data. Neurosurgery 2018;83(Issue 3):E125–7.

110. Selden NR, Ghogawala Z, Harbaugh RE, et al. The future of practice science: challenges and opportunities for neurosurgery. Neurosurg Focus FOC 2013;34(1):E8.

Exoscopic Cerebrovascular Neurosurgery

Omer Doron, MD, David J. Langer, MD, Jason A. Ellis, MD*

KEYWORDS

• Brain surgery • Endoscope • Exoscope • Microscope • Microsurgery • Surgical education

KEY POINTS

• Advancements in high resolution operative field magnification have been the driving force for refinements in cerebrovascular surgery visualization.
• The exoscope offers advantages over the standard operating microscope in the areas of magnification, resolution, lighting, ergonomics, operative team cohesiveness, and microsurgical training.
• Overcoming the learning cure for use of the exoscope is feasible with dedicated practice.

INTRODUCTION

The operative microscope (OM) was first introduced in the early 20th century, although it only became popularized for use in neurosurgery in the 1960s.[1] Pioneering neurosurgeons including Theodore Kurze, Raymond Donaghy, M. Gazi Yasargil, and others were among the first to use the OM in cerebrovascular neurosurgery. Allowing for improved magnification, illumination, and stereoscopic visualization of the surgical field, the OM vastly improved the safety and effectiveness of neurovascular surgery. It is an understatement to say that the OM was a revolutionary tool in this field.[2]

Steady improvements during the ensuing decades ushered in improved microscope ergonomics, smoother mechanics, better optics, and advanced digital image processing. These advances coupled with the integration of additional tools such as neuronavigation, fluorescence imaging, and video angiography have made the OM an indispensable tool in neurovascular surgery. Despite the OM being such a transformative tool in neurosurgery, it has several deficiencies that have created space for newer technology to be advanced.[3,4]

In 2008, the extracorporeal telescope system or exoscope was first introduced.[5] While several variations exist, the device concept is that of a scope positioned outside of the body and projecting its view of the surgical field onto a monitor.[6] The surgical exoscope is essentially the operative field visualization technology that has picked up whereby the OM left off. Thus, it can be thought of as the technological successor to the OM in neurovascular surgery. In this article, we explore how the exoscope has built on the remarkable achievements of the OM to further improve surgical field visualization, operator comfort, robotic and other technology integration, as well as education in cerebrovascular microsurgery.

THE EXOSCOPIC ADVANTAGE

The hallmarks of exoscopic microneurosurgery include its agile nature, easy maneuverability, unparalleled optics, and provision of operative field views that are of high quality and standardized for all within the operating theater. These advantageous features shine even brighter in cerebrovascular neurosurgery, the subspecialty considered an early adopter of this technology.[7]

Multiple exoscope systems for use in neurosurgery are currently available including the VITOM 3D (Karl Storz SE & Co. KG, Tuttlingen, Germany), KINEVO (Carl Zeiss Meditec AG, Oberkochen, Germany), Modus V (Synaptive Medical, Toronto, Canada), and ORBEYE (Olympus, Tokyo, Japan). The VITOM (Karl Storz, Tuttlingen, Germany)

Department of Neurosurgery, Lenox Hill Hospital, Zucker School of Medicine at Hofstra/Northwell, 130 East 77th Street, Black Hall Bldg, Third Floor, New York, NY 10075, USA
* Corresponding author.
E-mail address: Jellis2@northwell.edu

Neurosurg Clin N Am 33 (2022) 483–489
https://doi.org/10.1016/j.nec.2022.05.008
1042-3680/22/© 2022 Elsevier Inc. All rights reserved.

serves as a mounted endoscope with upgraded optics that can be positioned using a pneumatic arm. In contrast, the Modus V (Synaptive Medical, Toronto, Canada) and the ORBEYE (Olympus, Tokyo, Japan) integrate a camera built into an arm that is attached to a base and can be manually manipulated with projection onto a high-definition screen. The ORBEYE (Olympus, Tokyo, Japan) offers 3D-4 K capability while the Modus V (Synaptive Medical, Toronto, Canada) offers robotic arm technology with the integration of navigation and additional software enhancements such as tractography. Finally, the KINEVO (Carl Zeiss AG, Oberkochen, Germany) can be used either as a microscope or an exoscope and it has a number of add-ons that improve visualization and enable additional planning.

Exoscope Versus Microscope

Over the last decade, since the exoscope was first introduced, technological advancements have improved not only the camera hardware and optics but also the viewing screen fidelity. Magnification power has increased, thanks to the development of ultrahigh-definition 3D camera technology. This has also enabled wide operative field views over long focal distances. Additional practical considerations such as the ease of storage due to smaller footprint and cost generally compares favorably with microscopes.[8,9]

Exoscope Versus Endoscope

First-generation exoscopes were often little more than mounted endoscope cameras used in an extracorporeal fashion. Bringing the endoscope "out of the body cavity" enlarged the field of view, lengthened the working distance, and unconstrained the camera from bony and soft tissue anatomy. This enabled "over the corner" views by tilting and rotating the exoscope with far greater freedom compared with both endoscopes and microscopes.[10,11] The extracorporeal location of exoscopes also eliminates the need to routinely clean the lens during surgery as is so often necessary in traditional endoscopic surgery.

ERGONOMICS

An immediate advantage offered by the use of exoscopes in microvascular neurosurgery is improved surgeon ergonomics, allowing for a more physiologic posture throughout the surgery. The OM with the required use of an eyepiece typically required the surgeon's head to be outside of a physiologically neutral body axis position. This configuration requires flexion of the operator's

cervical spine, which in long cases is known to worsen fatigue and compromise the surgeon's performance.[12,13] In cerebrovascular neurosurgery this effect is intensified as the duration of the microsurgical portion in these cases may be prolonged.[8] This leads to muscle and eye-strain with less control of hand movements and worsened overall stability. As head bending from a neutral position can result in up to four times increased load on the cervical spine,[6] this may lead to loss of lordosis and compensatory hyperkyphosis at the thoracic level. For the assisting surgeon, body position relative to the surgical field may be even worse, resulting in significant discomfort and limiting their ability to participate in microsurgical manipulation.

The OM was designed to allow "through-the-lens" imaging, with light being delivered from the operative field to the operator's face. The exoscope was transformative in that it "uncoupled" this connection, enabling a "sight-line" strategy via a digital screen. This enables the surgeon to operate using physiologic posture throughout the case with a head up and neutral position (**Fig. 1**).

In a simulation study conducted by Hafez and colleagues[8] modeling a bypass procedure, 2 hundred 1-mm chicken wing vessels were anastomosed either in an exoscopic or a microscopic approach (100 samples each). The authors stated that the exoscope improved comfort over the microscope and allowed for more unconstrained movements with a more relaxed posture. Importantly they note that this ergonomic superiority was more apparent during long working sessions. Nossek and colleagues[12] described the use of the Orbeye in 5 STA-MCA bypass cases and emphasized that such long cases requiring precise focus require surgeon comfort which is facilitated by a neutral sitting position. Use of an associated foot pedal that allows control of magnification and focus was also noted to improve the performance of the microvascular anastomosis.

Shimizu and colleagues reported a similar experience for microvascular decompression (MVD) in a case series using the retrosigmoid approach in the supine position.[14] The authors indicate the flexibility and small size of the ORBEYE improved posture and comfort even when the operative visual axis was approximately horizontal.

During microvascular anastomosis, we have noted that the extreme angles at which the exoscope camera can be placed relative to the surgical field allow the operator to inspect the entirety of the suture line including the back wall with minimal manipulation of the vessel or contortion of the surgeon's body. Hafez and colleagues[15] performed a comparative laboratory study and showed that

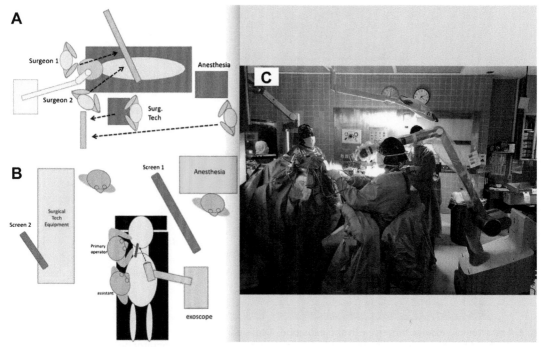

Fig. 1. Operating room set-up in a variety of cases. Typical setup for a bypass or clipping has the operator and assistant facing the screen with the exoscope between them (*A*). Alternatively, the setup for carotid endarterectomy allows the operator and assistant to stand side by side with the exoscope base contralateral (*B*). In sitting position cases, only the primary operator has access to the deep field, however, operator neck position remains neutral while the exoscope camera is positioned in a nearly perpendicular orientation to the occiput (*C*).

both the OM and exoscope allow for effective bypass suturing. However, noteworthy observations include that: 1. suturing time was shorter with the OM, presumably a result of the operator learning curve using the less familiar exoscope and 2. stitch distribution was better using the exoscope, supporting the idea it provides a better circumferential view and resolution of the suture line (**Fig. 2**A, B).

For carotid endarterectomy (CEA), several publications have demonstrated the utility of achieving extreme exoscope angles that would be ergonomically unfavorable using an OM.[7,16] This is especially the case in the setting of high cervical carotid bifurcations. Ellis and colleagues,[16] presented a series of 18 CEA cases comparing the use of the OM and exoscope as subjectively assessed by 2 surgeons. The authors concluded that the exoscope contributes to improved neck dissection (due to improved lighting and field of view), plaque resection, and suturing of the arteriotomy (attributed to the highly magnified, ultrahigh-resolution view which enables easy delineation of the vessel wall). In this study, the ability to inspect the ICA lumen after endarterectomy even in high bifurcation cases was thought to be a significant benefit conferred by the exoscope (**Fig. 2**C).

This advantageous combination of a wide field of view coupled with maneuverability through "tough" viewing angles was also demonstrated in aneurysm surgery. In one report of aneurysm clipping with the use of exoscopic visualization, it was noted that table position adjustments were required less frequently than with a traditional OM.[8,17] It was also noted that the exoscope angle allowed improved illumination under the sphenoid wing facilitating safe drilling.

OPTICS

The exoscope offers magnified, high-resolution views of the operative field that generally surpass that offered by most microscopes. Exoscopic magnification up to 25 times is achievable by most systems. In vascular procedures, the exoscope's high resolution facilitates dissection within subarachnoid planes, helps in the identification of vessel wall components, and may facilitate safer microsurgical manipulation of tissue (**Fig. 3**).[6,12]

Despite steady improvements in the OM over the years, the field of view remains relatively narrow and tissue desiccation from light source heating remains problematic. The need for constant refocusing with most movements is also an issue

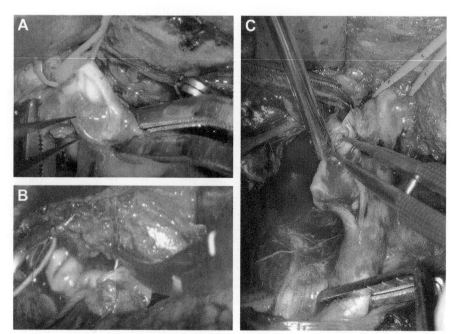

Fig. 2. Extracranial vascular surgery with the exoscope. These panels demonstrate the variety of possible operating angels achievable using the exoscope all while maintaining the neutral operator neck position. Distal anastomosis of a vein graft to the V3 vertebral artery segment between C1 and C2 is shown (*A*). Seamless transition to the proximal anastomosis of the vein graft to the external carotid artery is facilitated by the exoscope (*B*). Here the agility of the exoscope is highlighted as it allows the inspection of the distal lumen of the ICA in "high bifurcation" carotid endarterectomy surgery (*C*).

for practitioners using the OM. Assistant visualization of the operative field from an observer eyepiece is another source of concern when using the OM as this view is not stereoscopic and is at a different angle compared with the primary surgeon. In addition, integration of the OM with other platforms and creating an image layered with information such as neuronavigation or anatomic heads-up display is not possible without looking outside the eyepiece.

For cerebral bypass cases, whereby a highly magnified field is critical, Nossek and colleagues [12] reported "clear and crisp" visualization of all critical vessels when using an exoscope. This was primarily praised during the preparation of the donor and recipient vessels as well as for arteriotomy. It was also noted that the improvements in magnification and 3D capability allowed for ease of micro-anastomosis using interrupted 10 to 0 sutures. Specifically, the authors found that improved lighting allowed for better identification of the vessel walls (**Fig. 4**).

Noro and colleagues,[17] compared a mouthpiece–controlled OM (OPMI PENTERO 900; Carl Zeiss Meditec AG) and robotic arm–controlled 3D digital Aeos exoscope (Aesculap Inc) for the clipping of 2 unruptured right-sided middle cerebral artery bifurcation aneurysms.

They noted that the eyepiece often had to be adjusted on the OM, requiring the removal of one hand from the surgical field to adjust the view. The wider field of view enabled by the exoscope allowed the operator to continue the dissection with minor foot-pedal adjustments. Interestingly, in this report, the Aeos exoscope's ability to offer additional contrast and color modes to view the surgical field with the coloration of structures was thought to be beneficial. They found this tool provided an increased distinction between closely related anatomic structures, especially at deeper locations and through narrow surgical corridors.

OPERATING ROOM COMMUNICATION AND WORKFLOW

The exoscope provides a real-time image transmitted to several screens throughout the operating room. This enables surgeons, assistants, surgical technicians, and other operating room staff to share identical operative views simultaneously. Thus, the exoscope has been noted to be a tool that "democratizes" the operating room. This is considered quite valuable in cerebrovascular neurosurgery, especially in cases whereby the entire OR teams should be highly vigilant, coordinated, and efficient such as when bleeding or other complications have

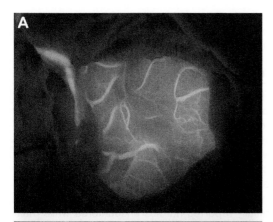

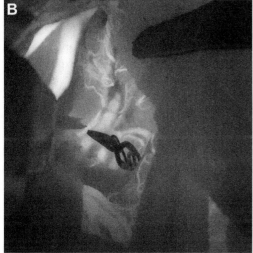

Fig. 3. Exoscopic video angiography. Here, ICG angiography after completion of an EC-IC bypass anastomosis is shown (A). Similarly, here ICG angiography shows complete occlusion of a right MCA aneurysm with the preservation of parent vessel filling (B).

occurred. Khalessi and colleagues[7] described this in the setting of an intraoperative aneurysm rupture. Using the exoscope, all team members became aware at once allowing easy augmentation of the team's coordinated workflow including rapid passing of instruments and unobstructed assistance to obtain vascular control. For aneurysms, the low profile of the exoscope and the space between the scope and the field were described as particularly helpful for passing long-handled instruments, such as clip appliers.[17]

Similarly, during AVM resection with the use of an ORBEYE,[7] the exoscope was found to be particularly useful when significant intraoperative bleeding was encountered. It was noted that the large screen with a wide field-of-view allowed clear visualization of the operative field allowing the surgeon and assistant to work simultaneously to clear the field and continue the AVM resection.

The identical view provided by the utilization of the exoscope conceptually allows for "four hand" surgery (see **Fig. 4**). This advantage was described both for donor vessel preparation in cerebral bypass surgery,[12] as well as for intracerebral hemorrhage evacuation.[18] Four hand microsurgery has been described for ICH evacuation using the exoscope which allows for microsurgical manipulation of the hematoma while retracting obstructing brain parenchyma with greater ease compared with visualization with a traditional OM.

Lastly, the positive impact of the exoscope on workflow is accentuated in cases whereby neuronavigation is a key part of the procedure. By enabling a "picture-in-picture" mode, the operator may gain an immediate understanding of the relationship between the magnified surgical field and the neuroanatomical location being probed. These features become increasingly important in the resection of deep-seated lesions such as cavernomas as well as in intracerebral hematoma.[19] With a shift toward more minimally invasive approaches with less anatomic cues apparent, real-time neuronavigational feedback is increasingly necessary to safely perform vascular neurosurgery. The ease of using either a navigation wand or a hand-held ultrasound probe while not stopping to take the eyes off of the field or moving the scope away from the field are clear advantages afforded by the exoscope.

EDUCATIONAL BENEFITS

In the current era whereby vascular microneurosurgical exposure has become scarce for trainees, tools that facilitate efficient microsurgical training have become even more vital. For cerebrovascular neurosurgery, perhaps one of the most important advantages conferred by the use of the exoscope is its ability to serve as an educational tool. A systematic review found that most of the studies described a significant benefit to the exoscope as a teaching platform.[20] Evaluating trainee's experience, Nossek and colleagues[12] found that using an exoscope improved learner participation throughout the procedure and enabled more hands-on involvement of the assistant. The exoscope, facilitated by the identical viewing perspective of the primary surgeon and trainee/assistant, allows for seamless transitioning between the primary operators.[8,20] By allowing comfortable posture of the assistant working alongside the primary surgeon, the exoscope facilitated opportunities for microsurgical experience to be gained by the trainee safely.[18] This con whereby surgeon and assistant have the same point of view improved understanding of anatomic relations and dissection techniques by the trainee.

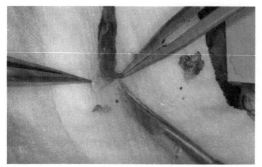

Fig. 4. "Four hand surgery." Easy utilization of an assistant for microsurgical manipulation is demonstrated with the use of the exoscope. Such fine maneuvering by an assistant is often cumbersome, uncomfortable, or impossible using the standard operating microscope. In this case, both operators are seen "cleaning up" the distal tip of the harvested superficial temporal artery.

PITFALLS

The introduction of a new learning curve for senior neurosurgeons who have spent decades mastering the use of the OM is undoubtedly a major challenge to a more widespread utilization of the exoscope. Operating in a heads-up fashion, facing a screen and not an eyepiece while establishing clear, unobstructed surgical "sight lines" to the monitors, necessitates the recalibration of not only the surgeon but the entire operating room team.[6,12,16]

Burkhardt and colleagues[21] found that half of the surgeons they surveyed found it more difficult to assist with the VITOM 3D as compared with the OM. In their study, scrub nurses also found their positioning uncomfortable approximately 75% of the time. However, this wasn't reported with the ORBEYE. Surgical techs did identify that instruments often needed to be passed in front of the assistant surgeon in some cases, which may be undesirable.[7]

As the exoscope has necessarily been liberated from the operator's face, the mouthpiece has been abandoned. Undoubtedly, mouth-piece trained neurosurgeons may find it difficult to transition over to a foot pedal.[12]

Older literature indicated that some may develop headaches as a result of operating in 3D. However, newer series[7,22] presumably using more advanced 3D technology suggest this issue has largely been resolved. Nonetheless, similar to "simulator sickness," this phenomenon is expected to be mitigated by repeated exposure. Visual difficulty due to eyestrain has also been reported with the use of 3D displays and seems to be related to the length of time spent viewing.[22]

This was experienced during longer procedures and may require the introduction of strategies such as planned breaks.

Future Directions

The exoscope has clear advantages over the OM for surgical field visualization, improved team communication, ease of maintenance/storage/use, and surgical education. While early adopters widely praise these attributes of the exoscope, it is likely that widespread utilization in neurovascular surgery awaits the next generation of cerebrovascular surgeons currently in training. The initially reported hurdles encountered while making the transition from OM to exoscope typically fit within the realm of a "learning curve" rather than lack of feasibility.

As more experience is gained and the exoscope becomes more widely used, it is expected that continued seamless integration of surgical adjuncts is warranted. Further integration of robotics, automation, augmented reality, hands-free real-time neuronavigation are actively being refined with new exoscope hardware and software. The exoscope is well-positioned to become an integral tool in the cerebrovascular neurosurgeon's armamentarium.

CLINICS CARE POINTS

- Operative field magnification, resolution, lighting, ergonomics, operative team cohesiveness, and microsurgical training are all facilitated by the use of the exoscope in cerebrovascular surgery
- Both new and seasoned microneurosurgeons have embraced this technology with the knowledge that transitioning from the operative microscope will require focused training

DISCLOSURE

The authors have nothing to disclose.

REFERENCES

1. Yaşargil MG, Krayenbühl H. The use of the binocular microscope in neurosurgery. Bibl Ophthalmol 1970; 81:62–5.
2. Kriss TC, Kriss VM. History of the operating microscope: from magnifying glass to microneurosurgery. Neurosurgery 1998;42:899–907.

3. Wing-Yee CW. Evolution and clinical application of microsurgery. BMC Proc 2015;9(Suppl 3):A53.

4. Wårdell K. Neuroengineering challenges in neurosurgery. Int J Artif Organs 2019;42:386.

5. Mamelak AN, Nobuto T, Berci G. Initial clinical experience with a high-definition exoscope system for microneurosurgery. Neurosurgery 2010;67:476–83.

6. Langer DJ, White TG, Schulder M, et al. Advances in Intraoperative Optics: A Brief Review of Current Exoscope Platforms. Oper Neurosurg (Hagerstown) 2020;19:84–93.

7. Khalessi AA, Rahme R, Rennert RC, et al. First-in-man clinical experience using a high-definition 3-dimensional exoscope system for microneurosurgery. Onsurg 2019;16(6):717–25.

8. Hafez A, Haeren RHL, Dillmann J, et al. Comparison of Operating Microscope and Exoscope in a Highly Challenging Experimental Setting. World Neurosurg 2021;147:e468–75.

9. Herlan S, Marquardt JS, Hirt B, et al. 3D Exoscope System in Neurosurgery-Comparison of a Standard Operating Microscope with a New 3D Exoscope in the Cadaver Lab. Oper Neurosurg (Hagerstown) 2019;17:518–24.

10. Nagatani K, Takeuchi S, Feng D, et al. [High-Definition Exoscope System for Microneurosurgery:Use of an Exoscope in Combination with Tubular Retraction and Frameless Neuronavigation for Microsurgical Resection of Deep Brain Lesions]. No Shinkei Geka 2015;43:611–7.

11. Panchal S, Yamada Y, Nagatani T, et al. A practice survey to compare and identify the usefulness of neuroendoscope and exoscope in the current neurosurgery practice. Asian J Neurosurg 2020; 15(3):601–7.

12. Nossek E, Schneider JR, Kwan K, et al. Technical aspects and operative nuances using a high-definition 3-dimensional exoscope for cerebral bypass surgery. Onsurg 2019;17(2):157–63.

13. Kwan K, Schneider JR, Du V, et al. Lessons learned using a high-definition 3-dimensional exoscope for spinal surgery. Onsurg 2019;16(5):619–25.

14. Shimizu T, Toyota S, Nakagawa K, et al. Retrosigmoid approach in the supine position using OR-BEYE: A consecutive series of 14 cases. Neurol Med Chir (Tokyo) 2021;61:55–61.

15. Hafez A, Elsharkawy A, Schwartz C, et al. Comparison of Conventional Microscopic and Exoscopic Experimental Bypass Anastomosis: A Technical Analysis. World Neurosurg 2020;135:e293.

16. Ellis JA, Doron O, Schneider JR, et al. Technical aspects and operative nuances using a high-definition 4K-3-dimensional exoscope for carotid endarterectomy surgery. Br J Neurosurg 2021;1–6. https://doi.org/10.1080/02688697.2021.1982865.

17. Haeren R, Hafez A, Lehecka M. Visualization and Maneuverability Features of a Robotic Arm Three-Dimensional Exoscope and Operating Microscope for Clipping an Unruptured Intracranial Aneurysm: Video Comparison and Technical Evaluation. Oper Neurosurg (Hagerstown) 2022;22:28–34.

18. Murakami T, Toyota S, Suematsu T, et al. Four hands surgery for intracerebral hemorrhage using orbeye: Educational values and ergonomic advantages – A technical note. Asian J Neurosurg 2021;16(3):634–7.

19. Scranton RA, Fung SH, Britz GW. Transulcal parafascicular minimally invasive approach to deep and subcortical cavernomas: Technical note. J Neurosurg 2016;125:1360–6.

20. Ricciardi L, Chaichana KL, Cardia A, et al. The Exoscope in Neurosurgery: An Innovative "Point of View". A Systematic Review of the Technical, Surgical, and Educational Aspects. World Neurosurg 2019;124:136–44.

21. Oertel JM, Burkhardt BW. Vitom-3D for Exoscopic Neurosurgery: Initial Experience in Cranial and Spinal Procedures. World Neurosurg 2017;105:153–62.

22.. Fiani B, Jarrah R, Griepp DW, et al. The Role of 3D Exoscope Systems in Neurosurgery: An Optical Innovation. Cureus 2021;13:e15878.

Endoscopic Techniques in Vascular Neurosurgery

Aneek Patel, BS[a], Hussam Abou-Al-Shaar, MD[a], Arka N. Mallela, MD, MS[a], Hanna Algattas, MD[a], Michael M. McDowell, MD[a], Georgios A. Zenonos, MD[a], Eric W. Wang, MD[b], Carl H. Snyderman, MD, MBA[b], Paul A. Gardner, MD[a,*]

KEYWORDS

- Endoscopic endonasal approach • Aneurysm clipping • Paraclinoid • Nasoseptal flap
- Reconstruction • Skull base • Multidisciplinary

KEY POINTS

- Endoscopes can be used as a primary visualization tool to provide unique corridors for treating vascular lesions (eg, the endoscopic endonasal approach) or as an adjunct to standard microscopic approaches (endoscope assisted).
- Anatomically favorable aneurysms for endoscopic endonasal surgery include medially projecting paraclinoidal internal carotid artery (ICA) aneurysms, low-lying basilar, mid-basilar, and ventral posterior-inferior cerebellar artery or vertebrobasilar junction aneurysms.
- Endoscopic endonasal vascular surgery poses a steep learning curve that requires multidisciplinary collaboration and shared expertise. Success leverages existing microsurgical vascular techniques along with a strong understanding of endonasal anatomy, endoscopic techniques and instrumentation, and advanced skull base reconstruction techniques.
- The endoscopic endonasal approach provides direct access to the ventral skull base, from the subfrontal anterior fossa to the parasellar region to the clivus. This direct corridor can be used for anatomically favorable lesions as long as it allows for adequate vascular control and improved access compared with an open approach.
- Endoscopes should be readily available during microscopic treatment of vascular lesions and can provide added visualization to ensure completeness of treatment of aneurysms on the deep side of arteries (ie, ventral ICA, medial ophthalmic/carotid cave, and so forth), confirm preservation of hidden perforating arteries, and inspect cavernous malformation cavities to ensure completeness of resection.

 Video content accompanies this article at http://www.neurosurgery.theclinics.com

INTRODUCTION

Most of the intracranial aneurysms and vascular lesions (arteriovenous malformations, dural arteriovenous fistulas (dAVFs), and cavernous malformations) can be safely accessed either endovascularly or through open microscopic approaches with excellent outcomes. However, for those that are not well suited to endovascular treatment, there are regions of the ventral skull base best accessed endonasally and there are certain vascular lesions of the proximal anterior and posterior circulation with specific characteristics—be it location, size, and in cases of aneurysms, aneurysm projection, and neck features—for which open transcranial approaches can be

[a] Department of Neurological Surgery, University of Pittsburgh Medical Center, 200 Lothrop Street, PUH B-400, Pittsburgh, PA, 15213, USA; [b] Department of Otolaryngology, University of Pittsburgh Medical Center, 200 Lothrop Street, EEINS Suite 500, Pittsburgh, PA, 15213, USA
* Corresponding author. Department of Neurological Surgery, University of Pittsburgh Medical Center, 200 Lothrop Street, Suite PUH B-400, Pittsburgh, PA 15213.
E-mail address: gardpa@upmc.edu

Neurosurg Clin N Am 33 (2022) 491–503
https://doi.org/10.1016/j.nec.2022.06.005
1042-3680/22/© 2022 Elsevier Inc. All rights reserved.

unfavorably challenging. In those instances, the midline corridor of the endoscopic endonasal approach (EEA) can often provide a safe and more direct route with increased visibility of both the pathology itself as well as sites of proximal and distal vascular control, minimizing the exposure and manipulation of major vessels and neural elements.

The concept of an anterior midline corridor for vascular lesions first manifested itself in the 1980s through the use of a transoral approach to posterior circulation aneurysms.[1,2] Although the approach minimized contact with critical skull base structures and tissue exposure, the technique had a high rate of perioperative complications. In addition, it often led to palatal insufficiency and retropharyngeal pseudomeningoceles.[3] To reduce such morbidity, Ogilvy and colleagues[4] successfully clipped several posterior circulation aneurysms in 1996 using a transfacial transclival approach that reflected the nose laterally, removed the septum, and involved bilateral ethmoidectomies and maxillectomies. However, postoperative meningitis rates were still high due to the rudimentary skull base reconstruction methods available at the time.

The EEA confers the same benefits of other midline trajectory approaches and provides direct visualization of certain vascular lesions, bolstered by more effective skull base reconstruction using vascularized flaps. The use of EEA to address midline lesions along the skull base has increased in recent decades; as experience with the approach has grown, technical innovations have expanded EEA's access past the posterior fossa into the craniocervical junction, allowing for access from the crista galli all the way down to C2.[5,6] The EEA approach was first reported for aneurysm surgery in 2006 by Kassam and colleagues, who used it for a large vertebral artery (VA) aneurysm followed by a superior hypophyseal aneurysm in 2007.[7,8] Since then, the application of and experience with EEA for cerebrovascular surgery has slowly grown, allowing for a clearer understanding of the types of vascular lesions well suited for this approach and best practices preoperatively, intraoperatively, and postoperatively, to ensure optimal outcomes for patients while minimizing complications.

Each aneurysm, dAVF, cavernous malformation, and arteriovenous malformation (AVM) should be treated in a tailored case-by-case fashion based on the anatomy of the lesion and its surroundings, through the best modality, whether endoscopic, microscopic, endovascular, or radiosurgical. Because of the limited experience with EEA for vascular lesions, most reports describe its

utilization for aneurysm surgery with only scarce literature (case reports) on its use for dAVF, AVM, and cavernous malformations. This paper is designed to delineate which aneurysms and vascular lesions are best addressed using an endoscope, especially via the unique EEA corridor, as well as for additional visualization during microsurgery.

Nature of the Problem

Aneurysms

Despite advances in endovascular technology, certain intracranial aneurysms remain best managed with clipping due to vessel location and aneurysm morphology. In addition, certain aneurysms of both the anterior and posterior circulations can be particularly difficult to access, as they are largely hidden when approached through traditional transcranial microscopic corridors. Endoscopes can be used to improve this visualization during inspection after transcranial clipping or to allow entirely different corridors (endonasal) for clipping. Paraclinoid internal carotid artery (ICA) aneurysms that project inferomedially, for instance, can require completely blind clipping through transcranial approaches (which can be evaluated by adding endoscopic assistance) and allow for direct visualization and clipping endonasally.[6]

The aforementioned illustrates the first challenge, visualization; given the anatomic location of such proximal ICA aneurysms, visualization from a lateral approach often requires opening of the falciform ligament into the optic nerve sheath and mobilization or retraction of the optic nerve for even partial view of the associated delicate neurovascular structures at an unfavorable angle.[9–11] Structures that must be carefully addressed frequently include the ophthalmic artery, superior hypophyseal artery, optic apparatus, and pituitary stalk. The same issue holds true for mid-basilar/anterior inferior cerebellar artery (AICA) or distal/ventral posterior inferior cerebellar artery (PICA) aneurysms where clipping often ends up partially blind from a lateral approach.

The second challenge is vascular control. Achieving proximal control of the ICA through an anterolateral transcranial approach may require an anterior clinoidectomy and, for many ophthalmic or superior hypophyseal artery aneurysms, might require cervical ICA exposure, which in itself does not account for other collaterals via ICA/external carotid artery (ECA) connections.[12] Transcavernous dissection can be performed to achieve more proximal control, but this necessitates manipulation of cranial nerves. Both challenges of visualization and proximal control can be mitigated through the EEA, which allows for direct midline visualization of these aneurysms with no additional manipulation of major neurovascular elements as well as the immediate availability of a large length of proximal parasellar and paraclival cavernous ICA that can be exposed for proximal control.

There are specific sites along the posterior circulation that pose similar challenges during lateral transcranial approaches. Vascular lesions near the ventral pons and medulla, in particular, are difficult to access through lateral approaches due to their relationship ventral to cranial nerves, the brainstem, and a significant degree of perforators whose location and course vary in each patient. Low-lying basilar apex and basilar trunk aneurysms are poorly visualized through subtemporal or anterolateral approaches due to obscuration by the posterior clinoid process and caudal clivus.[13] Superior cerebellar artery (SCA), AICA, and ventromedial PICA aneurysms all pose similar visualization challenges and lack either proximal, distal, or contralateral vascular access necessary for true control.[6,14] For such posterior vascular aneurysms, the endoscopic endonasal transclival approach offers a microsurgical clipping option through an anatomically superior corridor.

The angle of aneurysm projection is just as critical as the location in aneurysm surgery. Aneurysms whose anatomic sites are readily accessible with good proximal and distal control can still be challenging to clip if the aneurysm points toward or away from the angle of approach, preventing a clear view of and access to the neck while simultaneously being able to screen for perforating vessels. For this reason, proximal circulation aneurysms that project from the deep aspect of a vessel relative to the approach can prove difficult to clip through lateral open transcranial approaches but could be more amenable to the midline trajectory of EEA or at very least require endoscopic inspection to ensure adequate treatment.[15]

Cavernous Malformations

Cavernous malformations (also known as cavernomas, cavernous angiomas, and cavernous hemangiomas) are the second most common intracranial vascular lesion, among which approximately 20% are located within the brainstem—predominantly in the pons.[16] Brainstem cavernous malformations (BCMs) are particularly difficult to treat because they are embedded within eloquent brainstem parenchyma.[17] However, surgical resection is often necessary, in the subacute phase following hemorrhage, due to their high rehemorrhage risk compared with supratentorial

cavernous malformations and their symptomatic compression of critical brainstem structures and nuclei.[18] When such BCMs approach the pial surface—as they commonly do—surgical resection is often indicated, and the discussion turns to selecting the most direct approach that minimizes retraction of surrounding eloquent parenchyma.[19]

BCMs approaching the pial surface of the ventral pons can be approached through several microsurgical approaches, including a retrosigmoid approach or transpetrosal approach.[20] However, these trajectories inherently have relatively lateral trajectories and therefore cannot completely minimize retraction or even transgression of surrounding parenchyma. In addition, a transpetrosal approach requires significant bony drilling for adequate visualization while still having limited maneuverability.[19,21] Although a retrosigmoid approach through the middle cerebellar peduncle could allow for a safe window between cranial nerves V and VII, this narrow window commonly requires a piecemeal resection of the BCM and limits access both rostrally and caudally to these lesions.[22] Therefore, for ventral, midline, pontine, or medullary BCMs, a direct ventral approach such as that afforded by a transclival EEA should be considered. Midline ventral midbrain cavernous malformations, unlike cavernous malformations of the lower brainstem, can be approached subfrontally or transventricularly, but such approaches are not optimal because they are not directly ventral and therefore lead to unnecessary damage to surrounding parenchyma, including critical fiber tracts and cranial nerves.[23] In appropriate cases, a transtuberculum/transplanum or transclival with pituitary transposition EEA could potentially provide optimal, safe access to midbrain cavernous malformations (**Fig. 1**).[24] However, the decision to approach a BCM endonasally should not be made without careful evaluation of the descending motor tracts (such as with high-definition fiber tracking) to ensure that they would not be transgressed by an anterior approach.[25]

Cases of EEA for optochiasmatic and retrochiasmatic cavernous malformations have also been described; given the rarity of such lesions, very few cases of this approach have been documented. Cavernous malformations of the optic pathway are most commonly addressed through anterolateral or midline transcranial approaches.[26] However, it is critical to closely study the relationship of the optic pathway with the lesion, as such transcranial approaches may risk excessive retraction and manipulation of critical neurovascular structures and injury to small perforators, especially if the cavernous malformation is inferior to the chiasm or retrochiasmatic. Meng and

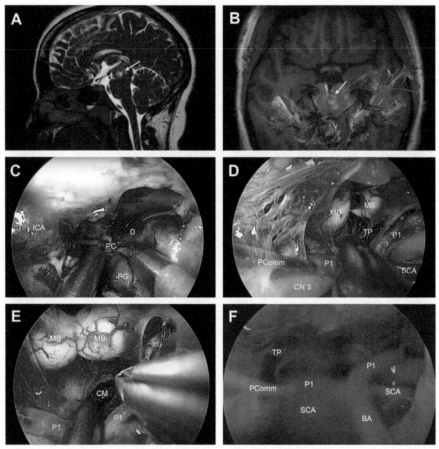

Fig. 1. A 25-year-old woman presented with sudden-onset diplopia and headaches. (*A*) Fast imaging employing steady-state acquisition (FIESTA) MRI demonstrated a midline mesencephalic cavernous malformation (*arrow*). (*B*) High-definition fiber tracking was performed to confirm that a direct anterior approach would not disrupt descending motor tracts. (*C*) Pituitary hemitransposition was performed to gain access to the interpeduncular cistern. The medial cavernous sinus is dissected and the lateral attachment of the diaphragma to the distal dural ring is cut to release the gland and stalk, respectively. (*D*) Thalamoperforating arteries were carefully dissected, and (*E*) the cavernous malformation was resected in a piecemeal fashion. (*F*) ICG angiography confirmed patency of the basilar artery, PCAs, and thalamoperforating arteries. BA, basilar artery; CM, cavernous malformation; CN, cranial nerve; D, diaphragma sellae; ICA, internal carotid artery; MB, mammillary body; P1, posterior cerebral artery; PC, posterior clinoid; PComm, posterior communicating artery; PG, pituitary gland; SCA, superior cerebellar artery; TP, thalamoperforating arteries.

colleagues described a case of an orbitochiasmatic cavernous malformation that was successfully resected endonasally with no complications.[27] Such an approach, for directly midline suprasellar vascular malformations, affords the same benefits of direct access and visualization as it does for similarly located aneurysms. Conversely, cavernous malformations that displace the optic chiasm or apparatus inferiorly or originate on the superior aspect of these structures should not be approached endonasally, as they would require transgression or retraction of the chiasm.

It should be noted, of course, that the application of EEA for any midline cavernous malformation has not been well studied and is largely

limited to case reports and small case series; however, EEA offers a promising, direct approach for midline or ventral cavernous malformations that is growing in use as centers expand their technical experience and comfort with EEAs.

Dural Arteriovenous Fistulas

High-risk dAVFs are traditionally treated via endovascular embolization.[28] However, in the case that endovascular treatment fails or that the vascular anatomy of the lesion is too complex, too narrow, or distal to readily reach endovascularly, surgical intervention remains the definitive treatment modality by disconnecting venous drainage as it exits the fistula.[29] Anterior fossa dAVFs, notably, are

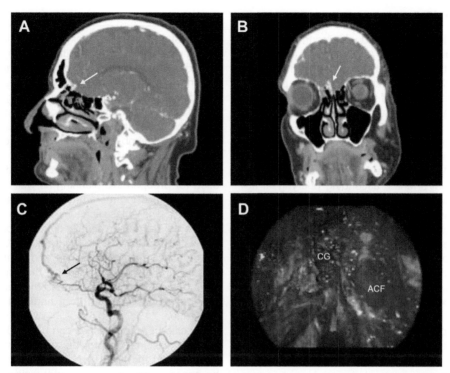

Fig. 2. A middle-aged man presents with new headache and is found to have an anterior fossa dAVF, depicted on (*A, B*) preoperative CT angiography and (*C*) digital subtraction angiography. Given its midline position, the dAVF was completely resected through an EEA that minimized disruption of surrounding neurovascular structures. (*D*) Intraoperative, endoscopic endonasal view showing the bipolar coagulation of the fistula just deep to its attachment to the midline dural attachment of the falx where the crista galli (CG) had been. ACF, anterior cranial fossa dura; CG, crista galli (removed). *Arrow* is pointed at the dAVF.

particularly difficult to access endovascularly due both to the tortuosity and narrow calibers of the ophthalmic and ethmoidal arteries as well as the small but significant risk of central retinal artery occlusion.[30] For such lesions, a low bifrontal craniotomy can provide wide exposure of the dAVF in a safe and highly effective manner.[31] Although an endonasal approach has not been largely used as a surgical corridor for venous disconnection of skull base dAVFs, EEA can provide access to such anterior fossa and clival dAVFs (**Fig. 2**). In addition, EEA does allow the potential for endovascular venous access via direct puncture that cannot otherwise be gained. Particularly for carotid-cavernous fistulas, EEA can provide a corridor for a direct puncture of the cavernous sinus to deploy embolic agents.[32] Karas and colleagues have recently extended this endonasal direct puncture technique to paracavernous dAVFs as well, directly puncturing the superior ophthalmic vein that could not otherwise be accessed endovascularly.[33]

Arteriovenous Malformations

The management of AVMs depends on their location, Spetzler-Martin grade, and patient characteristics. The management paradigm includes surgical resection, stereotactic radiosurgery, endovascular embolization, or a combination of the aforementioned techniques.[34] Wide exposure and access is necessary for safe and complete AVM resection. As such, only pure midline AVMs would be amenable to EEA. For osseous-based AVMs growing into the clivus, an extended subfrontal approach can be used in such cases to provide adequate access for resection. However, this approach is limited posteriorly by the optic chiasm and laterally by the cavernous sinus, making it difficult to access portions of the AVM in the lower third of the clivus. In the specific case of a midline clival AVM extending throughout the entirety of the clivus with minimal lateral extension, an EEA can potentially be used to gain clear exposure to the clivus along its length for successful resection.[35] It should again be noted that this application has not been well studied beyond case reports and small series but offers a strong alternative to a subfrontal approach in properly selected patients. Theoretically, small and focal AVMs of the subfrontal region (eg, gyrus rectus) would be ideal for endonasal access.

CASE EXAMPLE

A 4-year-old girl presented with recurrent, severe epistaxis due to a clival AVM that was diagnosed at 18 months of age. At that time, she had been treated with nasal packing followed by polyvinyl alcohol embolization of the right internal maxillary artery (IMAX), which was the predominant initial supply of the AVM. Two years later, however, she presented with a life-threatening episode of epistaxis; repeat angiography at that time revealed that the AVM was now being supplied by both IMAXs, facial arteries, ascending pharyngeal arteries, ICAs, and ophthalmic arteries. At that time, endovascular management was performed by the sequential embolizations of 4 feeding vessels. However, she continued to have significant episodes of life-threatening epistaxis, leading to 7 additional endovascular interventions as well as Gamma Knife radiosurgery. Given the yet recurrent epistaxis, further imaging was performed and revealed a persistent AVM supply from both VAs, right supraclinoid ICA via a large posterior communicating artery (PComm) feeding the left ophthalmic artery and several branches of the ECA.

Surgical resection was planned for the AVM, given the failure of adequate endovascular or radiosurgical management. A pterional craniotomy was first performed to remove right VA feeders (via the right PComm). Despite successful removal of retrograde filling into the VA and into the ICA, the patient continued to have recurrent epistaxis episodes. A subfrontal approach to address the upper third of the clivus was then chosen; feeders emerging from the ophthalmic artery were identified and coagulated distal to the artery to preserve vision. However, most of the AVM was lower along the clivus, and therefore this surgery did not fully resolve the epistaxis episodes.

A staged endoscopic approach was then performed to avoid large craniofacial surgery in a young patient. Given the extent of the lesion and need for additional maneuverability, a sublabial and anterior nasal septal incision was also made to provide additional access into the sphenoid sinus. Draining veins in the nasopharyngeal mucosa were cauterized and endoscopic exposure down to C1 was achieved. In 2 stages, the clivus and ventral skull base were drilled down to expose and coagulate individual vessels that had formed within bony channels; this process extended caudally to C1 and laterally to the pterygoid plates. Sequentially, and with the use of intraoperative angiography, all feeders were obliterated. Postoperatively, the patient recovered fully with no subsequent epistaxis episodes.[35]

Anatomy

Successful cerebrovascular surgery relies on a strong understanding of vascular anatomy that fluidly adapts to the anatomic variations of individual patients. Given the distinct view and approach corridor of endoscopic endonasal surgery, it is useful to consider and refer to cerebrovascular anatomy, as it appears endonasally. Labib and colleagues described the widely accepted classification scheme for the ICA segments from an endoscopic endonasal perspective that can be used for preoperative planning as well as intraoperatively by using more readily identifiable landmarks.[36] The classification includes 6 ICA segments: parapharyngeal, petrous, paraclival, parasellar, paraclinoid, and intradural ICA, each with distinct anatomic borders and relationships to adjacent landmarks. Saliently, the supraclinoidal/intradural segment describes the segment of ICA between the distal dural ring and the ICA bifurcation.[37]

Specific EEA approaches can be used to reach vascular lesions or provide control at certain points along the ICA. The lacerum segment can be accessed through a transpterygoid approach and lies immediately medial to the Vidian canal; if further exposure is required inferiorly, the eustachian tube (ET) can be resected or mobilized, with the parapharyngeal segment lying lateral to the ET.[38] The paraclival segment can be identified along the lateral margins of the clival recess in the sphenoid sinus, and, as is the case with the parasellar segment just distal to it, can be accessed through wide sphenoidotomy.[39] Exposure of these segments is afforded by carefully removing the bone overlying the cavernous ICA, if needed, from foramen lacerum to the medial opticocarotid recess, providing unparalleled proximal control of the cavernous and/or paraclinoidal ICA.[40] Continuing more distally/superiorly, the anterior communicating artery (AComm) can be endoscopically accessed through a transtuberculum/transplanum approach, although the relationship with the optic chiasm and variable proximal control make this anatomy less ideal for EEA, which provides little or no clear advantage over craniotomy for most aneurysms in this location.[41]

The posterior circulation can be accessed along the V4 segment of the VA to the vertebrobasilar junction and up to the basilar apex (depending on the height).[42] A transclival EEA can directly reach these vascular segments and provides unparalleled access to the midbasilar artery without the need to substantially manipulate cranial nerves and vasculature along the skull base.[43] More caudally and laterally, the anterior medullary segment of PICA at the level of the inferior olive can be reached through a "far-medial" approach—a supracondylar, transjugular tubercle approach accomplished by drilling above the hypoglossal canal to laterally expand the surgical corridor and gain increased degrees of surgical freedom during aneurysm surgery (Videos 1 and 2).[44]

Preoperative Planning

Preoperative planning of EEA cerebrovascular surgery must always be a joint effort between neurosurgery and otolaryngology, with clear communication and alignment on the approach and contingencies. Careful study of preoperative imaging is necessary to ensure the vascular relationship with the skull base. Computed tomography (CT) angiography with sagittal and coronal reconstructions is usually much more useful for this than digital subtraction angiography, as it best shows the bony/vascular/neural relationships. Fast imaging employing steady-state acquisition or constructive interference in steady state MRI can also reveal key paraclinoidal relationships such as ICA-optic nerve and location of the aneurysm relative to the distal dural ring and cavernous sinus. A clear plan for proximal and distal vascular control is essential before the surgery begins. In the case of an intraoperative vascular injury, the surgical team should be able to gain rapid control of bleeding and address the injury; this is particularly critical for endoscopic surgery, in which a narrow corridor can limit instrumentation, visualization, and maneuverability (Video 3).

For anterior circulation aneurysms, proximal control can often be planned along an exposed portion of parasellar or paraclival ICA; in the event of an intraoperative bleed, this segment can be temporarily clipped to allow the team to assess and address the situation. During the draping process, a clear corridor of access to the neck should be confirmed to allow for manual cervical ICA compression if needed. For AComm aneurysms, the ipsilateral A1 segment of the anterior cerebral artery can be used for proximal control planning and can sometimes be readily accessed endonasally, depending on the relative relationship of the optic nerve and A1.[45] Proximal control of aneurysms of the basilar apex or trunk can be achieved near the vertebrobasilar junction; the transclival EEA allows for a wide resection of the clivus augmented inferiorly by resecting the medial jugular tubercle using the "far-medial" approach that provides excellent exposure of proximal control sites.[46]

Given the potential for significant retrograde bleeding in large vessels, distal control planning is equally critical. Exposure of the vessel distal to the vascular lesion with an acceptable clipping angle can at times be difficult endoscopically; this can be compounded by calcification of the caroticoclinoidal ring, which needs to be recognized and planned for preoperatively.[39] In the case that no clear distal control can be achieved or seems difficult during preoperative planning (large aneurysm, lateral curve of ICA), a pterional or "eyebrow" supraorbital craniotomy with transsylvian approach can be done at the beginning of the surgery in the event that such distal control becomes emergently necessary.[8]

Reconstruction planning should also be discussed well before the surgery, taking into account the expected dural defect size, adding in the proximity and prominence of the clip to the dural reconstruction, and the anticipation of rare postoperative radiation therapy (AVM). A multilayered reconstruction, including fat to buttress the clip, and centered around a vascularized nasoseptal flap, such as a nasoseptal flap, can provide significantly lower cerebrospinal fluid (CSF) leak rates and rapid healing but must be planned for and clearly communicated in advance.[47] Extended flaps are typically recommended, given the area that needs to be covered to ensure proximal aneurysm clips are well covered.

Preparation and Patient Positioning

Endoscope-assisted microsurgery does not require any specific planning other than ensuring that endoscopic screens are easily visible immediately to the side of the microscope. A separate endoscope system provides excellent visualization, but there are also integrated systems such as the Kinevo with Qevo (Zeiss) that provide greater ease of use intraoperatively, thereby lowering the barrier to use.

For a purely EEA, the patient should be positioned supine in 3-pin radiolucent head fixation. In order to provide an optimal working angle for the primary surgeon, the patient's head should be turned approximately 15° toward the surgeon and the neck laterally flexed away from the operative side in order to further tilt the nasal corridor toward the surgeon. The patient's neck should be extended approximately 10° to 15° in order to allow freedom of movement of pistol-grip instruments.[48] The head of the bed is elevated 15 to 20° to minimize bleeding. The nostrils are packed with oxymetazoline-soaked cottonoids or other nasal decongestant before the midface is prepped with betadine, taking care to protect the eyes. The abdomen and thigh opposite to the femoral sheath should also be prepared and draped for a possible fat or fascia lata graft; alternatively, a radial sheath can also be used.[49] A microscope should be, at least, available, if not draped in the room, in the event that the surgery emergently requires an open transcranial approach. Blood should be available in the room as well as adenosine (0.3 mg/kg) and indocyanine green (ICG) dye. Anesthesia should also prepare by placing defibrillator pads, if adenosine is used.

Procedural Approach

The following general framework can be used for the aforementioned aneurysms that are well indicated for endonasal clipping, with adaptations based on the location of the aneurysm as well as the patient's specific anatomy. The same general approaches can be used for cavernous malformations, dAVFs, and AVMs depending on their anatomic location and supply.

- Preparation as described earlier, with calibration of stereotactic neuronavigation, somatosensory evoked potentials, brainstem auditory evoked potentials, and cranial nerve monitoring, as needed, throughout the case (not necessary for paraclinoidal aneurysms; consider abducens nerve monitoring for basilar/vertebrobasilar junction lesions).
- Harvest vascularized nasoseptal flap. The size of the nasoseptal flap should be sufficient to cover a much wider area than the dural defect in the event that foreign objects such as clips need to be covered by the reconstruction.[50] The harvested flap can be stored in the nasopharynx for anterior circulation aneurysms or in the maxillary sinus for posterior circulation aneurysms or lower brainstem vascular malformations requiring a transclival approach.[51] A rhinopharyngeal flap can also be used to bolster the reconstruction and fill any defects not covered by the nasoseptal flap in the case of transclival approaches.[52]
- For a standard paraclinoidal or basilar apex aneurysm, a wide sphenoidotomy and posterior ethmoidectomy should be performed to allow for a 2-surgeon, 4-handed technique. A binasal technique, in which the dissecting surgeon is controlling 2 different instruments in either nostril, is necessary in endoscopic endonasal cerebrovascular surgery to optimize instrumentation, maneuverability, and visualization.[53]
- A transplanum/transsellar approach can be used for anterior circulation aneurysms as

well as midline mesencephalic cavernous malformations, whereas a transclival approach can be used for posterior circulation aneurysms as well as midline pontine/medullary cavernous malformations and clival dAVFs. A pituitary transposition is usually necessary for control of the basilar apex, even if low-lying.[54]

- Particularly for aneurysm surgery, proximal and distal control sites should be exposed before attempting to expose and clip the aneurysm. A 0° endoscope can be used for most of the approach, although a 45° can also be used to visualize lateral borders, to look under the pituitary gland, or to inspect clipped aneurysms with tangential trajectories, whether endonasally or transcranially.[55]
- For ventral BCMs, the location of durotomy can normally be identified by mild discoloration of the brainstem and should be confirmed via stereotactic neuronavigation.[56]
- Endoscopy-specific aneurysm clipping instruments that accommodate the narrow corridor of approach are needed. An elongated, single-shaft clip applier should be used (Lazic, Mizuho America, Inc, CA, USA). Curved clips may be superior to traditional straight clips depending on the angle of projection of the aneurysm in relation to the trajectory of approach. In general, given the relatively narrow corridor, more creativity with clip placement may be necessary, although medial paraclinoidal aneurysms tend to be directly in line with the nasal corridor.
- Endoscopic ICG videoangiography and/or intraoperative Doppler should be used to confirm complete aneurysm occlusion, complete dAVF/AVM resection, and the flow of parent vessels. Doppler should be performed before clipping to provide a clear comparison. If visualization of the aneurysm/dAVF/AVM or adjacent vessels is in question, a preclipping ICG run may also be considered. Endoscopic ICG visualization is currently commercially available (Karl Storz, Tuttlingen, Germany), allowing the same ability to evaluate vascularity with an endoscope as with microscopes.
- A multilayered reconstruction should be used to reduce the likelihood of CSF leak and/or flap necrosis. An intradural graft matrix should be wrapped around the clip, followed by a fat and/or fascial graft to support and cover the clip, followed by the previously harvested nasoseptal flap, ideally covering any exposed fat or clip.[57]

INTRAOPERATIVE COMPLICATION MANAGEMENT

In the event of an intraoperative vascular injury or rupture, the surgical team must act in a swift and preplanned manner to rapidly regain control of the situation (see Video 3). Such planning and experience are particularly crucial in endoscopic endonasal cerebrovascular surgery, where the already narrow endonasal corridor can limit maneuverability and visualization. For this reason, wide exposures should always be planned, when possible, in order to allow for a 2 surgeon, 4-hand technique.[40] An endoscope holder could prove disastrous in such a situation where dynamic and expert endoscopy is key to maintain a view.

Unlike a microscope, the endoscope is immersed in the surgical field as an instrument itself. Therefore, it can get surrounded by blood during a bleed, preventing visibility. Intuitively, the endoscope should be pulled back slightly, whereas a large-bore suction and gentle cottonoid tamponade is used in order to reestablish visualization. Frequent flushing of the field with water by the endoscopist surgeon can allow the dissecting surgeon to focus on localization of the bleeding. Once general visualization is reestablished and blood flow reduced by tamponade or proximal clipping, it should be determined if the rupture site can be occluded by the clip construct. If so, a permanent clip should be attempted. If this is not the case, repair of the rupture should be considered. Small tears in an artery may be amenable to closure via careful bipolar cauterization. If a site of proximal and distal control relative to the rupture can be readily identified and accessed, temporary clips should be placed. At this point, in the case of aneurysm surgery, the bleeding should be sufficiently quelled, allowing the team to shift focus to permanently clipping the aneurysm.

When undergoing temporary clipping, the mean arterial blood pressure should be kept slightly elevated (target 80–90 mm Hg) in order to allow for some level of collateral perfusion unless the elevated pressure is preventing maintenance of visualization.[58] If temporary clipping for vascular control cannot be readily established, manual cervical compression, transient adenosine-induced cardiac arrest, or rapid ventricular pacing can also be considered.[59] Care should be taken to avoid the instinct of merely packing off the bleeding blindly, as this can lead to uncontrolled intracerebral hemorrhage. In general, with such a deep field, the "blood is better out than in."

Alternatives to clipping can include compression with crushed muscle and/or cottonoids until hemostasis is achieved. These materials can similarly be incorporated into the clip construct as needed, especially in the setting of a neck rupture (see Video 3).[60] If hemostasis cannot be appropriately reestablished during the intraoperative rupture of vascular lesions, the parent vessel (eg, ICA) can be sacrificed as a last-resort option. Endovascular access can be particularly useful for gaining both proximal and distal control of the aneurysm through balloon occlusion if control sites cannot be clearly visualized and/or accessed surgically. For high-risk vascular lesions, balloon test occlusion (BTO) of the ICA should be performed as part of the preoperative workup in order to determine if ICA sacrifice would be tolerated.[61]

With lesions such as osseous AVMs, repeated staged surgery may be necessary due to blood loss and/or length of surgery. In general, however, for intradural vascular lesions, this technique is not a good option.

Recovery and Rehabilitation

Several intraoperative steps can substantially reduce the occurrence of postoperative complications. Namely, the surgical team should ensure complete aneurysm occlusion or AVM/dAVF resection; this can be done intraoperatively through careful white light endoscopic inspection, near-infrared, endoscopic ICG videoangiography, microvascular Doppler ultrasonography, or postoperatively through CT angiography or digital subtraction angiography. Endoscopic ICG videoangiography (Karl Storz, Tuttlingen, Germany) is a powerful, increasingly available means of ensuring both aneurysm occlusion as well as flow of parent vessels.[62] In a study of 295 consecutive aneurysm clippings that used intraoperative microscopic ICG video angiography, the need for additional clipping or clip replacement was identified in nearly one-sixth of the patients, therefore substantially reducing the rate of reoperation or further interventions.[63]

Patients should be closely monitored for the most common complication after EEA, a postoperative CSF leak, most of which occur during the first postoperative week or just after packing removal.[64] The use of vascularized nasoseptal flaps and lumbar drainage have been proved to substantially lower CSF leak rates in these high flow settings.[65,66] However, endoscopic clipping poses additional risk of flap necrosis or CSF leak by nature of direct pressure or transmitted pulsations from the clip onto the flap. A protuberant clip could push against and tent the flap, interfering with healing and adhesion in the short-term and potentially eroding through the flap in the long-term; this can be accounted for by using a multilayer reconstruction with fascia and fat padding the reconstruction up to the level of the flap as needed. An inlay of collagen graft should be placed directly around the clip, followed by a fascial or fat graft that is then covered by a pedicled nasoseptal flap regardless of dural defect size.[40] Lumbar drainage should be used and short-term Diamox administration can be considered as a further supplement for healing.

Outcomes

Although endonasal endoscopic cerebrovascular surgery is still a relatively new technique lacking comprehensive outcome studies, it provides a safe and effective option for appropriately selected lesions as discussed earlier. It should be noted that open cerebrovascular surgery itself is largely a safe treatment route with excellent outcomes; the intent of developing EEA for cerebrovascular surgery is not to offer a superior alternative for all patients, but rather to expand the armamentarium and anatomic access corridors for cerebrovascular surgery for specific well-selected patients.

The success of EEA cerebrovascular surgery largely depends on the experience of the skull base team performing the operation. Endoscopic endonasal surgery has a steep learning curve due to the novel endoscopic anatomy, maneuvering, and instrumentation it requires. Snyderman and colleagues have broken down different surgeries using EEA into a graded training program of 5 distinct levels of difficulty, with endoscopic endonasal vascular surgery included in the fifth and most difficult level that should not be attempted until expertise in all prior levels of EEA difficulty is achieved.[67] Such a training program is particularly salient for the application of EEA to other vascular malformations, including ventral cavernous malformations, anterior fossa dAVFs, and clival AVMs, for which most of the EEA applications that have been reported are case reports and case series from institutions with extensive, multidisciplinary expertise in endoscopic endonasal techniques. Given that microsurgical techniques remain the safe standard of practice for such lesions when surgical resection is indicated, "level 5" expertise should be reached before attempting this approach for such lesions. Moreover, this learning curve should be approached as a comprehensive skull base team that includes neurosurgeons and otolaryngologists rather than as individual endeavors.

SUMMARY

The endoscopic endonasal approach offers a safe and effective corridor to certain cerebrovascular lesions that are poorly approached, visualized, or controlled through traditional microscopic open approaches. In particular, medially projecting paraclinoid, low-lying basilar apex/trunk aneurysms, proximal SCA, AICA, and ventromedial PICA aneurysms can be exposed well through endoscopic techniques. EEA can also provide direct ventral access to appropriately indicated midline AComm aneurysms, midline brainstem cavernous malformations, and clival AVMs and dAVFs. Although effective, however, the endonasal approach to vascular lesions remains a novel application of the technique that requires a strong understanding of endoscopic anatomy and a substantial level of endoscopic technical expertise shared among all members of the skull base team.

CLINICS CARE POINTS

- Inferomedially projecting paraclinoidal aneurysms can be difficult to access via open approaches due to the need for neurovascular manipulation but can be readily approached endonasally.

- Posterior circulation aneurysms at the vertebrobasilar junction, ventromedial PICA, proximal SCA/AICA, or posterior cerebral artery with a low basilar apex are suitable candidates for EEA clipping.

- Low, midline, and ventral BCMs with little lateral extension can be approached via EEA rather than traditional, inherently lateral microsurgical approaches in order to minimize damage to eloquent brainstem parenchyma.

- The angle of aneurysm projection is a critical determinant of whether or not an aneurysm can be clipped endoscopically.

- Proximal and distal control should always be planned for and exposed before attempting aneurysm clipping. In the event of an intraoperative rupture, proximal control should first be established through temporary trapping before determining the need for distal control and permanently clipping the aneurysm. Rapid ventricular pacing or transient adenosine-induced cardiac arrest can also be considered if proximal control cannot be readily accessed. ICA sacrifice is the last resort in such cases (BTO of the ICA should be done preoperatively in any relatively high-risk EEA aneurysm case).

- Intraoperative ICG videoangiography and Doppler can detect the need for additional clipping and reduce the need for reoperation.

- The use of multilayered reconstruction centered around the vascularized nasoseptal flaps reduces the risk of postoperative CSF leak and/or flap necrosis. A multilayered reconstruction technique should be used to prevent the clip from tenting or eroding through the flap.

- Anterior dAVF or ventral BCMs that displace the motor tracts laterally are both additional rare indications for endoscopic vascular management.

- Endoscopes provide added visualization during microscopic treatment of vascular lesions including confirming clipping of aneurysms on the deep side of arteries (ie, ventral ICA, medial ophthalmic/carotid cave, and so forth), preservation of hidden perforating arteries, and inspection of cavernous malformation cavities to ensure completeness of resection.

DISCLOSURE

The authors have nothing to disclose.

SUPPLEMENTARY DATA

Supplementary data related to this article can be found online at https://doi.org/10.1016/j.nec.2022.06.005.

REFERENCES

1. Archer DJ, Young S, Uttley D. Basilar aneurysms: a new transclival approach via maxillotomy. J Neurosurg 1987;67(1):54–8.
2. Crockard HA, Koksel T, Watkin N. Transoral transclival clipping of anterior inferior cerebellar artery aneurysm using new rotating applier: Technical note. J Neurosurg 1991;75(3):483–5.
3. Hitchcock E, Cowie R. Transoral-transclival clipping of a midline vertebral artery aneurysm. J Neurol Neurosurg Psychiatry 1983;46(5):446–8.
4. Ogilvy CS, Barker Ii FG, Joseph MP, et al. Transfacial transclival approach for midline posterior circulation aneurysms. Neurosurgery 1996;39(4):736–42.
5. Liu JK, Patel J, Goldstein IM, et al. Endoscopic endonasal transclival transodontoid approach for ventral decompression of the craniovertebral junction: operative technique and nuances. Neurosurg Focus FOC 2015;38(4):E17.
6. Patel A, Abou-Al-Shaar H, McDowell MM, et al. Endoscopic Endonasal Aneurysm Treatment. In: PA G, CH S, B J, editors. Vascular challenges in skull base surgery. 1st edition. Thieme Medical Publishers, Inc.; 2021.
7. Kassam AB, Mintz AH, Gardner PA, et al. The expanded endonasal approach for an endoscopic transnasal clipping and aneurysmorrhaphy of a large vertebral artery aneurysm: technical case report. Neurosurgery 2006;59(1 Suppl 1):ONSE162–165 [discussion: ONSE162-165].
8. Kassam AB, Gardner PA, Mintz A, et al. Endoscopic endonasal clipping of an unsecured superior hypophyseal artery aneurysm. Technical note. J Neurosurg 2007;107(5):1047–52.
9. Barami K, Hernandez VS, Diaz FG, et al. Paraclinoid Carotid Aneurysms: Surgical Management, Complications, and Outcome Based on a New Classification Scheme. Skull base 2003;13(1):31–41.
10. Kutty RK, Kumar A, Yamada Y, et al. Visual Outcomes after Surgery for Paraclinoid Aneurysms: A Fujita Experience. Asian J Neurosurg 2020;15(2):363–9.
11. Szentirmai O, Hong Y, Mascarenhas L, et al. Endoscopic endonasal clip ligation of cerebral aneurysms: an anatomical feasibility study and future directions. J Neurosurg 2016;124(2):463–8.
12. Yamada Y, Ansari A, Sae-Ngow T, et al. Microsurgical treatment of paraclinoid aneurysms by extradural anterior clinoidectomy: the fujita experience. Asian J Neurosurg 2019;14(3):868–72.
13. Wong AK, Wong RH. Keyhole clipping of a low-lying basilar apex aneurysm without posterior clinoidectomy utilizing endoscopic indocyanine green video angiography. Surg Neurol Int 2020;11:31.
14. Koutourousiou M, Vaz Guimaraes Filho F, Fernandez-Miranda JC, et al. Endoscopic endonasal surgery for tumors of the cavernous sinus: a series of 234 patients. World Neurosurg 2017;103:713–32.
15. Xiao LM, Tang B, Xie SH, et al. Endoscopic endonasal clipping of anterior circulation aneurysm: surgical techniques and results. World Neurosurg 2018;115:e33–44.
16. Li D, Wu Z-Y, Liu P-P, et al. Natural history of brainstem cavernous malformations: prospective hemorrhage rate and adverse factors in a consecutive prospective cohort. J Neurosurg JNS 2021;134(3):917–28.
17. Kearns KN, Chen C-J, Tvrdik P, et al. Outcomes of surgery for brainstem cavernous malformations. Stroke 2019;50(10):2964–6.
18. Abla AA, Lekovic GP, Turner JD, et al. Advances in the treatment and outcome of brainstem cavernous malformation surgery: A single-center case series of 300 surgically treated patients. Neurosurgery 2011;68(2):403–14.
19. Linsler S, Oertel J. Endoscopic endonasal transclival resection of a brainstem cavernoma: a detailed account of our technique and comparison with the literature. World Neurosurg 2015;84(6):2064–71.
20. Abou-Al-Shaar H, Labib MA, Spetzler RF. Brainstem Cavernous Malformations. In: Macdonald RL, editor. Neurosurgical operative atlas: vascular

neurosurgery. 3rd edition. Thieme Medical Publishers, Inc.; 2018.

21. Dong X, Wang X, Shao A, et al. Endoscopic endonasal transclival approach to ventral pontine cavernous malformation: case report. Front Surg 2021;8.

22. Kimball MM, Lewis SB, Werning JW, et al. Resection of a pontine cavernous malformation via an endoscopic endonasal approach: a case report. Oper Neurosurg 2012;71(suppl_1):onsE186–94.

23. Enseñat J, D'Avella E, Tercero A, et al, Endoscopic endonasal surgery for a mesencephalic cavernoma. Acta neurochirurgica 2015;157(1):53–5.

24. Ezequiel G, Andrew SV, Maximiliano N, et al. Endoscopic endonasal approach for brainstem cavernous malformation. Neurosurg Focus: Video FOCVID. 2019;1(2):V2.

25. Vaz-Guimaraes F, Gardnerl PA, Fernandez-Miranda JC, et al. Endoscopic endonasal skull base surgery for vascular lesions: a systematic review of the literature. J Neurosurg Sci 2016;60(4): 504–13.

26. Liu JK, Lu Y, Raslan AM, et al. Cavernous malformations of the optic pathway and hypothalamus: analysis of 65 cases in the literature. Neurosurg Focus FOC 2010;29(3):E17.

27. Meng X, Feng X, Wan J. Endoscopic endonasal transsphenoidal approach for the removal of optochiasmatic cavernoma: case report and literature review. World Neurosurg 2017;106:1053.e1011–4.

28. Katsaridis V. Treatment of dural arteriovenous fistulas. Curr Treat Options Neurol 2009;11(1):35–40.

29. Kiyosue H, Hori Y, Okahara M, et al. Treatment of intracranial dural arteriovenous fistulas: current strategies based on location and hemodynamics, and alternative techniques of transcatheter embolization. Radiographics 2004;2(6):1637–53.

30. Mack WJ, Gonzalez NR, Jahan R, et al. Endovascular management of anterior cranial fossa dural arteriovenous malformations. A technical report and anatomical discussion. Interv Neuroradiology : 2011;17(1):93–103.

31. Lawton MT, Chun J, Wilson CB, et al. Ethmoidal dural arteriovenous fistulae: an assessment of surgical and endovascular management. Neurosurgery 1999;45(4):805–11.

32. Tang CL, Liao CH, Chen WH, et al. Endoscope-assisted transsphenoidal puncture of the cavernous sinus for embolization of carotid-cavernous fistula in a neurosurgical hybrid operating suite. J Neurosurg 2017;127(2):327–31.

33. Karas PJ, North RY, Srinivasan VM, et al. Endoscopic endonasal transsphenoidal direct access and Onyx embolization of a dural arteriovenous fistula mimicking a carotid-cavernous fistula: case report. J Neurosurg 2021;135(3):722–6.

34. Kelly ME, Guzman R, Sinclair J, et al. Multimodality treatment of posterior fossa arteriovenous malformations. J Neurosurg 2008;108(6):1152–61.

35. Kassam AB, Thomas AJ, Zimmer LA, et al. Expanded endonasal approach: a fully endoscopic completely transnasal resection of a skull base arteriovenous malformation. Child's nervous Syst : ChNS 2007;23(5):491–8.

36. Labib MA, Prevedello DM, Carrau R, et al. A road map to the internal carotid artery in expanded endoscopic endonasal approaches to the ventral cranial base. Neurosurgery 2014;10(Suppl 3):448–71 [discussion: 471].

37. Fortes FSG, Pinheiro-Neto CD, Carrau RL, et al. Endonasal endoscopic exposure of the internal carotid artery: an anatomical study. Laryngoscope 2012; 122(2):445–51.

38. Kassam AB, Gardner P, Snyderman C, et al. Expanded endonasal approach: fully endoscopic, completely transnasal approach to the middle third of the clivus, petrous bone, middle cranial fossa, and infratemporal fossa. Neurosurg Focus FOC 2005;19(1):1–10.

39. Fernandez-Miranda JC, Tormenti M, Latorre F, et al. Endoscopic endonasal middle clinoidectomy: anatomic, radiological, and technical note. Oper Neurosurg 2012;71(suppl_2):ons233–9.

40. Gardner PA, Vaz-Guimaraes F, Jankowitz B, et al. Endoscopic endonasal clipping of intracranial aneurysms: surgical technique and results. World Neurosurg 2015;84(5):1380–93.

41. Froelich S, Cebula H, Debry C, et al. Anterior communicating artery aneurysm clipped via an endoscopic endonasal approach: technical note. Neurosurgery 2011;68(2 Suppl Operative):310–6 [discussion: 315-316].

42. Kassam A, Snyderman CH, Mintz A, et al. Expanded endonasal approach: the rostrocaudal axis. Part II. Posterior clinoids to the foramen magnum. Neurosurg focus 2005;19(1):E4.

43. Patel A, Abou-Al-Shaar H, Nuñez MA, et al. Vascular Anatomy of the Head and Neck/Circle of Willis. In: Gardner PA, Snyderman CH, Jankowitz B, editors. Vascular challenges in skull base surgery. 1st edition. Thieme Medical Publishers, Inc.; 2021.

44. Morera VA, Fernandez-Miranda JC, Prevedello DM, et al. Far-medial" expanded endonasal approach to the inferior third of the clivus: the transcondylar and transjugular tubercle approaches. Neurosurgery 2010;66(6 Suppl Operative):211–9. ; discussion 219-220.

45. Qin K, Wang Y, Tian G, et al. A comparative analysis of the endoscopic endonasal and pterional approaches for clipping anterior communicating artery aneurysms on three-dimensional printed models. Chin Med J 2021;134(17):2113–5.

46. Vaz-Guimaraes Filho F, Wang EW, Snyderman CH, et al. Endoscopic endonasal "far-medial" transclival approach: Surgical anatomy and technique. Oper Tech Otolaryngology-Head Neck Surg 2013;24(4): 222–8.

47. Hadad G, Bassagasteguy L, Carrau RL, et al. A novel reconstructive technique after endoscopic expanded endonasal approaches: vascular pedicle nasoseptal flap. Laryngoscope 2006;116(10): 1882–6.

48. Solari D, Villa A, De Angelis M, et al. Anatomy and surgery of the endoscopic endonasal approach to the skull base. Transl Med Unisa 2012;2:36–46.

49. Christian E, Harris B, Wrobel B, et al. Endoscopic endonasal transsphenoidal surgery: implementation of an operative and perioperative checklist. Neurosurg Focus FOC 2014;37(4):E1.

50. Pinheiro-Neto CD, Prevedello DM, Carrau RL, et al. Improving the design of the pedicled nasoseptal flap for skull base reconstruction: a radioanatomic study. The Laryngoscope 2007;117(9):1560–9.

51. Kassam AB, Thomas A, Carrau RL, et al. Endoscopic reconstruction of the cranial base using a pedicled nasoseptal flap. Neurosurgery 2008;63(1 Suppl 1):ONS44–52 [discussion: ONS52-43].

52. Champagne PO, Zenonos GA, Wang EW, et al. The rhinopharyngeal flap for reconstruction of lower clival and craniovertebral junction defects. J Neurosurg 2021;1–9.

53. Dehdashti AR, Ganna A, Witterick I, et al. Expanded endoscopic endonasal approach for anterior cranial base and suprasellar lesions: indications and limitations. Neurosurgery 2009;64(4):677–87 [discussion: 687-679].

54. Fernandez-Miranda JC, Gardner PA, Rastelli MM Jr, et al. Endoscopic endonasal transcavernous posterior clinoidectomy with interdural pituitary transposition. J Neurosurg 2014;121(1):91–9.

55. Felisati G, Lenzi R, Pipolo C, et al. Endoscopic expanded endonasal approach: preliminary experience with the new 3D endoscope. Acta Otorhinolaryngol Ital 2013;33(2):102–6.

56. Nayak NR, Thawani JP, Sanborn MR, et al. Endoscopic approaches to brainstem cavernous malformations: case series and review of the literature. Surg Neurol Int 2015;6:68.

57. Simal-Julián JA, Miranda-Lloret P, Pérez de San Román Mena L, et al. Impact of multilayer vascularized reconstruction after skull base endoscopic endonasal approaches. J Neurol Surg B Skull Base 2020;81(2):128–35.

58. Lawton MT. Seven aneurysms: tenets and techniques for clipping. New York: Thieme; 2011.

59. Powers CJ, Wright DR, McDonagh DL, et al. Transient adenosine-induced asystole during the surgical treatment of anterior circulation cerebral aneurysms: technical note. Neurosurgery 2010; 67(2 Suppl Operative):461–70.

60. Barrow DL, Spetzler RF. Cotton-clipping technique to repair intraoperative aneurysm neck tear: a technical note. Neurosurgery 2011;68(2 Suppl Operative):294–9 [discussion: 299].

61. Kikuchi K, Yoshiura T, Hiwatashi A, et al. Balloon test occlusion of internal carotid artery: angiographic findings predictive of results. World J Radiol 2014;6(8):619–24.

62. Fischer G, Rediker J, Oertel J. Endoscope- versus microscope-integrated near-infrared indocyanine green videoangiography in aneurysm surgery. J Neurosurg 2018;1–10.

63. Roessler K, Krawagna M, Dorfler A, et al. Essentials in intraoperative indocyanine green videoangiography assessment for intracranial aneurysm surgery: conclusions from 295 consecutively clipped aneurysms and review of the literature. Neurosurg focus 2014;36(2):E7.

64. Khan DZ, Marcus HJ, Horsfall HL, et al. CSF rhinorrhoea after endonasal intervention to the skull base (CRANIAL) - Part 1: multicenter Pilot Study. World Neurosurg 2021;149:e1077–89.

65. Patel MR, Stadler ME, Snyderman CH, et al. How to choose? Endoscopic skull base reconstructive options and limitations. Skull base 2010;20(6): 397–404.

66. Heiferman DM, Somasundaram A, Alvarado AJ, et al. The endonasal approach for treatment of cerebral aneurysms: a critical review of the literature. Clin Neurol Neurosurg 2015;134:91–7.

67. Snyderman C, Kassam A, Carrau R, et al. Acquisition of surgical skills for endonasal skull base surgery: a training program. Laryngoscope 2007; 117(4):699–705.

Cerebrovascular Anatomy
Laboratory Research, Education, Innovations, and Future Directions

Ali Tayebi Meybodi, MD[a],*, Arnau Benet, MD[b]

KEYWORDS

- Cerebrovascular surgery • Microanatomy • Surgical neuroanatomy • Neurosurgical anatomy
- Skull base surgery

KEY POINTS

- Understanding the history and evolution of surgical neuroanatomy is key to a solid foundation of meaningful microsurgical anatomic research.
- Cerebrovascular anatomic research is a rapidly growing field with great impact on the improvement of efficiency and safety of complex open cerebrovascular procedures.
- Surgical anatomy research in cerebrovascular and skull base includes four types of studies: (1) descriptive, (2) approach design and feasibility assessment, (3) analytical and comparative, and (4) technique optimization and modification.
- Cerebrovascular and skull base anatomic research can significantly promote educating cerebrovascular and skull base surgeons.

The foundation of the study of the art of operating must be laid in the dissecting room, and it is only when we have acquired dexterity on the dead subject, that we can be justified in interfering with the living
— *Robert Liston, Practical Surgery, 1837*

major advances in the field of cerebrovascular anatomic research have transformed the craft of cerebrovascular surgery into a modern art. In this review, we discuss the evolution, advances, limitations, and future directions of cerebrovascular and skull base anatomic research.

INTRODUCTION

Friedrich Tiedemann, the German anatomist, said "Doctors without anatomy are like moles. They work in the dark and the work of their hands are mounds." This is probably most true for neurosurgery. These words hold even more true for the cerebrovascular surgeon. It is with an in-depth understanding of surgical neuroanatomy that the vascular neurosurgeon could safely navigate the darkest corners of the brain "Labyrinth" and victoriously defeat the "Minotaur" of cerebrovascular pathology. Cerebrovascular anatomy, however, is far from a stagnant field. Over the past century,

SURGICAL NEUROANATOMY: EARLY DEVELOPMENT

In the land of Egypt ruled by the Ptolemaic dynasty during the third century BC, Herophilus of Chalcedon (325–255 BC) and his younger colleague Erasistratus of Ceos, performed several cadaveric dissections during 30 to 40 years. Following this period, human cadaver dissections were mostly stopped, to be resumed 1600 years later.[1] However, several notable figures, such as Galen of Pergamon (AD 129–200), contributed to the science of neuroanatomy in this period of relative dormancy.

[a] Department of Neurosurgery, Rutgers New Jersey Medical School, 90 Bergen Street, Suite 8100, Newark, NJ 07101-1709, USA; [b] Division of Neurosurgery, Barrow Neurological Institute, 350 West Thomas Road, Phoenix, AZ 85013, USA
* Corresponding author.
E-mail address: Tayebi.a77@gmail.com

Neurosurg Clin N Am 33 (2022) 505–515
https://doi.org/10.1016/j.nec.2022.05.003
1042-3680/22/© 2022 Elsevier Inc. All rights reserved.

Abbreviations	
BA	Basilar artery
PCA	Posterior cerebral artery
SCA	Superior cerebellar artery
VA	Vertebral Artery
III	Oculomotor nerve
VI	Abducens nerve
IAC	Internal auditory canal
GSPN	Greater superficial petrosal nerve
BAX	Basilar artery apex
CN	Cranial nerve
ICA	Internal carotid artery
MCA	Middle cerebral artery
PCoA	Posterior communicating artery
AChA	Anterior choroidal artery
LGB	Lateral geniculate body
Chor. plex.	Choroid plexus
tr.	Tract
LPChA	Lateral posterior choroidal artery
Hippo.	Hippocampus
BVR	Basal vein of Rosenthal

The fourteenth century marks the gradual resumption of human cadaveric dissections. Mondino de'Luzzi completed a dissection manual, *Anatomia Mondini*, in 1316.[2] Some 200 years later, Johannes Dryander published his *Anatomiae* in which he used his "layer" dissection techniques and illustrated the dura mater, cerebral cortex, and posterior fossa structures in this "first textbook of neuroanatomy" (**Fig. 1**).[3] Contemporarily, Andreas Vesalius' *De Humani Corporis Fabrica Libri Septem* in 1543 distilled his anatomic observations in seven volumes (**Fig. 2**).[4] Vesalius' depictions of brain anatomy were the best to date. The next major leap in gross neuroanatomy was taken by Thomas Willis (1621–1675), the English anatomist. His 1664 book *Cerebri Anatome* included more accurate illustrations of the anatomic features of the brain's basal surface and vasculature (**Fig. 3**).[5] Of note, Willis used the assistance of several colleagues in production of the illustrations in his book. Christopher Wren was a critical coworker of Willis not only because of his contributions to the illustrations, but also for the unique technique of intravascular infusion of India ink and alcohol to better delineate/preserve the brain.[2,5] One should also note the contributions of contemporary René Descartes (1596–1650) in his 1662 *De homine*. Humphrey Ridley (1653–1708) provided even more accurate and detailed depictions of basal vasculature of the brain, thanks to his opportunity to dissect on the freshly executed.[6]

Seeing anatomy as a fashionable art fueled the "anatomic experiences" during the fifteenth to seventeenth centuries.[2,7] During the eighteenth century, and especially with the incorporation of linear perspective into anatomic depictions, the "art of anatomy" began its metamorphosis toward the "science of anatomy." Felix Vicq d'Azyr (1748–1794) was a pioneer in comparative anatomy and a major contributor to modern neuroanatomy. Using a cadaveric fixation method originally developed by the Dutch anatomist Frederik Ruysch (1638–1731), he developed his own method of white matter dissection.[8] He dissected and described many cerebral structures, such as the fornix and the mammillothalamic tract in his 1786 *Traité d'anatomie et de physiologie* (**Fig. 4**).[9] Other notable figures of this era include Thomas Sömmerring (1755–1830) and Pierre Camper (1722–1789).

The eighteenth century is also known for several surgeons who expanded the frontiers of neurosurgery, such as Percival Pott (1714–88), John Hunter (1728–93), Benjamin Bell (1749–1806), and Lorenz Heister (1683–1758). This period is also notable for the expansion of the neurosurgical armamentarium. Finally, the dawn of nineteenth century witnessed the works of Sir Charles Bell (1774–1842) who combined precision and artistic illustration of brain dissections (**Fig. 5**).[10]

DAWN OF MODERN NEUROSURGERY: EVOLUTION OF NEUROSURGICAL ANATOMY

The nineteenth century should be considered the dawn of modern neurosurgery because of major progress in anesthesia, cerebral localization, and

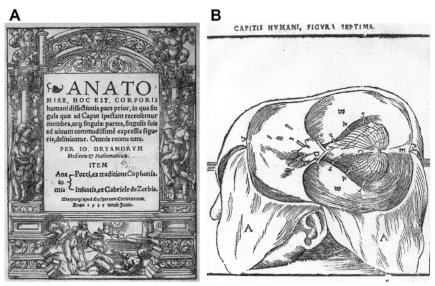

Fig. 1. (*A*) Title page and (*B*) the seventh figure of Dryander's *Anatomiae* depicting posterior fossa contents and cranial nerves. (Marpurgi: Apud Eucharium Ceruicornum, 1537; Source: https://www.archive.org).

neuropathology. Following the early observations of Gustav Theodor Fritsch and Eduard Hitzig, and Pierre Paul Broca in the 1860s, David Ferrier (1843–1928) and John Jackson (1835–1911) developed the concept of cerebral localization by ablation and stimulation studies, respectively.[11,12] These efforts were followed by others, such as Sir Rickman John Godlee (1859–1925), Sir William Gowers (1845–1915), Sir Victor Horsley (1857–1916), and Fedor Krause (1857–1937) to advance surgical techniques, among several other names.

Harvey W. Cushing, Walter E. Dandy, and Mahmut G. Yasargil

The early twentieth century is identified by Harvey Cushing (1869–1939) and Walter Dandy (1886–1946) as the fathers of modern neurosurgery. They introduced innovative approaches and techniques to treat brain lesions.[13–15] Exquisite, immensely didactic, and masterfully rendered illustrations by Dorcas Hager Padget elevated Dandy's work. Later, Mahmut G. Yasargil provided

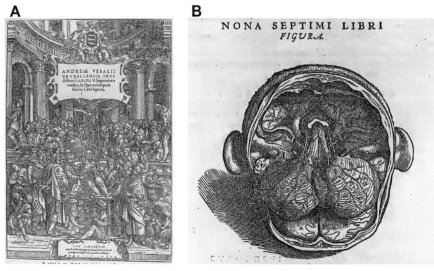

Fig. 2. (*A*) Title page and (*B*) the ninth figure of the seventh book of Vesalius, *De Humani Corporis Fabrica Libri Septem*. The illustration shows extracted cerebellum after removal of the supratentorial structures, depicting the brainstem and posterior fossa cranial nerves. (Basileae: Per Ioannem Oporinum, 1555; source: https://www.archive.org).

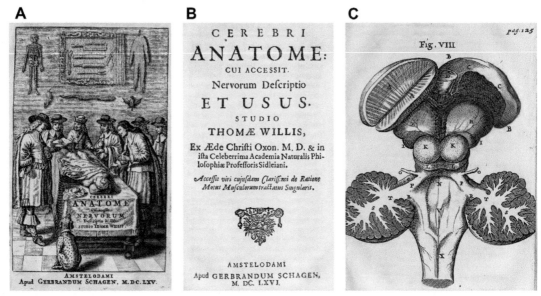

Fig. 3. (*A*) Frontispiece and (*B*) title page of Willis' *Cerebri Anatome*. (*C*) Depiction of the posterior aspect of corpus striatum, brainstem, and cerebellum. (Amstelodami: Apud Gerbrandum Schagen, 1666; source: https://www.archive.org).

a detailed microanatomic description of the skull base cisterns along with the relevant neurovascular anatomy and emphasized the importance of arachnoid dissection in accessing skull base cisterns to expose vascular lesions.[16] The notion of a cisternal roadmap to the brainstem and skull base was a breakthrough in cerebrovascular surgery and a starting point for further development of approaches to the once deemed inaccessible lesions of the brain. Yasargil worked with his mentor and colleague Professor Hugo Krayenbühl to provide detailed explanations of the pathoanatomy of cerebral aneurysms, arteriovenous malformations, and cerebral bypasses.

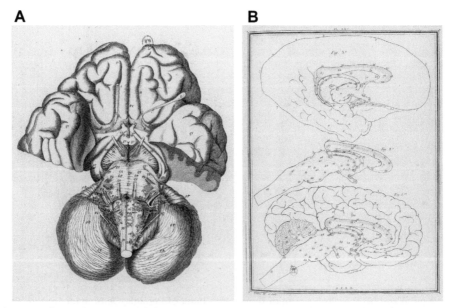

Fig. 4. Selections of Vicq d'Azyr's *Traité d'anatomie et de physiologie*. (*A*) Basal surface of the brain. (*B*) Medial surface of the brain, upper brainstem structures, and components of the limbic system. Note illustration of the mammillothalamic tract in *middle panel* (*a-b*). (Paris: Didot, 1786; source: https://gallica.bnf.fr).;;

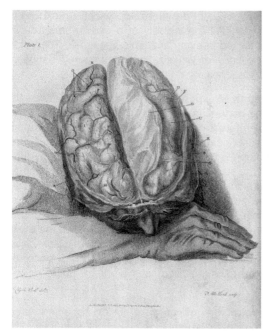

Fig. 5. Plate I from Bell's *The Anatomy of the Brain, explained in a series of engravings.* (The anatomy of the brain, explained in a series of engravings / By Charles Bell).

The Work and Legacy of Albert L. Rhoton Jr

Yasargil's descriptions and surgical anatomic illustrations, although elegant, lacked the anatomic clarity of exquisite cadaveric dissections. Given the worldwide drive to access deeper surgical targets, there was an enormous demand for detailed and surgically relevant anatomic descriptions. This gap was filled by Albert Rhoton. Beginning in the 1960s, he expanded his detailed neuroanatomic research focused mainly on surgical microneuroanatomy. His work was themed to be applied to neurosurgery. Through decades of microneuroanatomic research, Rhoton led a team of research fellows from all around the world to perfect the art of neurosurgical microanatomic depiction, research, and education. The interest for applied surgical neuroanatomic knowledge is reflected by the progressively increasing number of citations of his works over the past six decades. Not surprisingly, 8 of his 10 most-cited articles were on cerebrovascular anatomy.[17] Such attention may not be merely because of interest in cerebrovascular surgery per se, but may be caused by the growing appreciation of the importance of knowledge of cerebrovascular anatomy by the neurosurgical community. Rhoton will remain one of the most influential figures in neurosurgical anatomy and appropriately considered in alignment with such names as Vesalius, Willis, and Bell.[17]

CURRENT CEREBROVASCULAR ANATOMIC RESEARCH
Subtypes of Neurosurgical Anatomic Studies

Microanatomic neurosurgical research is generally categorized into four major research types: (1) descriptive, (2) approach designing and feasibility assessment, (3) analytical and comparative, and (4) technique optimization and modification studies. A brief discussion follows with some examples included as references.

Descriptive studies

Descriptive studies are the most basic type of anatomic studies and provide explanatory information about anatomic structures. This type of anatomic research may bring breakthroughs in structural knowledge as technology develops innovative techniques to assess tissue beyond the spectrum of current devices (eg, arachnoid trabecular and membranes seen with scanning electron microscope). The key to descriptive anatomic research is sufficient number of specimens to define "normal" anatomy; that is, the most frequently found pattern. Such studies may be further divided into qualitative, quantitative, and landmark identification studies. Qualitative studies reveal anatomic facts, such as shape, number, location, size, course, and variations of a structure and its relation to adjacent structures. Another use of qualitative descriptive studies is the help they provide with categorization of the anatomic structures and/or regions important to the surgeon. For example, segmentation of intracranial arteries helps the surgeon formulate a treatment plan based on the anatomic location of a particular vascular region.[18] Also, descriptive studies could help with rectification of an anatomic misunderstanding[19] or describe new structures.[20]

Quantitative studies provide measurements, such as diameters, lengths, distances, and angles. A major limitation of quantitative studies is the limited number of cadaveric specimens. Therefore, the confidence intervals of the ranges and averages of parameters reported are inherently high and such information may not be readily applicable to individual patients. Despite the limitations, quantitative descriptive studies are still useful when it comes to specific questions relevant to skull base anatomy. For instance, knowing the angle between the greater superficial petrosal nerve (GSPN) and the internal auditory canal (IAC) would help understanding performing a safe anterior petrosectomy.[21] Oftentimes, descriptive studies combine quantitative and qualitative results to provide a thorough description.

Landmark identification studies comprise the third subtype of descriptive studies. Although quantifying a specific anatomic area provides useful information, knowing the terrain via identification of landmarks is more informative and less subject to error. Using the example of anterior petrosectomy, knowing that the trajectory of the IAC roughly bisects the angle between the arcuate eminence and GSPN is more reliable and intraoperatively applicable than the IAC-GSPN angle.[22]

Landmarks could be of different types. An anatomic entity may serve as a surgical landmark. For example, the inferior nuchal line is used to identify the suboccipital vertebral artery.[23] However, anatomic entities are not the most common landmarks. Rather, different geometric entities (points, lines, triangle, rhomboids) construed from the relationships between anatomic entities are most commonly used as neurosurgical landmarks.

Approach designing studies

New approach designing studies are the second major type of anatomic research. The building blocks of such studies are the descriptive studies. Introduction of a new skull base approach requires in-depth understanding of the anatomy and is unlikely without proper cadaveric dissection experience. In such studies, the researcher uses various anatomic facts to design a new approach. Such approaches can vary from a minimally invasive approach to access a specific target to complex skull base approaches during which bone removal is maximized to minimize brain retraction. Alternatively, safe corridors could be explored and established to access intra-axial lesions, such as cavernous malformations of the brainstem. Historically, approach designing studies focused on a large anatomic region as the target.[24] More recently, such studies are more focused on specific anatomic targets and/or pathologic entities.[25]

Analytical and comparative studies

The expanding volume of approach designing studies led to the birth of analytical and comparative studies. These studies aim to compare different approaches to establish relative advantages and limitations of a specific approach in comparison with alternative plausible approaches. Several parameters could be used for comparison.

Visibility of structures Being able to see the surgical target is quintessential. For example, to clip a basilar artery apex (BAX) aneurysm, the surgeon primarily needs to see the BAX (ie, the basilar artery, and it's quadrifurcation). The pterional and subtemporal approaches could be used for this purpose. However, a sample question would be "How different are these approaches in exposing the BAX?" The visibility of a certain structure is assessed in every anatomic specimen. Then, the frequency of visualization is compared between approaches.

Length of exposure In skull base surgery, vessels and nerves are important structures to preserve. Therefore, the better they are exposed, the greater the surgical control over them. Although in some surgeries they are merely to be protected en route to the surgical target, in others, they are the actual surgical target (eg, in bypass surgeries). Therefore, the exposed length becomes of paramount importance. For example, aneurysms of the posterior cerebral artery could be approached via the pterional or subtemporal approaches. Therefore, it is important to know which approach is superior in terms of length of exposure along the posterior cerebral artery.

Surgical area of exposure In skull base and cerebrovascular surgery, the surgical field includes areas where the surgeon is directly operating on and adjacent areas that, although off-target, require active control. This region is delimited by the structures of interest. For example, in case of a BAX aneurysm, the surgical area of exposure is a polygon defined by distal-most points on ipsilateral and contralateral superior cerebellar and posterior cerebral arteries, the proximal-most visible point on the basilar trunk, and the most superior visible point in the interpeduncular fossa. The area of this polygon is calculated and compared between different surgical approaches (**Fig. 6**).

Angle of attack and surgical freedom During surgical dissection, the tip of the instrument touches the target while the handle is in the surgeon's hand. The maneuverability of a surgical instrument is limited by the surgical corridor. The structures making the corridor include the bony edges of the craniotomy, the brain in the periphery of the surgical corridor, and the neurovascular structures between the surgeon and the target. The ideal surgical corridor provides maximal visualization and instrument maneuverability with the shallowest surgical field. Therefore, measuring the maneuverability of a surgical instrument is a reasonable way to compare approaches. The simplest form of quantifying such maneuverability is the angle of attack. Maintaining the target as the vertex of the angle, the maximum angle reconstructed by placing the surgical probe at multiple points across the periphery of a surgical corridor constructs the angle of attack.[26]

The angle of attack has the limitation of measuring maneuverability in a single plane. To

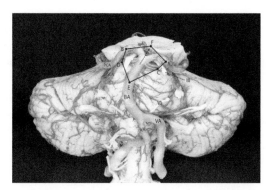

Fig. 6. Depiction of surgical area of exposure for operative approach to the basilar apex. Points A–D show the distal-most points exposed on ipsilateral and contralateral superior cerebellar and posterior cerebral arteries. Point E is the proximal-most exposed point on the basilar trunk. Point F is the most superior visible point in the interpeduncular fossa, on an imaginary line that was extended from the BAX along the same direction as the basilar trunk. (*From Tayebi Meybodi et al. Comprehensive Anatomic Assessment of the Pterional, Orbitopterional, and Orbitozygomatic Approaches for Basilar Apex Aneurysm Clipping. Oper Neurosurg (Hagerstown). 2018, 15(5):538-550* with permission).

overcome this limitation, the concept of surgical freedom was introduced in 2000.[27] The surgical freedom is the objective assessment of the maneuverability offered by a surgical approach to a specific target. To calculate the surgical freedom, the tip of a straight probe is placed on the target. Then, the probe is rested on several points across the periphery of the surgical corridor to create a polygonal pyramid. The spatial coordinates of the vertices of the base of this pyramid are recorded using a stereotactic navigation system. Surgical freedom is then calculated as the area of this base. Alternatively, the spatial maneuverability could be imagined as a spherical sector, hence the surgical freedom could be calculated as the surface area of its spherical dome (**Fig. 7**).[28] Recent studies, have used the volume of the surgical freedom to better represent the maneuverability.[29]

Technique development and feasibility assessment studies

Cerebrovascular and skull base surgery are technically demanding disciplines and there is no limit for improving the safety and efficiency. However, surgical simulation in the laboratory setting offers the highest fidelity to a live surgical procedure while avoiding patient harm. Questions and challenges encountered in the operating room could spark ideas that may seem unreasonable and

impossible to undertake on patients. Such problems make for the opportunity to assess the feasibility of novel techniques or optimize the existing ones.[30–32]

Laboratory Research and Cerebrovascular Surgery Education

Laboratory research could be effectively used for cerebrovascular surgery training. This goal is different from performing exploratory dissections and practicing with various surgical instruments, although inspiration may be nurtured while practicing the known techniques through an inquisitive attitude. A few aspects of laboratory research and education are discussed.

Technique demonstration

Technical nuances of surgical approaches are best learned doing hands-on work in the laboratory. The fundamental pedagogical advantage of surgical simulation is the possibility of an educational pause, the liberating feeling of harmless maneuvering, which leads to more aggressive and adventurous dissection off live-surgery limits, and the possibility to reevaluate a dissection afterward, to name a few. Such practice should be combined with operating room experience involving progressive autonomy. However, this ideal combination may not be always available. Therefore, learning through observation remains an important (although suboptimal) solution. Watching surgeries is certainly a great way to achieve this goal. However, surgical pictures and videos have limited educational value because they are often bloody and show the field through a narrow confusing corridor. Therefore, depictions of bloodless and clean operative simulations could play a significant role in teaching most complex surgeries and technical nuances (**Fig. 8**).

Aneurysm models

Clipping cerebral aneurysms is technically challenging. Intraoperative aneurysm rupture, suboptimal clipping leading to parent vessel compromise, and/or aneurysm residue are pitfalls potentially leading to serious complications. Creation of aneurysm models helps trainees face these challenges in a controlled milieu to perfect dexterity. Models are created using laboratory animals or static material.[33,34]

Microanastomosis training models

Learning microvascular anastomosis is an important technique in cerebrovascular surgery. Usually, the trainee starts with nonliving models, such as silicone tubes. Effective translation of learning from nonliving models to living models

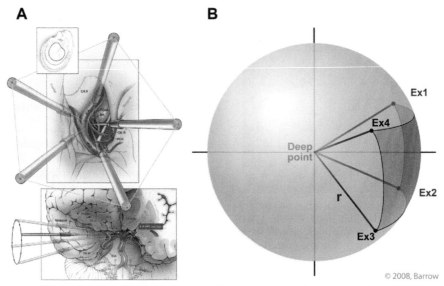

Fig. 7. (*A*) Artist's illustration showing the technique of reconstructing the polygon of surgical freedom for the basilar apex and ipsilateral and contralateral P1-P2 junctions during a pterional craniotomy and through the carotid-oculomotor triangle. (*B*) Spherical interpretation of surgical freedom. Deep point represents the surgical target. Ex1 to Ex4 represent extremum points around the surgical window. r = length of the surgical probe. The surgical freedom is the surface area of the spherical dome (*purple*). (Fig. [A], From *Tayebi Meybodi et al. Analysis of Surgical Freedom Variation Across the Basilar Artery Bifurcation: Towards a Deeper Insight into Approach Selection for Basilar Apex Aneurysms. Oper Neurosurg (Hagerstown). 2018, 15(6):692-700* with permission). (Fig. [B], Courtesy of *Barrow Neurological Institute, Phoenix, Arizona, USA.* Used with permission).

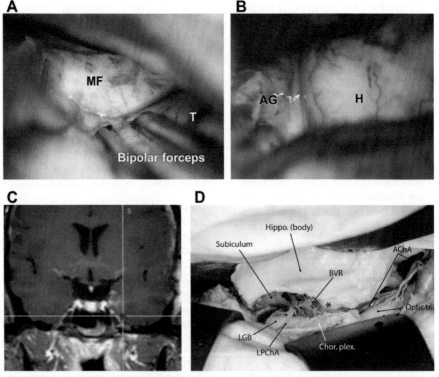

Fig. 8. (*A–C*) Depiction of amygdala and hippocampus during a subtemporal approach to mesial temporal region in a patient with amygdalohippocampal tumor showing limited view of middle fossa (MF), temporal lobe (T), amygdala (AG), and hippocampus (H) with neuronavigation confirmation. (*D*) Cadaveric simulation of subtemporal amygdalohippocampectomy showing clear visualization of temporal horn structures. * = intralimbic gyrus. (Courtesy of *Barrow Neurological Institute, Phoenix, Arizona, USA.* Used with permission).

has been shown.[35] Research could help optimization of existing models and designing new ones with increasing complexity.[36]

Limitations of Cerebrovascular Surgical Anatomy Research

Brain stiffness

Cadaveric research uses fresh or embalmed specimens. Although the fresh tissue may offer the highest fidelity to the living brain, the quality of the tissue rapidly decays rendering the specimen unusable and a biohazard. The embalming techniques stop structural breakdown of the brain at the cost of changing its physical properties, which limit the fidelity of surgical maneuvering (because of changes in tissue stiffness). Such difference limits the generalization of analytical findings to intraoperative settings. Efforts have been made to improve the fidelity of specimen stiffness to the living brain.[37]

Absence of pathology

One of the limitations of cadaveric research is the absence of the pathology of interest. The presence of a tumor, vascular malformation, or aneurysm could alter the regional anatomy and therefore deduced conclusions from studying a normal brain are less reliable. Reproduction of models including the pathology of interest could be tried to mitigate this limitation (**Fig. 9**).[38]

FUTURE DIRECTIONS

Surgical cerebrovascular anatomic research is rapidly growing. Despite major advances in the twentieth century, descriptive neurosurgical anatomy is continually expanding through better descriptions of the already known structures, finding new anatomic landmarks, and providing more robust approach analyses. Importantly, with the increasing use of minimally invasive skull base approaches, the need for most accurate descriptions and reliable anatomic landmarks is felt more than ever. Although early anatomists used rulers and calipers, future anatomists rely on the creation of blueprints to use the described anatomy to further develop minimally invasive neurosurgery. White matter dissection and the development of the human brain connectome (with the help of tractographic

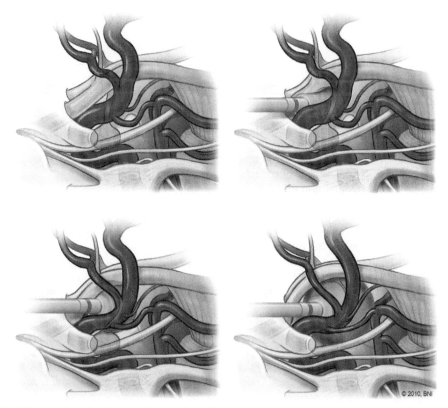

Fig. 9. Artist's illustration of technique for creation of a suprasellar lesion using progressive inflation of a Fogarty balloon. (Courtesy of *Barrow Neurological Institute, Phoenix, Arizona, USA.* Used with permission).

studies) may also bring about a breakthrough in anatomic discovery beyond the cerebral cortex, which is critical for intra-axial surgery.

Neurosurgical anatomy education is an infinite art with continuous development. Excellent static two-dimensional and three-dimensional (3D) images of cadaveric dissections are currently available. Recently, efforts have been made to provide accurate 3D-animated interactive models for enhancing anatomic understanding.[39] Combination of photogrammetry and cadaveric dissections is developing and could revolutionize skull base and cerebrovascular anatomic education.[40] Such models could be enhanced with augmented virtual reality technology to provide the most accurate and informative models for research and education.

On another aspect, training cerebrovascular surgeons could be boosted with research on optimizing practice models and training protocols. Developing new low-cost nonliving and living models for stepwise practicing on learning microvascular anastomosis and aneurysm clipping is a tangible need. Such training protocols could be augmented using a combination of 3D-printed models and improved living models of cerebrovascular pathologies (eg, aneurysms). Obviously, optimization of the training protocols requires dedicated laboratory research.

SUMMARY

Since ancient times, neurosurgical anatomic research has evolved immensely. Current cerebrovascular surgical microanatomy research is expanding faster than ever, empowered by almost two centuries of descriptive anatomy and boosted by the finest dissection works in the last six decades. Research is being conducted in the fields of descriptive, analytical, approach designing, feasibility assessment, and education. Incorporation of novel cadaveric specimen preparations, incorporation of advanced radiologic techniques, virtual and augmented reality, photogrammetry, and advanced 3D printing into cadaveric research help increase accuracy, reliability, and clinical applicability of cerebrovascular anatomic research.

DISCLOSURE

The authors have nothing to disclose.

REFERENCES

1. Wiltse LL, Pait TG. Herophilus of Alexandria (325-255 B. C.). The father of anatomy. Spine (Phila Pa 1976) 1998;23(17):1904–14.

2. Cavalcanti DD, Feindel W, Goodrich JT, et al. Anatomy, technology, art, and culture: toward a realistic perspective of the brain. Neurosurg Focus 2009; 27(3):E2.

3. Hanigan WC, Ragen W, Foster R. Dryander of Marburg and the first textbook of neuroanatomy. Neurosurgery 1990;26(3):489–98.

4. Vesalius A. Andreae Vesalii Bruxellensis De humani corporis fabrica libri septem. Nieuwendijk: De Forel; 1975. 659 i.e. 663 p., 1 fold. leaf of plates.

5. Willis T, Feindel W. The anatomy of the brain and nerves. Special. Classics of Medicine Library; 1978. xvi, 2, 192 p., 14 leaves of plates (4 fold.).

6. Ridley H. The anatomy of the brain, containing its mechanisms and physiology: together with some new discoveries and corrections of ancient and modern authors upon that subject. London: Samuel Smith; 1695.

7. Schumacher GH. Theatrum anatomicum in history and today. Int J Morphol 2007;25(1):15–32.

8. Boling W, Olivier A, Civit T. The French contribution to the discovery of the central area. Neurochirurgie 1999;45(3):208–13.

9. Vicq d'Azyr F. Traité d'anatomie et de physiologie—avec des planches colorës représentant au naturel les divers organes de 'Homme et des Animaux. Paris: F.A. Didot; 1786.

10. Bell C. The anatomy of the brain explained in a series of engravings. T.N. Longman and O. Rees, and T. Cadell and W. Davies; 1802:vii, 87 p., 12 leaves of plates; London.

11. Pearce JM. Sir David Ferrier MD, FRS. J Neurol Neurosurg Psychiatr 2003;74(6):787.

12. Swash M. John Hughlings Jackson (1835-1911): an adornment to the London Hospital. J Med Biogr 2015;23(1):2–8.

13. Kretzer RM, Coon AL, Tamargo RJ, et al. Dandy's contributions to vascular neurosurgery. J Neurosurg 2010;112(6):1182–91.

14. Cohen-Gadol AA, Spencer DD, Harvey W. Cushing and cerebrovascular surgery: part II, Vascular malformations. J Neurosurg 2004;101(3):553–9.

15. Cohen-Gadol AA, Spencer DD, Harvey W. Cushing and cerebrovascular surgery: part I, Aneurysms. J Neurosurg 2004;101(3):547–52.

16. Yasargil MG, Kasdaglis K, Jain KK, et al. Anatomical observations of the subarachnoid cisterns of the brain during surgery. J Neurosurg 1976;44(3): 298–302.

17. Farhadi DS, Jubran JH, Zhao X, et al. The neuroanatomic studies of Albert L. Rhoton Jr. in historical context: an analysis of origin, evolution, and application. World Neurosurg 2021;151:258–76.

18. Rodríguez-Hernández A, Rhoton AL, Lawton MT. Segmental anatomy of cerebellar arteries: a proposed nomenclature. Laboratory investigation. J Neurosurg 2011;115(2):387–97.

19. Eduardo Corrales C, Mudry A, Jackler RK. Perpetuation of errors in illustrations of cranial nerve anatomy. J Neurosurg 2017;127(1):192–8.

20. Tayebi Meybodi A, Little AS, Vigo V, et al. The pterygoclival ligament: a novel landmark for localization of the internal carotid artery during the endoscopic endonasal approach. J Neurosurg 2019;130(5): 1699–709.

21. Tanriover N, Sanus GZ, Ulu MO, et al. Middle fossa approach: microsurgical anatomy and surgical technique from the neurosurgical perspective. Surg Neurol 2009;71(5):586–96 [discussion: 596].

22. Garcia-Ibanez E, Garcia-Ibanez JL. Middle fossa vestibular neurectomy: a report of 373 cases. Otolaryngol Head Neck Surg 1980;88(4):486–90.

23. Tayebi Meybodi A, Zhao X, Borba Moreira L, et al. The inferior nuchal line as a simple landmark for identifying the vertebral artery during the retrosigmoid approach. Oper Neurosurg (Hagerstown) 2020;18(3):302–8.

24. Pellerin P, Lesoin F, Dhellemmes P, et al. Usefulness of the orbitofrontomalar approach associated with bone reconstruction for frontotemporosphenoid meningiomas. Neurosurgery 1984;15(5):715–8.

25. Figueiredo EG, Deshmukh P, Nakaji P, et al. The minipterional craniotomy: technical description and anatomic assessment. Neurosurgery 2007;61(5 Suppl 2):256–64 [discussion: 264-5].

26. Gonzalez LF, Crawford NR, Horgan MA, et al. Working area and angle of attack in three cranial base approaches: pterional, orbitozygomatic, and maxillary extension of the orbitozygomatic approach. Neurosurgery 2002;50(3):550–5 [discussion: 555-7].

27. Spektor S, Anderson GJ, McMenomey SO, et al. Quantitative description of the far-lateral transcondylar transtubercular approach to the foramen magnum and clivus. J Neurosurg 2000;92(5):824–31.

28. Jittapiromsak P, Deshmukh P, Nakaji P, et al. Comparative analysis of posterior approaches to the medial temporal region: supracerebellar transtentorial versus occipital transtentorial. Neurosurgery 2009;64(3 Suppl):ons35–42 [discussion: ons42-3].

29. Houlihan LM, Naughton D, Preul MC. Volume of surgical freedom: the most applicable anatomical measurement for surgical assessment and 3-dimensional modeling. Front Bioeng Biotechnol 2021;9: 628797.

30. Youssef AS, Uribe JS, Ramos E, et al. Interfascial technique for vertebral artery exposure in the suboccipital triangle: the road map. Neurosurgery 2010; 67(2 Suppl Operative):355–61.

31. Rennert RC, Strickland BA, Radwanski RE, et al. Running-to-interrupted microsuture technique for vascular bypass. Oper Neurosurg (Hagerstown) 2018;15(4):412–7.

32. Rubio RR, Vigo V, Gandhi S, et al. An anatomical feasibility study for revascularization of the ophthalmic artery. Part II: intraorbital segment. World Neurosurg 2020;133:401–8.

33. Tenjin H, Okano Y. Training model for cerebral aneurysm clipping. Interdiscip Neurosurg 2017;10: 114–8. https://doi.org/10.1016/j.inat.2017.07.018.

34. Marbacher S, Marjamaa J, Abdelhameed E, et al. The Helsinki rat microsurgical sidewall aneurysm model. J Vis Exp 2014;(92):e51071.

35. Mokhtari P, Meybodi AT, Lawton MT, et al. Transfer of learning from practicing microvascular anastomosis on silastic tubes to rat's abdominal aorta. World Neurosurg 2017. https://doi.org/10.1016/j.wneu.2017. 08.132.

36. Byvaltsev VA, Akshulakov SK, Polkin RA, et al. Microvascular anastomosis training in neurosurgery: a review. Minim Invasive Surg 2018. https://doi.org/ 10.1155/2018/6130286.

37. Benet A, Rincon-Torroella J, Lawton MT, et al. Novel embalming solution for neurosurgical simulation in cadavers. J Neurosurg 2014;120(5):1229–37.

38. Garcia-Garcia S, Gonzalez-Sanchez JJ, Gandhi S, et al. Contralateral transfalcine versus ipsilateral anterior interhemispheric approach for midline arteriovenous malformations: surgical and anatomical assessment. World Neurosurg 2018;119:e1041–51.

39. Nowinski WL, Chua BC, Marchenko Y, et al. Three-dimensional reference and stereotactic atlas of human cerebrovasculature from 7Tesla. Neuroimage 2011;55(3):986–98.

40. Rodriguez Rubio R, Chae R, Vigo V, et al. Immersive surgical anatomy of the pterional approach. Cureus 2019;11(7):e5216.

UNITED STATES POSTAL SERVICE® Statement of Ownership, Management, and Circulation
(All Periodicals Publications Except Requester Publications)

1. Publication Title	2. Publication Number	3. Filing Date
NEUROSURGERY CLINICS OF NORTH AMERICA	010 – 548	9/18/2022

4. Issue Frequency	5. Number of Issues Published Annually	6. Annual Subscription Price
JAN, APR, JUL OCT	4	$447.00

7. Complete Mailing Address of Known Office of Publication (Not printer) (Street, city, county, state, and ZIP+4®)

ELSEVIER INC.
230 Park Avenue, Suite 800
New York, NY 10169

Contact Person
Malathi Samayan

Telephone (Include area code)
91-44-4299-4507

8. Complete Mailing Address of Headquarters or General Business Office of Publisher (Not printer)

ELSEVIER INC.
230 Park Avenue, Suite 800
New York, NY 10169

9. Full Names and Complete Mailing Addresses of Publisher, Editor, and Managing Editor (Do not leave blank)

Publisher (Name and complete mailing address)

DOLORES MELONI, ELSEVIER INC.
1600 JOHN F KENNEDY BLVD. SUITE 1800
PHILADELPHIA, PA 19103-2899

Editor (Name and complete mailing address)

STACY EASTMAN, ELSEVIER INC.
1600 JOHN F KENNEDY BLVD. SUITE 1800
PHILADELPHIA, PA 19103-2899

Managing Editor (Name and complete mailing address)

PATRICK MANLEY, ELSEVIER INC.
1600 JOHN F KENNEDY BLVD. SUITE 1800
PHILADELPHIA, PA 19103-2899

10. Owner (Do not leave blank. If the publication is owned by a corporation, give the name and address of the corporation immediately followed by the names and addresses of all stockholders owning or holding 1 percent or more of the total amount of stock. If not owned by a corporation, give the names and addresses of the individual owners. If owned by a partnership or other unincorporated firm, give its name and address as well as those of each individual owner. If the publication is published by a nonprofit organization, give its name and address.)

Full Name	Complete Mailing Address
WHOLLY OWNED SUBSIDIARY OF REED/ELSEVIER, US HOLDINGS	1600 JOHN F KENNEDY BLVD. SUITE 1800 PHILADELPHIA, PA 19103-2899

11. Known Bondholders, Mortgagees, and Other Security Holders Owning or Holding 1 Percent or More of Total Amount of Bonds, Mortgages, or Other Securities. If none, check box ▸ ☐ None

Full Name	Complete Mailing Address
N/A	

12. Tax Status (For completion by nonprofit organizations authorized to mail at nonprofit rates) (Check one)
The purpose, function, and nonprofit status of this organization and the exempt status for federal income tax purposes:
☒ Has Not Changed During Preceding 12 Months
☐ Has Changed During Preceding 12 Months (Publisher must submit explanation of change with this statement)

PS Form 3526, July 2014 [Page 1 of 4 (see instructions page 4)] PSN: 7530-01-000-9931 PRIVACY NOTICE: See our privacy policy on www.usps.com.

---

13. Publication Title			14. Issue Date for Circulation Data Below
NEUROSURGERY CLINICS OF NORTH AMERICA			JULY 2022

15. Extent and Nature of Circulation			Average No. Copies Each Issue During Preceding 12 Months	No. Copies of Single Issue Published Nearest to Filing Date
a. Total Number of Copies (Net press run)			132	121
b. Paid Circulation (By Mail and Outside the Mail)	(1)	Mailed Outside-County Paid Subscriptions Stated on PS Form 3541 (Include paid distribution above nominal rate, advertiser's proof copies, and exchange copies)	52	44
	(2)	Mailed In-County Paid Subscriptions Stated on PS Form 3541 (Include paid distribution above nominal rate, advertiser's proof copies, and exchange copies)	0	0
	(3)	Paid Distribution Outside the Mails Including Sales Through Dealers and Carriers, Street Vendors, Counter Sales, and Other Paid Distribution Outside USPS®	47	45
	(4)	Paid Distribution by Other Classes of Mail Through the USPS (e.g., First-Class Mail®)	0	0
c. Total Paid Distribution (Sum of 15b (1), (2), (3), and (4))		▸	99	89
d. Free or Nominal Rate Distribution (By Mail and Outside the Mail)	(1)	Free or Nominal Rate Outside-County Copies included on PS Form 3541	17	14
	(2)	Free or Nominal Rate In-County Copies Included on PS Form 3541	0	0
	(3)	Free or Nominal Rate Copies Mailed at Other Classes Through the USPS (e.g., First-Class Mail)	0	0
	(4)	Free or Nominal Rate Distribution Outside the Mail (Carriers or other means)	0	0
e. Total Free or Nominal Rate Distribution (Sum of 15d (1), (2), (3) and (4))		▸	17	14
f. Total Distribution (Sum of 15c and 15e)		▸	116	103
g. Copies not Distributed (See Instructions to Publishers #4 (page #3))		▸	16	18
h. Total (Sum of 15f and g)		▸	132	121
i. Percent Paid (15c divided by 15f times 100)		▸	85.34%	86.4%

* If you are claiming electronic copies, go to line 16 on page 3. If you are not claiming electronic copies, skip to line 17 on page 3.

16. Electronic Copy Circulation	Average No. Copies Each Issue During Preceding 12 Months	No. Copies of Single Issue Published Nearest to Filing Date
a. Paid Electronic Copies ▸		
b. Total Paid Print Copies (Line 15c) + Paid Electronic Copies (Line 16a) ▸		
c. Total Print Distribution (Line 15f) + Paid Electronic Copies (Line 16a) ▸		
d. Percent Paid (Both Print & Electronic Copies) (16b divided by 16c × 100) ▸		

☐ I certify that 50% of all my distributed copies (electronic and print) are paid above a nominal price.

17. Publication of Statement of Ownership

☒ If the publication is a general publication, publication of this statement is required. Will be printed
in the ___OCTOBER 2022___ issue of this publication.   ☐ Publication not required.

18. Signature and Title of Editor, Publisher, Business Manager, or Owner	Date
Malathi Samayan - Distribution Controller *Malathi Samayan*	9/18/2022

I certify that all information furnished on this form is true and complete. I understand that anyone who furnishes false or misleading information on this form or who omits material or information requested on the form may be subject to criminal sanctions (including fines and imprisonment) and/or civil sanctions (including civil penalties).

PS Form 3526, July 2014 (Page 3 of 4) PRIVACY NOTICE: See our privacy policy on www.usps.com

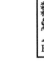

Printed and bound by CPI Group (UK) Ltd, Croydon, CR0 4YY

08/05/2025

01864723-0018